Botanical Influences on Illness

A Sourcebook of Clinical Research

Botanical Influences on Illness

A sourcebook of clinical research

Melvyn R. Werbach, M.D.
Michael T. Murray, N.D.

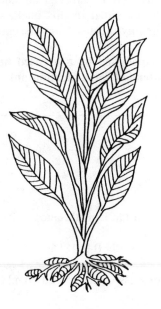

III THIRD LINE PRESS
Tarzana, California

Printed in the United States of America

ISBN 0-9618550-4-5

Library of Congress Catalog Card Number: 94-060010

ACKNOWLEDGMENTS

I am blessed with a devoted wife and two wonderful sons. Thank you, Gail, Adam and Kevin for being there. Also, my gratitude to my parents for making everything possible for me, and to Gail's parents for making it possible for her to enter my life.

Melvyn R. Werbach, M.D.

Most of all, I would like to acknowledge my wife, Gina. Her love, support and patience are the major blessings in my life. Also, I want to give a very heartfelt thanks to my parents, Cliff and Patty Murray; and my parents-in-law, Robert and Kathy Bunton, for their incredible love, support, and true friendship.

Michael T. Murray, N.D.

DEDICATION

To the researchers, physicians, and scientists who over the years have striven to better understand the use of natural medicines. The evolution in understanding that is occurring in medicine is largely a result of long, hard hours of study and research by individuals who never experience the public spotlight. Without their work, this book would not exist, and medical progress would halt.

BOTANICAL INFLUENCES ON ILLNESS:

A SOURCEBOOK OF CLINICAL RESEARCH

TABLE OF CONTENTS

INTRODUCTION

Botanical medicine refers to the use of plants or plant substances as medicinal agents. While the medicinal use of plants has existed since the dawn of time, the scientific investigation of herbal remedies is a recent development, and our knowledge of how plants actually affect human physiology remains largely a mystery. As of today, even though investigators are intent on proving whether or not medicinal applications of plants and plant substances are effective and, if so, what their mechanisms of action may be, many practitioners remain content to accept empirical evidence of a plant's efficacy.

Botanical Influences on Illness seeks to demonstrate the growing scientific basis for the medicinal application of botanicals. The bulk of the text consists of a series of chapters covering the major illnesses for which a reasonable amount of scientific literature exists. Individual plants and plant substances are discussed first, followed by any notable mixtures of two or more botanical ingredients. Our emphasis in the selection of abstracts is on studies of clinical interest, namely those that have investigated the efficacy of preventive and therapeutic interventions. We have attempted to approach the subject in an unbiased manner by selecting studies with negative, as well as positive, outcomes and by including warnings of known contraindications and side effects.

In each chapter, following the listing of a botanical agent, we present a series of statements concerning that agent, each of which is followed by selected abstracts from the literature which either substantiate or refute it. **None of these statements is a therapeutic recommendation!** When available, abstracts from review articles have been included to provide the perspective of acknowledged experts. Randomized, double-blind controlled studies are emphasized; however, because such studies are often unavailable, uncontrolled studies (open trials), observational (epidemiological) studies, animal experiments, *in vitro* studies and even informal clinical observations are included.

Abstracts are presented in the order of their year of publication, with the latest papers listed first. As it is not possible to include all studies, preference has been given to the best, the most relevant, and the most recent.

While *Botanical Influences on Illness* provides information that can be used to make therapeutic decisions, it is meant to be used as a sourcebook, not as a treatment manual, and therefore assumes that the reader who wishes to utilize botanical medicines either has an appropriate professional background or is under the guidance of a trained professional.

It is our hope that you will come away from this book with a deeper appreciation of the state of this rapidly evolving field as it exists today — and that the professional reader will be better able, not only to utilize botanical medicines in practice, but to answer the many questions concerning these important natural substances being asked by an increasingly sophisticated public.

MODERN BOTANICAL MEDICINE - AN OVERVIEW

I. GOVERNMENT REGULATION OF HERBAL PRODUCTS

The term 'herb' refers to a plant used for medicinal purposes. Medical doctors and pharmacists trained in the United States are usually taught that the use of herbs is merely a reflection of folklore, outdated theories, and myth. Yet, even today, for many of the people of the world, herbs are the only medicines available or are preferred to synthetic drugs. In 1985, the World Health Organization estimated that perhaps 80% of the world's population rely on herbs for their primary health care needs.[1] This widespread use of herbal medicines is not restricted to developing countries as it has been estimated that 30% to 40% of all medical doctors in France and Germany rely on herbal preparations as their primary medicines.[2]

Throughout the world, but especially in Europe and Asia, there has been a tremendous renaissance in the use and appreciation of herbal medicine. In Germany, estimates show that over $4 billion dollars are spent on herbal products each year. In Japan, the figure is thought to be even higher. Herbal products are a major business in the United States as well with an estimated annual sales figure of $1.3 billion dollars for 1992 and climbing.[3] However, it is interesting to note that while annual sales of ginseng products in the U. S. in 1992 was roughly $10 million dollars, over 3 million pounds (roughly $100 million dollars) of American ginseng were exported.[4,5]

The rebirth of herbal medicine, especially in developed countries, is largely based on a renewed interest by scientific researchers. During the last 10 to 20 years there has been an explosion of scientific information concerning plants, crude plant extracts, and various substances from plants as medicinal agents. Plants still play a major role in modern pharmacy.

For the past 25 years about 25% of all prescription drugs in the United States have contained active constituents obtained from plants. Digoxin, codeine, colchicine, morphine, vincristine, and yohimbine are some popular examples. Many over-the-counter preparations also are composed of plant compounds as well. It is estimated that more than $11 billion dollars of plant based medicines are purchased each year in the U.S. alone and $43 billion dollars worldwide.[6]

Pharmacognosy, the study of natural drugs and their constituents, plays a major role in current drug development. Unfortunately, the standard path of the approval of a plant-based drug in the U.S. is a process that typically takes 10 to 18 years at a total cost of roughly $230 million dollars.

Because a plant cannot be patented, plants are screened for biological activity and then the so-called 'active' constituents (compounds) are isolated. In the United States, if the compound is powerful enough, the drug company will begin the process to procure Food and

Drug Administration (FDA) approval. Because of the expense and lack of patent protection, very little research has been done during this century on whole plants or crude plant extracts as medicinal agents, *per se*, by the large American pharmaceutical firms.

In contrast, European policies have made it economically feasible for companies to research and develop herbs as medicines. In Germany, herbal products can be marketed with drug claims if they have been proven to be safe and effective[7] and the legal requirements for herbal medicines are identical to those of all other drugs. Whether the herbal product is available by prescription or OTC is based upon its application and safety of use. Herbal products sold in pharmacies are reimbursed by insurance if they are prescribed by a physician.

The proof required by a manufacturer in Germany to illustrate safety and effectiveness for an herbal product is far less than the proof required by the FDA for drugs in the United States. In Germany, a special commission (Commission E) developed a series of 200 monographs on herbal products similar to the OTC monographs in the U.S.[7] An herbal product is viewed as safe and effective if a manufacturer meets the quality requirements of the monograph or produces additional evidence of safety and effectiveness that can include data from existing literature, anecdotal information from practicing physicians, as well as limited clinical studies.

The best single illustration of the difference in the regulatory issues of herbal products in the United States compared to Germany is *Ginkgo biloba*. In Germany, as well as France, extracts of *Ginkgo biloba* leaves are registered for the treatment of cerebral and peripheral vascular insufficiency.[8] Ginkgo products are available by prescription and OTC purchase. Ginkgo extracts are among the top three most widely prescribed drugs in both Germany and France with a combined annual sales figure of more than $500 million dollars. In contrast, in the United States, extracts, which are identical to those approved in Germany and France, are available as 'food supplements'.

No medicinal claims are allowed for most American herbal products because the FDA requires the same standard of absolute proof as is required for new synthetic drugs. The FDA has rejected the idea of establishing an independent Expert Advisory Panel for the development of monographs similar to Germany's Commission E monographs, as well as other ideas to create a suitable framework for the marketing of herbal products in the United States. Currently, herbal products continue to be sold as 'food supplements' and manufacturers are prohibited from making any therapeutic claims for their products.

II. FORMS OF HERBAL PRODUCTS

Commercial herbal preparations are available in several different forms: bulk herbs; teas; tinctures; fluid extracts; and tablets or capsules.[9] It is important for physicians, pharmacists, health food store personnel, and anyone else who routinely recommends herbs to understand the differences of these forms, as well as methods of expressing strengths of herbal products.

One of the major developments in the herb industry involves improvements in extraction and concentration processes. An **extract** is defined as a concentrated form of the herb obtained by mixing the crude herb with an appropriate solvent (such as alcohol and/or water).

When an herbal tea bag is steeped in hot water, it is actually a type of herbal extract known as an **infusion**. The water is serving as a solvent in removing some of the medicinal properties from the herb. **Teas** often are better sources of bioavailable compounds than the powdered herb, but are relatively weak in action compared to tinctures, fluid extracts, and solid extracts. These forms are commonly used by herbal practitioners for medicinal effects.

Tinctures are typically made using an alcohol and water mixture as the solvent. The herb is soaked in the solvent for a specified amount of time, depending on the herb. This soaking is usually from several hours to days; however some herbs may be soaked for much longer periods of time. The solution is then pressed out, yielding the tincture.

Fluid extracts are more concentrated than tinctures. Although they are most often made from hydroalcoholic mixtures, other solvents may be used (vinegar, glycerine, propylene glycol, etc.). Commercial fluid extracts usually are made by distilling off some of the alcohol, typically by using methods that do not require elevated temperatures, such as vacuum distillation and counter-current filtration.

A **solid extract** is produced by further concentration of the extract by the mechanisms described above for fluid extracts as well as by other techniques such as thin layer evaporation. The solvent is completely removed leaving a viscous extract (soft solid extract) or a dry solid extract depending upon the plant, portion of the plant, or solvent used or if a drying process was used. The dry solid extract, if not already in powdered form, can be ground into course granules or a fine powder. A solid extract also can be diluted with alcohol and water to form a fluid extract or tincture.

Strengths of Extracts

The potencies or strengths of herbal extracts are generally expressed in two ways. If they contain known active principles, their strengths are commonly expressed in terms of the content of these active principles. Otherwise, the strength is expressed in terms of their concentration. For example, tinctures are typically made at a 1:5 concentration. This means one part of the herb (in grams) is soaked in five parts liquid (in milliliters of volume). This means that there is five times the amount of solvent (alcohol/water) in a tincture as there is herbal material.

A 4:1 concentration means that one part of the extract is equivalent to, or derived from, 4 parts of the crude herb. This is the typical concentration of a solid extract. One gram of a 4:1 extract is concentrated from 4 grams of crude herb.

Since a tincture is typically a 1:10 or 1:5 concentration while a fluid extract is usually 1:1, a solid extract is typically at least 4 times as potent when compared to an equal amount of fluid extract and 40 times as potent as a tincture if they are produced from the same quality of herb.

Typically, one gram of a 4:1 solid extract is equivalent to 4 ml of a fluid extract (1/7th of an ounce) and 40 ml of a tincture (almost 1 1/2 ounces). Some solid extracts are concentrated as high as 100:1, meaning it would take nearly 100 grams of crude herb, or 100 ml of a fluid extract (approximately 3.5 ounces), or 1,000 ml of a tincture (almost 1 quart) to provide an equal amount of herbal material in 1 gram of a 100:1 extract.

In the past, the quality of the extract produced often was difficult to determine as many of the active principles of the herbs were unknown. However, recent advances in extraction processes, coupled with improved analytical methods, have reduced this problem of quality control.[10] The concentration method of expressing the strength of an extract does not accurately measure potency since there may be great variation among manufacturing techniques and raw materials. By using a high quality herb (an herb high in active compounds), it is possible to have a more potent dried herb, tincture, or fluid extract compared to the solid extract that was made from a lower quality herb. Standardization is the solution to this problem.[11]

Standardized extracts (also referred to as guaranteed potency extracts) refer to an extract guaranteed to contain a 'standardized' level of active compounds. Stating the content of active compounds rather than the concentration ratio allows for more accurate dosages to be made. Presently, most of the standardized extracts distributed in the United States are actually manufactured in Europe. They are typically available in dry powdered form in either capsules or tablets.

III. TECHNIQUES USED IN THE PRODUCTION OF HERBAL PRODUCTS

There is a tremendous range of sophistication in the processing of herbs - from crude herb to highly concentrated standardized extracts. Nonetheless, there are some common stages. This section describes some of the processes in the production of herbal products and the machines that perform the functions.[12]

Collection/Harvesting

When plants are collected from their natural habitat they are said to be 'wild-crafted'. When they are grown utilizing commercial farming techniques they are said to be 'cultivated'. Collection of plants from cultivated sources ensures that the plant collected is the one that is desired. When an herb is wild-crafted, there is a much greater chance that the wrong herb will be picked, a situation that could lead to serious consequences. The use of analytical techniques (discussed below) can be employed to guarantee the plant collected is the one desired.

In the United States marketplace, herbs from all over the world are marketed. The collectors of the herbs vary from uneducated natives and self-proclaimed 'herbalists' to skilled botanists.

The mode of harvesting varies from hand labor to very sophisticated equipment. The mode is not as important as the time. A plant should be harvested when the part of the plant being used contains the highest possible level of active compounds. Again, this is ensured by the use of analytical techniques.

Drying

After harvesting, most herbs have a moisture content of 60% to 80% and cannot be stored without drying. Otherwise, important compounds would break down or micro-organisms would contaminate the material.

The majority of herbs require relatively mild conditions for drying. Commercially, most plants are dried within a temperature range of 100 to 140 degrees F. During drying the plant material must not be damaged or suffer losses that would prevent it from conforming to accepted standards. With proper drying, the herb's moisture content will be reduced to less than 14%.

Garbling

Garbling refers to the separation of the portion of the plant to be used from other parts of the plant, dirt, and other extraneous matter. This step is often done during collection. Although there are machines that perform garbling, usually garbling is performed by hand.

Grinding

Grinding or mincing an herb means mechanically breaking down either leaves, roots, seeds, or other parts of a plant into very small units ranging from larger course fragments to fine powder. Grinding is employed in the production of crude herbal products as well as in the initial phases of extracts.

Often the material has to be prechopped or minced before feeding it into a grinder. In the process of grinding, a number of machines can be used, but the most widely used is the hammer mill. These machines are simple in design. The hammers, arranged radially, follow the rotation of the shaft to which they are attached, breaking up the material that is fed into the machine from above. On the walls of the chamber is a grid, which determines the size of the material that is passed through it. Other types of grinders include knife mills and teeth mills.

Extraction

The process of extraction is used in making tinctures, fluid extracts, and solid extracts. Extraction in the context of this module refers to separating by physical or chemical means the desired material from a plant with the aid of a solvent. In the United States health food industry, most extracts utilize alcohol and water mixtures as solvents to remove soluble compounds from the herb. The exceptions are liposterolic extracts, which are produced either through the use of lipophilic solvents or with the aid of hypercritical carbon dioxide.

Most extracts that are produced by small manufacturers use maceration procedures. The simplest process consists of soaking the herb in the alcohol/water solution for a period of time and then filtering. Typically, this process will yield a lower quality extract at a higher price because the solvent, typically alcohol, cannot be reused. It is, in essence, sold to the customer. Since tinctures are 1:5 concentrates, this means 80% of the bottle is alcohol and water and only 20% herbal material. Tinctures are not as cost effective or as stable as solid extracts.

Larger manufacturers utilize more elaborate techniques to ensure that the herb is fully extracted and the solvent is reused. For example, countercurrent extraction is often used. In this process, the herb enters into a column of a large perculator composed of several columns. The material to be extracted is pumped through the different columns at a given temperature and flow speed where it continuously mixes with solvent. The extract rich solvent then passes into another column, while fresh solvent once again comes into contact with herbal material as it is passed into a new chamber. In this process, complete extraction of health promoting compounds can be performed. The extract rich solvent is then concentrated by techniques described below.

Concentration

After extraction of the herb, the resulting solutions can be concentrated into fluid extracts or solid extracts. In large manufacturing operations, techniques and machines, such as thin layer evaporators, are utilized that ensure the extracted plant components are not damaged. These machines work by evaporating the solvent and leaving the plant compounds. The solvent vapors pass into a condenser whereby they return to a liquid and can be reused. The result is separation of the extracted materials from the solvent so that the final product is a pure extract and the solvent can be used again and again.

Drying of Extracts

Although there are still a number of liquid form extracts on the market (tinctures, fluid extracts, and soft extracts), the preferred method is to dry the extract to a solid form. The main reason is greater chemical stability and reduced cost (alcohol is often more expensive than the herb). Tinctures, and fluid and soft extracts are easily contaminated by bacteria and other micro-organisms. Liquid forms of extracts also promote reactions, which break down the herbal compounds.

A number of drying techniques are employed including freeze-drying and spray-drying (atomization). The result is a dried powdered extract that can then be put into capsules or tablets.

Excipients

The same excipients used in the manufacture of drug preparations as well as vitamin and mineral supplements often are used in the production of tablets and capsules containing herbs or herbal extracts. Many manufacturers will provide a list of excipients contained in their products.

Analytical Methods

Improvements in analytical methods have definitely led to improvements in harvesting schedules, cultivation techniques, storage, activity, stability of active compounds, and product purity. All of these gains have resulted in tremendous improvements in the quality of herbal preparations now available.

For example, optimal activity and quality collection should be done at a time when the active ingredient is present in the greatest amount. Improvements in analysis have led to more precise harvesting of many herbs.

Methods currently utilized in evaluating herbs and their extracts include:

    organoleptic
    microscopic
    physical
    chemical/physical
    biological

Organoleptic means the 'impression of the organs'. Organoleptic analysis involves the application of sight, odor, taste, touch, and occassionally even sound, to identify the plant. Obviously, the initial sight of the plant or extract is so specific it identifies itself. If this is not enough, perhaps the plant or extract has a characteristic odor or taste. Organoleptic analysis represents the simplest, yet the most human, form of analysis.

Microscopic evaluation is indispensable in the initial identification of herbs, as well as in identifying small fragments of crude or powdered herbs, and in the detection of adulterants (e.g., insects, animal feces, mold, fungi, etc.). Every plant possesses a characteristic tissue structure, which can be demonstrated through study of tissue arrangement, cell walls, and configuration when properly mounted using the appropriate stains, reagents and media.

In crude plant evaluation, physical methods often are used to determine the solubility, specific gravity, melting point, water content, degree of fiber elasticity, and other physical characteristics.

Various chemical/physical methods also are used to determine percentage of active principles, alkaloids, flavonoids, enzymes, vitamins, essential oils, fats, carbohydrates, protein, ash, acid-insoluble ash, or crude fiber present.

The final analytical process requires more precise assays to determine quality. Sophisticated techniques, such as high pressure liquid chromatography and nuclear magnetic resonance, are often used to separate out molecules. The readings from these machines provide a chemical 'fingerprint' as to the nature of chemicals contained in the plant or extract. These techniques are invaluable in the effort to identify herbs, as well as standardize extracts.

The plant or extract can then be evaluated by various biological methods, mostly animal tests, to determine pharmacological activity, potency, and toxicity.

IV. QUALITY CONTROL IN HERBAL PRODUCTS

Quality control is a term that refers to processes involved in maintaining the quality or validity of a product. Regardless of the form of herbal preparation, some degree of quality control should exist. Currently, there is yet no organization or government body in the United States that certifies an herb as labeled correctly.

Without quality control, there is no assurance that the herb contained in the bottle is the same as what is stated on the outside. The widespread disregard for quality control in the health food industry has tarnished the reputation of many important medicinal herbs. For example, it has been estimated that because of supplier errors in collection, more than 50% of the Echinacea sold in the United States since 1908 and through 1991 was actually *Parthenium integrifolium*.[13] This highlights the importance of using the Latin name, since both of the above-mentioned herbs are referred to as "Missouri snakeroot," as well as the need for proper plant identification based upon organoleptic, microscopic, and chemical analysis.

Recent chemical analysis of commercially available feverfew (*Tanacetum parthenium*) and taheebo (*Tabebuia avellanedae*) for active components, parthenolide and lapachol respectively, have also shown need for concern. Analysis of over 35 different commercial preparations of feverfew indicated a wide variation in the amounts of parthenolide in commercial preparations.[14] The majority of products contained no parthenolide or only traces. Analysis of 12 commercial sources of taheebo could identify lapachol (in trace amounts) in only 1 product.[15]

Perhaps the best example of problems that can result when there is lack of quality control is *Panax ginseng.*

Panax ginseng and Quality Control

Panax ginseng contains at least 13 different steroid-like compounds, collectively known as ginsenosides. These compounds are believed to be the most important active constituents of *Panax ginseng.* The usual concentration of ginsenosides in mature ginseng roots is between 1% and 3%. However, independent research and published studies have clearly documented a tremendous variation in the ginsenoside content of commercial preparations.[16,17] In fact, the majority of products on the market contain only trace amounts of ginsenosides, and many formulations contain no ginseng at all. The lack of quality control has led to several problems, ranging from toxic reactions (discussed below) to absence of medicinal effect. The widespread disregard for quality control in the herbal industry has done much to tarnish the reputation of ginseng, as well as other important botanicals.

The problem of quality control is exemplified by a 1979 article entitled 'Ginseng Abuse Syndrome' that appeared in the *Journal of the American Medical Association.*[18] In this article, a number of side effects are reported, including hypertension, euphoria, nervousness, insomnia, skin eruptions, and morning diarrhea.

Given the extreme variation in quality of ginseng in the American marketplace and the use both of non-official parts of the plant and of adulterants it is not surprising that side effects were noted. None of the commercial preparations used in the trial had been subjected to controlled analysis. Furthermore, the species of ginseng used included *Panax ginseng, Panax quinquefolius, Eleutherococcus senticosus,* and *Rumex hymenosepalus* in a variety of different forms, i.e., roots, capsules, tablets, teas, extracts, cigarettes, chewing gum, and candies.

It is virtually impossible to derive any firm conclusions from the data presented in the *JAMA* article, especially in light of the fact that studies performed on standardized extracts of *Panax ginseng* have demonstrated the absence of side effects, as well as no mutagenic or teratogenic effects.[19,20] These findings further support the superiority of using herbal products that were produced using quality control measures.

The 'Hairy Baby' Story

To further illustrate the problems that can occur without proper plant identification and standardization, it was reported in another *JAMA* article that a 30-year-old woman took Siberian ginseng (mistakenly identified in the article as *Panax ginseng*) at a dose of two 650 mg tablets twice daily during nine months of pregnancy and two weeks of breast feeding.[21] She had experienced repeated premature uterine contractions during late pregnancy and had noted increased and thicker hair growth on her head, face, and pubic area. The woman gave birth to a full-term baby boy who was noted to have thick black pubic hair over the entire forehead along with other signs suggestive of androgenization. The authors of the report went on to warn physicians of the dangers of ginseng.

At first glance, this case report appears to be quite alarming. However, when examining the scenario more closely a different picture is presented. First of all, animal and human studies with *Eleutherococcus senticosus* have shown it to be extremely safe. In fact, in the animal studies eleutherococcus extract actually prevented the teratogenic effects of xenobiotics and, in a human study of 1,770 pregnant women, it was shown that eleutherococcus improved pregnancy outcome. There were no signs of androgenic effects in either the animal or human studies.[22]

The *JAMA* article caught the attention of Dr. Dennis Awang (Head, Natural Products Bureau of Drug Research, Health Protection Branch, Health and Welfare, Canada). Upon examination of the product the woman had taken, Dr. Awang discovered that the product did not contain Siberian ginseng, but was *Periploca sepium*.[23]

Does this mean the woman's reaction was due to *Periploca sepium*. Not necessarily. Studies in animals have determined that *Periploca sepium*, like Siberian ginseng, does not produce an androgenic response.[24] The most likely explanation for the 'hairy baby', was that it had nothing to with the herbal product being used.

Addressing the Quality Control Problem

The solution, at present, is for manufacturers and suppliers of herbal products to adhere to quality control standards and good manufacturing practices. With improvements in the identification of plants by laboratory analysis, consumers should at least be guaranteed that the right plant is being used. Physicians and other health care providers should ask for information from the suppliers of herbal products on their quality control process. What do they do to guarantee the validity of their product? As more physicians, pharmacists, retailers, and consumers begin asking for quality control from the suppliers, it is possible more quality control processes will be utilized by manufacturers.

Currently, only a few manufacturers adhere to complete quality control and good manufacturing procedures including microscopic, physical, chemical/physical, and biological analyses. Companies supplying standardized extracts currently offer the greatest degree of quality control, hence these products typically offer the highest quality.

Most standardized extracts are currently made in Europe under strict guidelines set forth by individual members of the European Economic Council (EEC) as well as those proposed by the EEC.[7,14] Included are guidelines for acceptable levels of impurities such as parasites (bacterial counts), pesticides, residual solvents, heavy metals, and product stability.

The production of standardized extracts serves as a model for quality control processes for all forms of herbal preparations. In general, it is believed that if the active components of a particular herb are known, whatever form the herb product is, the herb should be analyzed to ensure that it contains these components at an acceptable/standardized level. More accurate dosages can then be given. Products also should be subjected to bacteriological counts.

In many countries, numerous standardized extracts fulfill requirements for marketing as drugs. These extracts have typically gone through the following quality control steps:

1. Selection of suitable plant material.
2. Botanical investigation using organoleptic and microscopic techniques.
3. Chemical analysis using appropriate laboratory equipment.

4. Screening for biological activity.
5. Analysis of active fractions of crude extracts.
6. Isolation of active principles.
7. Determination of chemical structure of active principles.
8. Comparison with compounds of similar structure.
9. Analytical method developed for formulation.
10. Detailed pharmacological evaluation.
11. Studies performed to determine activity and toxicity of formulation.
12. Studies on absorption, distribution, and elimination of herbal compounds.
13. Clinical trials performed to determine activity in humans.
14. Registration by national drug authorities.

V. SOME UNDERLYING CONCEPTS IN MODERN BOTANICAL MEDICINE

Patients often will ask "what advantages do herbal medicines possess over synthetic drugs"? As a rule, botanical preparations are less toxic than their synthetic counterparts and offer less risk of side effects. Obviously, there are exceptions to this rule. In addition, the mechanism of action of an herb is often to correct the underlying cause. In contrast, a synthetic drug is often designed to alleviate the symptom or effect without addressing the underlying cause. An example of this would be the effect of H2-receptor antagonists versus deglycyrrhizinated licorice (DGL) in the treatment of peptic ulcers. While the drug acts on inhibiting the release of stomach acid, DGL acts to increase the quality and quantity of protective mucoid substances, as well as promote healing. In head to head comparative studies, DGL has proven to be as effective as cimetidine (Tagamet®) and ranitidine (Zantac®), but without side effects. (See: 'PEPTIC ULCER')

In many respects the pharmacological investigation of herbal medicine is just beginning. In addition to possessing currently understood actions, many herbs possess actions that are not at all consistent with modern understanding. For example, many herbs appear to impact body control mechanisms to aid in the normalization of numerous body processes. When there is an elevation in a certain body function the herb will have a lowering effect, and when there is decrease in a certain body function it will have a heightening effect. This action is totally baffling to orthodox pharmacologists, but not to experienced herbalists who frequently use the term 'adaptogenic'. Another term that often is used is 'general tonic'. In this connotation the term refers to an herb that improves the general tone or function of the entire organism.

Herbalists also will use a qualifier to describe an herb that appears to have more targeted effects. For example, hawthorn (Crataegus oxyacantha) is referred to as a 'heart' tonic, Silymarin from Silybum marianum is referred to as liver 'tonic', and dong quai (Angelica sinensis) is called a 'uterine' tonic.

Adaptogenic Activity

An 'adaptogen' is defined as a substance that (1) must be innocuous and cause minimal disorders in the physiological functions of an organism, (2) must have a nonspecific action (i.e., it should increase resistance to adverse influences by a wide range of physical, chemical, and biochemical factors), and (3) usually has a normalizing action irrespective of the direction of the pathologic state.

Perhaps the best known example of an adaptogen or general tonic is *Panax ginseng*, also known as Chinese or Korean ginseng. Perhaps the most famous medicinal plant of China, *Panax ginseng* has been used alone or in combination with other herbs for virtually every condition imaginable, reflecting a broad range of nutritional and medicinal properties.

Since the 1950's, a great amount of research has been conducted worldwide to determine whether the properties attributed to *Panax ginseng* belong in the realm of legend or fact. Unfortunately, inconsistent results (due mostly to different procedures in the preparation of extracts, use of nonofficial parts of the plant, use of adulterants, and lack of quality control in the ginseng used) have made determination of ginseng's true properties difficult. Nonetheless, enough good research does exist to indicate that *Panax ginseng* possesses activity consistent with its near legendary status, especially when high quality extracts, standardized for active constituents, are used.

According to tradition and scientific evidence, *Panax ginseng*, as well as Siberian ginseng (*Eleutherococcus senticosus*) and many other herbs, possess this kind of equilibrating, tonic, antistress action.

VI. SAFETY ISSUES

In the 1970s, when herbs began their rise in popularity, numerous articles appeared in medical journals and the lay press questioning the safety of herbal products. Since then, herb usage has increased dramatically, but toxicity reports have not. In a June 1992 article appearing in the *Food and Drug Law Journal*, the results of an extensive review on herbal safety conducted by the Herbal Research Foundation, a nonprofit organization composed of some of the leading experts on pharmacognosy, pharmacology, and toxicology, confirmed there is no substantial evidence that toxic reactions to herbal products are a major source of concern.[25] The review was based on reports from the American Association of Poison Control Centers and the Center of Disease Control.

Although there are numerous herbs in the environment that can definitely cause significant toxicity, the herbs commonly used in the United States for health purposes are usually quite safe. Nonetheless, it is important for health care providers to be aware of any possible adverse reaction with herbal product use. It is, therefore, essential that they have a good understanding of the more popular herbal products.

REFERENCES

1. Farnsworth N et al. Medicinal plants in therapy. Bull World Health Org 63:965-81, 1985.
2. Interview. An interview with Prof. H. Wagner. HerbalGram 17:16-17, 1988.
3. Unpublished data from the American Herbal Products Association.
4. Deveny K. Garlic and ginseng supplements become potent drugstore sellers. The Wall Street Journal 10/1/92 pB1,B5.
5. Market Report. HerbalGram 26:40, 1992.
6. Principe PP. The economic significance of plants and their constituents as drugs. Econ Med Plant Res 3:1-17, 1989.
7. Keller K. Legal Requirements for the use of phytopharmaceutical drugs in the Federal Republic of Germany. J Ethnopharamacol 32:225-9, 1991.
8. Kleijnen J, Knipschild P. Drug Profiles - Ginkgo biloba. Lancet 340:1136-9, 1993.

9. Bonati A. *Formulation of Plant Extracts into Dosage Forms.* In: *The Medicinal Plant Industry.* Wijeskera ROB (ed). CRC Press, Boca Raton, FL, 1991:107-14.

10. Karlsen J. *Quality Control and Instrumental Analysis of Plant Extracts.* In: *The Medicinal Plant Industry.* Wijeskera ROB (ed). CRC Press, Boca Raton, FL, 1991:99-106.

11. Bonati A. *How and why should we standardize phytopharmical drugs for clinical validation.* *J Ethnopharmacol* 32:195-7, 1991.

12. Bombardelli E. *Technologies for the Processing of Medicinal Plants.* In: *The Medicinal Plant Industry.* Wijeskera ROB (ed). CRC Press, Boca Raton, FL, 1991:85-98.

13. Awang DVC, Kindack DG. *Echinacea.* *Can Pharm J* 124:512-6, 1991.

14. Heptinstall S et al. *Parthenolide content and bioactivity of feverfew (Tanacetum parthenium (L.) Schultz-Bip.). Estimation of commercial and authenticated feverfew products.* *J Pharm Pharmacol* 44:391-5, 1992.

15. Awang DVC. *Commercial taheebo lacks active ingredient.* *Can Pharm J* 121:323-6, 1988.

16. Liberti LE, Marderosian AD. *Evaluation of commercial ginseng products.* *J Pharm Sci* 67:1487-9, 1978.

17. Soldati F, Sticher O. *HPLC separation and quantitative determination of ginsenosides from Panax ginseng, Panax quinquefolium and from ginseng drug preparations.* *Planta Med* 39(4):348-57, 1980.

18. Siegel RK. *Ginseng abuse syndrome.* *JAMA* 241:1614-5, 1979.

19. Hikino H. *Traditional remedies and modern assessment: The case of ginseng.* In: *The Medicinal Plant Industry.* Wijeskera ROB (ed). CRC Press, Boca Raton, FL, 1991:149-66.

20. Shibata S et al. *Chemistry and pharmacology of Panax.* *Econ Medicinal Plant Res* 1:217-84, 1985.

21. Koren GS et al. *Maternal ginseng use associated with neonatal androgenization.* *JAMA* 264:2866, 1990.

22. Farnsworth NR et al. *Siberian ginseng (Eleutherococcus senticosus): current status as an adaptogen.* *Econ Medicinal Plant Res* 1:156-215, 1985.

23. Awang DVC. *Maternal use of ginseng and neonatal androgenization.* *JAMA* 265:1828, 1991.

24. Waller DP et al. *Lack of androgenicity of Siberian ginseng.* *JAMA* 267:2329, 1992.

25. McCaleb RS: *Food ingredient safety evaluation.* *Food Drug Law Journal* 47:657-65, 1992.

CONCISE MATERIA MEDICA

A 'materia medica' refers to a book containing guidelines on the prescription and medical use of botanical preparation. This section is designed to provide a concise pharmacological description of 26 of the most important herbs in the industrialized Western countries:

Aloe vera
Bilberry (*Vaccinium myrtillus*)
Bromelain (from *Ananas comosus*)
Centella asiatica (Gotu Kola)
Cranberry (*Vaccinium macrocarpon*)
Curcumin (from *Curcuma longa*)
Dong Quai (*Angelica sinensis*)
Echinacea spp.
Ephedra sinica (Ma Huang)
Feverfew (*Tanacetum parthenium*)
Garlic (*Allium sativum*)
Ginger (*Zingiber officinale*)
Ginkgo biloba
Goldenseal (*Hydrastis canadensis*)
Gugulipid (from *Commiphora mukul*)
Hawthorn (*Crataegus* spp.)
Licorice (*Glycyrrhiza glabra*)
Panax ginseng
Procyanidolic Oligomers (leukocyanidins; pycnogenols)
Sarsaparilla (*Smilax sarsaparilla*)
Saw Palmetto (*Serenoa repens*)
Siberian Ginseng (*Eleutherococcus senticosus*)
Silymarin (from *Silybum marianum*)
St. John's Wort (*Hypericum perforatum*)
Tea Tree oil (from *Melaleuca alternifolia*)
Valerian (*Valeriana officinalis*)

Note: The 'possible applications' listed below coincide with individual chapter headings.

Aloe vera

Possible applications:

    Topical:
        Wound Healing
    Internal:
        Acquired Immunodeficiency Syndrome

Bronchial Asthma
Cancer
Diabetes Mellitus
Immunodepression

Aloe vera products, both for internal and external use, are widely used in the United States. Despite this widespread use and acceptance, there are very few controlled studies on *Aloe vera*. From the information currently available, it can be concluded that *Aloe vera* can be used topically in the treatment of minor burns, cuts, and abrasions.

The use of aloe orally, other than for its well-accepted laxative effect, has not been fully studied. Preliminary and anecdotal studies indicate that *Aloe vera* juice may have 'tonic' and anti-ulcer effects on the gastrointestinal tract.

The polysaccharide component of *Aloe vera*, acemannan, possesses significant immune enhancing and antiviral activity. Preliminary studies indicate it may be useful as an adjunct to current AIDS therapy (i.e., AZT).

Aloe vera gel can be applied liberally for topical applications. A wide range of products are available on the market; however, simply pure *Aloe vera* gel is sufficient.

Aloe vera juice can be consumed orally as a beverage or tonic. As detailed information is currently lacking as to the optimal dose for these types of products it is recommended that no more than 1 quart be consumed in any one day.

The dose of acemannan being used in HIV/AIDS patients is 800-1,600 mg. per day. This would correspond to a dose of approximately 1/2 to 1 liter per day for most *Aloe vera* juice products. However, it appears that there may be great variation in the amount of acemannan from one manufacturer to the next.

Bilberry or European blueberry (*Vaccinium myrtillus*)

Possible applications:

Atherosclerosis
Cataract
Diabetes Mellitus
Dysmenorrhea
Inflammation
Neuralgia and Neuropathy
Peptic Ulcer
Peripheral Vascular Disease
Pregnancy-related Illness (varicose veins)
Retinopathy
Vascular Fragility
Visual Dysfunction

Bilberry, or European blueberry, is a shrubby perennial plant that grows in the woods and forest meadows of Europe. The fruit is a blue-black berry that differs from an American blueberry in that its meat also is blue-black.

The active components of bilberries are its flavonoids, specifically its anthocyanosides. Anthocyanosides are extremely powerful antioxidants and vascular stabilizers. Bilberry extracts have been widely used in Europe in the treatment of various vascular disorders, as well as in several eye diseases. Clinical studies have demonstrated a positive effect in the treatment of capillary fragility, blood purpuras, various disturbances of blood flow to the brain (similar to *Ginkgo biloba*), venous insufficiency, varicose veins, and blood in the urine not caused by infection.

Perhaps the most significant therapeutic applications for bilberry extracts are in the field of ophthalmology. Interest in bilberry anthocyanosides was first aroused when it was observed during World War II that British Royal Air Force pilots reported improved night visual acuity on bombing raids after consuming bilberries. Subsequent studies showed that the administration of bilberry extracts to healthy subjects resulted in improved night visual acuity, quicker adjustment to darkness, and faster restoration of visual acuity after exposure to glare.

Apparently, bilberry anthocyanosides have an affinity for the part of the retina responsible for vision. This affinity is consistent with several of the clinical effects observed including positive results in macular degeneration, cataracts, retinitis pigmentosa, diabetic retinopathy, and night-blindness.

The standard dose for bilberry extracts is based on its anthocyanoside content, as calculated by its anthocyanidin percentage. The dosage for a bilberry extract standardized for an anthocyanidin content of 25% is 80 to 160 mg three times daily.

Extensive toxicological investigation has demonstrated that bilberry extracts are usually without toxic effects. Administration to rats of dosages as high as 400 mg/kg produces no apparent side effects, and excess levels are usually quickly excreted through the urine and bile.

Bromelain

Possible applications:

> Atherosclerosis
> Cancer
> Dysmenorrhea
> Infection
> Inflammation
> Osteoarthritis
> Peripheral Vascular Disease
> Rheumatoid Arthritis
> Scleroderma
> Sports Injuries
> Wound Healing

Bromelain is a mixture of sulfur-containing protein-digesting enzymes (proteolytic enzymes or proteases) obtained from the stem of the pineapple plant (*Ananas comosus*). Bromelain was introduced as a medicinal agent in 1957, and since that time more than 200 scientific papers on its therapeutic applications have appeared in medical literature.

Bromelain has been reported in these scientific studies to exert a wide variety of beneficial effects, including reducing inflammation in cases of arthritis, sports injury or trauma and prevention of swelling (edema) after trauma or surgery. Bromelain has been shown to be effective in a number of other health conditions including angina, indigestion, and upper respiratory tract infections.

Several mechanisms may account for bromelain's anti-inflammatory effects, including the inhibition of proinflammatory compounds. Bromelain also blocks the production of kinins. Kinins are compounds produced during inflammation that increase swelling and cause pain.

The standard dosage of bromelain is based on its m.c.u. (milk clotting unit) or g.d.u. (gelatin-digesting unit) activity. The most beneficial range of activity appears to be 1,800 to 2,000 m.c.u. or g.d.u. Unless bromelain is being used as a digestive aid, administration should be on an empty stomach (before or between meals), the typical dosage being 250 to 750 mg. three times per day.

Although no significant side effects have been noted, as with most therapeutic agents, allergic reactions may occur in sensitive individuals or with prolonged occupational exposure. Other possible, but unconfirmed, reactions include nausea, vomiting, diarrhea, metrorrhagia, and menorrhagia.

Centella asiatica (Gotu kola)

Possible applications:

> Alcoholic Liver Disease
> Periodontal Disease
> Peripheral Vascular Disease
> Scleroderma
> Vascular Fragility
> Wound Healing

> *Note: Do not confuse gotu kola with cola nut. Gotu kola is not related to the cola nut (Cola nitida or C. acuminata), nor does it contain any caffeine.*

Centella has been utilized as a medicine in India and Indonesia since prehistoric times with use centered around its ability to heal wounds and relieve leprosy. Modern research has substantiated its efficacy in both of these applications.

Regarding wound healing, the outcome of Centella's complex actions is a balanced effect on cells and tissues participating in the process of healing, particularly connective tissues. This action makes Centella useful in a wide range of conditions where enhancing wound healing is required. In the United States, the most popular use of *Centella asiatica* has been in the treatment of cellulite and varicose veins.

Numerous studies have demonstrated that the total triterpenoid fraction of *Centella asiatica* (TTFCA) is effective in the treatment of venous insufficiency due to its ability to enhance the connective tissue structure of the perivascular sheath, reduce sclerosis or hardening, and improve the blood flow through the affected limbs.

Significant improvement in symptomatology (such as feelings of heaviness in the lower legs, numbness, nighttime cramps, etc.), physical findings (swelling, spider veins, skin ulcers, vein distensibility, etc.), and functional capacity (improved venous blood flow) were observed in approximately 80% of patients in the clinical trials.

Using TTFCA or extracts standardized for triterpenoid acids may produce more reliable results compared to crude preparations. The concentration of triterpenoids in centella can vary between 1.1% and 8%, with most samples yielding a concentration between 2.2-3.4% percent. To achieve a similar dosage of triterpenoids compared to TTFCA with the crude plant would require 2 to 4 grams per day, although it is not known if this would still correlate with the clinical efficacy noted for TTFCA.

Clinical studies using TTFCA indicate extremely good tolerance when used orally, as no significant side effects have been reported. Topical application can result in contact dermatitis.

Cranberry (*Vaccinium macrocarpon*)

Possible applications:

Infection
Kidney Stones

The drinking of cranberry juice has long been a recommendation in the treatment of urinary tract infections. Cranberry juice has been shown to be quite effective in several clinical studies. In one study, 16 ounces of cranberry juice per day produced beneficial effects in 73% of the subjects with active urinary tract infections. Furthermore, withdrawal of the cranberry juice in the people who benefitted resulted in recurrence of bladder infection in 61%.

Although many people believe the action of cranberry juice is due to acidifying the urine and the antibacterial effects of a cranberry component hippuric acid, these are probably not the major mechanisms of action. In order to acidify the urine at least 1 quart of cranberry juice would have to be consumed at one sitting. In addition, the concentration of hippuric acid in the urine as a result of drinking cranberry juice is not sufficient to inhibit bacteria. A positive effect of cranberry juice in the treatment of bladder infection was noted when only 16 ounces of cranberry juice per day was consumed. This data would indicate that another mechanism is more likely.

Recent studies have shown components in cranberry juice to reduce the ability of E. coli to adhere, or stick to, the lining of the bladder and urethra. In order for bacteria to infect they must first adhere to the mucosa. By interfering with adherence, cranberry juice greatly reduces the likelihood of infection. This is the most likely explanation of cranberry juice's positive effects in bladder infections.

Cranberry juice also has been shown to reduce the amount of ionized calcium in the urine by more than 50% in patients with recurrent kidney stones.

The dosage of cranberry extract should be based on the equivalent of 16 ounces of cranberry juice daily. There is no known toxicity as a result of cranberry ingestion.

Curcumin

Possible applications:

> Atherosclerosis
> Cancer
> Gallbladder Disease
> Inflammation
> Rheumatoid Arthritis

Tumeric (*Curcuma longa*) is one of the most widely used spices in India. It is used as a food color and flavor, an ingredient in many medicinal preparations, and as a cosmetic. Curcumin, the yellow pigment of turmeric, is a very powerful, yet safe, anti-inflammatory agent. In addition to its use in inflammation, turmeric and curcumin have also demonstrated significant protective effect against cancer development in experimental studies with animal models of cancer, and there is early data from human studies to back-up this research.

For medicinal effects, curcumin is recommended at a dose of 250 to 500 mg three times a day. Combining curcumin with bromelain may enhance its absorption and activity.

Dong Quai (*Angelica sinensis*)

Possible applications:

> Dysmenorrhea
> Menopausal Symptoms

In Asia, dong quai's reputation is perhaps second only to ginseng. Predominantly regarded as a 'female' remedy, dong quai has been used in such conditions as painful menstruation, menopausal symptoms, and to assure a healthy pregnancy and easy delivery. Scientific investigation has shown dong quai produces a balancing effect on estrogen activity and a tonic effect on the uterus.

Three times a day dosages are as follows:

> Dried root (or as tea): 1-2 gram
> Tincture (1:5): 3-5 ml.
> Fluid extract (1:1): 0.5-2 ml.
> Solid extract (4:1): 125-500 mg.

Dong quai is generally quite safe; however, because it does contain photoreactive substances, overexposure to sunlight should be avoided.

Echinacea angustifolia and *Echinacea purpurea* (purple cornflower)

Possible applications:

> Cancer
> Candidiasis
> Immunodepression
> Infection

Wound Healing

Echinacea is a North American herb which was used extensively by the native Americans. In fact, Echinacea was used by the American Indians against more illnesses than any other plant. Today, Echinacea is still one of the most widely used botanicals. Its primary clinical applications have been in cases of infections or when immune system enhancement is desired. Numerous studies have shown that Echinacea has profound immunostimulatory effects resulting in enhanced T-cell mitogenesis, macrophage phagocytosis, antibody binding, and natural killer cell activity, as well as increased levels of circulating neutrophils.

Root extracts of Echinacea also have been shown to possess interferon-like activity, as well as direct antiviral activity against many viruses including influenza, herpes, and vesicular stomatitis viruses.

Numerous clinical investigations have confirmed Echinacea's immune enhancing effects.

Echinacea contains many so-called 'active constituents' including polysaccharides, flavonoids, alkamides, and essential oils. Various forms of echinacea have been shown to be effective. Echinacea can, therefore, be given in any of the following forms and dosages three times daily:

Dried root (or as tea): 0.5 to 1 g
Freeze-dried plant: 325 to 650 mg
Juice of aerial portion of *E. purpurea* stabilized in 22% ethanol: 1 to 2 ml
Tincture (1:5): 2 to 4 ml (1 to 2 tsp)
Fluid extract (1:1): 1 to 2 ml (0.5 to 1 tsp)
Solid (dry powdered) extract (6.5:1 or 3.5% echinacoside): 100 to 250 mg

Echinacea is regarded as an extremely safe herb with no reported toxicity.

Ephedra sinica (Ma Huang)

Possible applications:

Bronchial Asthma
Obesity

Ephedra's medicinal use in China dates from approximately 2800 B.C. It was used primarily in the treatment of the common cold, asthma, hayfever, bronchitis, edema, arthritis, fever, hypotension, and hives. Western medicine's interest in ephedra began in 1923 with the demonstration that the isolated alkaloid ephedrine possessed a number of pharmacological effects. Ephedrine was synthesized in 1927 and since this time both ephedrine and pseudoephedrine have been used extensively in over-the-counter cold and allergy medications.

The dosage of Ephedra is dependent on the alkaloid content. The average total alkaloid content of *Ephedra sinica* is 1 to 3%. For asthma and as a weight-loss aid the dose of Ephedra should have an ephedrine content of 12.5-25.0 mg and be taken two to three times daily. For the crude herb this would require a dose of 500 to 1,000 mg 3 times per day. Standardized preparations are preferred as they are more dependable for therapeutic activity. For example, *Ephedra sinica* extracts are available that have a standardized alkaloid content of 10%. The dosage of a 10% alkaloid content extract would be 125 to 250 mg 3 times daily.

Ephedra preparations can produce the same side effects that ephedrine can, i.e. increased blood pressure and heart rate, insomnia, and anxiety. The U.S. Food and Drug Administration advisory review panel on nonprescription drugs recommended that ephedrine not be taken by patients with heart disease, high blood pressure, thyroid disease, diabetes, or difficulty in urination due to enlargement of the prostate gland. Nor should ephedrine be used in patients on antihypertensive or antidepressant drugs. These warnings are appropriate for Ephedra preparations.

Feverfew (*Tanacetum parthenium*)

Possible applications:

>Allergy
>Dysmenorrhea
>Headache
>Inflammation
>Rheumatoid Arthritis

Feverfew has been used for centuries to relieve fever, migraines, and arthritis. Physician John Hill, in his book The Family Herbal (1772) noted, "In the worst headache this herb exceeds whatever else is known." Recently, there has been a great increase in interest in feverfew for the treatment of headaches due to positive results in double-blind studies.

Feverfew works in the treatment and prevention of migraine headaches by inhibiting the release of blood vessel dilating substances from platelets (serotonin and histamine), inhibiting the production of inflammatory substances (leukotrienes, serine proteases, etc.), and re - establishing proper blood vessel tone.

Its efficacy is dependent upon adequate levels of parthenolide, the active ingredient. The preparations used in the clinical trials had a parthenolide content of 0.4%. The dosage of feverfew used in the London Migraine Clinic study was one capsule containing 25 mg of the freeze-dried pulverized leaves twice daily. In the another study it was one capsule containing 82 mg of dried powdered leaves once daily. While these low dosages might be effective in preventing an attack, a higher dose (1 to 2 grams) may be necessary during an acute attack.

Feverfew is well-tolerated and no serious side effects have been reported. However, chewing the leaves can result in small ulcerations in the mouth and swelling of the lips and tongue. This side effect occurs in about 10% of users.

Garlic (*Allium sativum*)

Possible applications:

>Acquired Immunodeficiency Syndrome
>Allergy
>Atherosclerosis
>Cancer

Candidiasis
Cardiac Arrhythmia
Diabetes Mellitus
Hypertension
Immunodepression
Infection

Garlic has been used throughout history throughout the world for the treatment of a wide variety of conditions, especially infections. Garlic's antibiotic activity was noted by Pasteur in 1858 and garlic was used by Albert Schwietzer in Africa for the treatment of dysentery.

More recent research has shown garlic to have broad-spectrum antimicrobial activity against many types of bacteria, viruses, worms, and fungi. Garlic is especially active against Candida albicans, reportedly being more potent than nystatin, gentian violet, and six other reputed antifungal agents. In addition to its antibiotic activity, garlic also has been shown to enhance various aspects of immune function. These effects support the historical use of garlic in the treatment of a variety of infectious conditions.

Perhaps the best known popular use of garlic is its cardiovascular applications. Clinical studies have shown garlic to impact many key factors involved in atherosclerosis, including an ability to lower blood pressure, LDL-cholesterol, triglycerides, and platelet aggregation while simultaneously increasing HDL-cholesterol and fibrinolysis.

Commercial preparations concentrated for alliin appear to be the most effective. Because alliin is relatively odorless until it is converted to allicin in the body, these preparations are also more socially acceptable. The compound alliin is converted to allicin by the enzyme alliinase, which is activated when garlic is crushed.

A variety of commercial garlic preparations exist on the market. For best results, products standardized for alliin content are preferred. The dosage should provide a daily dose of 8 mg alliin or a total allicin potential of 4,000 mcg.

For the vast majority of individuals, garlic is nontoxic at the dosages commonly used. For some, however, it causes allergic contact dermatitis (eczema) and irritation to the digestive tract.

Ginger (*Zingiber officinale*)

Possible applications:

Atherosclerosis
Headache
Inner Ear Dysfunction
Nausea and Vomiting
Osteoarthritis
Pain ('rheumatic')
Pregnancy-related Illness (nausea and vomiting)
Rheumatoid Arthritis

Historically, the majority of complaints for which ginger was used concerned the gastrointestinal system. It is generally regarded as an excellent carminative (a substance that promotes the elimination of intestinal gas) and intestinal spasmolytic (a substance that relaxes and soothes the intestinal tract).

A clue to ginger's success in eliminating gastrointestinal distress is offered by recent double-blind studies which demonstrated that ginger is very effective in preventing the symptoms of motion sickness, especially seasickness. In fact, several studies have shown ginger to be superior to diphenhydramine, a commonly used drug for this symptom complex. Ginger reduces all symptoms associated with motion sickness including dizziness, nausea, vomiting, and cold sweating.

Ginger also has been used to treat the nausea and vomiting associated with pregnancy. Recently, the benefit of ginger was confirmed in hyperemesis gravidarum, the most severe form of pregnancy-related nausea and vomiting.

Ginger possesses some anti-inflammatory effects which may be beneficial in the treatment of migraine headaches and arthritic conditions.

Most clinical studies have used powdered ginger root at a dose of 1 gram per day. The dose of ginger root extracts should approximate this dosage. There does not appear to be any toxicity associated with ginger root ingestion.

Ginkgo biloba

Possible applications:

> Allergy
> Atherosclerosis
> Bronchial Asthma
> Cardiac Arrhythmia
> Cerebrovascular Disease
> Dementia
> Depression
> Diabetes Mellitus
> Eczema
> Glaucoma
> Impotence
> Inner Ear Dysfunction
> Multiple Sclerosis
> Neuralgia and Neuropathy
> Peripheral Vascular Disease
> Retinopathy
> Vascular Fragility

Ginkgo biloba is the world's oldest living tree species. It is the sole survivor of the family Ginkgoaceae. The ginkgo tree can be traced back more than 200 million years to the fossils of the Permian period and for this reason often is referred to as "the living fossil." Once common in North America and Europe, the ginkgo was destroyed in all regions of the world, except China, during the ice age. Ginkgo has long been cultivated in China as a sacred tree and medicine.

Ginkgo biloba's medicinal use can be traced back to the oldest Chinese materia medica (2800 B.C.). The ginkgo leaves have been used in traditional Chinese medicine for their ability to 'benefit the brain', relieve the symptoms of asthma and coughs, and help the body eliminate filaria, the worm that causes elephantitis.

Ginkgo leaf extracts are now among the leading prescription medicines in both Germany and France. The extracts account for 1.0% and 1.5% of total prescription sales in Germany and France respectively. Over 100,000 physicians worldwide combined to write more than 10,000,000 prescriptions in 1989.

Ginkgo biloba extract (GBE) may be the most important plant-derived medicine available. It offers significant benefit to many elderly people with impaired blood flow to the brain or cerebral insufficiency. The symptoms of cerebral insufficiency include short-term memory loss, vertigo, headache, ringing in the ears, and depression. These symptoms are often referred to as 'symptoms of aging'.

GBE has been extensively studied and appears to work primarily by increasing blood flow to the brain, resulting in an increase in oxygen and glucose utilization. However, this explanation is quite simplistic as GBE exerts profound, widespread tissue effects including membrane stabilizing, antioxidant, and free radical scavenging effects. Its vascular effects are primarily a result of direct stimulation of the release of endothelium-derived relaxing factor (EDRF) and prostacyclin. In addition, GBE inhibits enzymes in a way that leads to smooth muscle cell relaxation in the wall of the vessel. GBE also exerts a profound effect on platelet function including inhibition of platelet aggregation, adhesion, and degranulation.

Because of the multitude of vascular effects, GBE offers effective treatment for the signs, symptoms, and underlying pathophysiology of arterial insufficiency. GBE has been confirmed by more than 50 double-blind studies to be effective in cerebral, as well as peripheral arterial, insufficiency. GBE may offer significant protective action against the development of Alzheimer's disease, hearing loss, and strokes.

The usual dosage of the *Ginkgo biloba* extract standardized to contain 24% ginkgoflavonglycosides is 40 mg three times a day.

GBE is safe to use as there have been no reports of significant adverse reactions at the prescribed dose. Mild adverse reactions, although quite rare, have been reported and include gastrointestinal upset and headache.

Goldenseal (*Hydrastis canadensis*)

Possible applications:

> Alcoholic Liver Disease
> Cancer
> Infection

Goldenseal was used extensively by the American Indian as an herbal medication and clothing dye. Its medicinal use centered around its ability to soothe the mucous membranes that line the respiratory, digestive, and genito-urinary tracts in inflammatory conditions induced by allergy or infection.

The medicinal value of goldenseal (as well as barberry and Oregon grape root) is thought to be due to its high content of alkaloids, of which berberine has been the most widely studied. The broad antibiotic effects of berberine, combined with its anti-infective and immune stimulating actions, support the historical use of berberine containing plants in infections of the mucous membranes, i.e., the linings of the oral cavity, throat, sinuses, bronchi, genito-urinary tract, and gastrointestinal tract.

Goldenseal's historical use also is supported by several clinical studies that have shown berberine is successful in the treatment of acute diarrhea. Berberine has been found effective against diarrheas caused by *E. coli* (traveler's diarrhea), *Shigella dysenteriae* (shigellosis), *Salmonella paratyphi* (food poisoning), *Giardia lamblia* (giardiasis), and *Vibrio cholerae* (cholera). Berberine also has the ability to inhibit the adherence of bacteria (group A streptococci) to host cells.

For best results, goldenseal extracts standardized for berberine or hydrastine content are preferred. For an extract standardized at 5% hydrastine, the dosage would be 250 to 500 mg three times daily.

Goldenseal and other berberine-containing plants are generally nontoxic at the recommended dosages even during long-term therapy, however, berberine-containing plants are not recommended for use during pregnancy and higher dosages may interfere with B vitamin metabolism.

Gugulipid (*Commiphora mukul*)

Possible applications:

> Acne Vulgaris
> Atherosclerosis

Gugulipid is the extract of the oleoresin (gum guggul or guggulu) of the mukul myrrh tree (*Commiphora mukul*), which is native to India, standardized for guggulsterones. The active components of gugulipid are two compounds, Z-guggulsterone and E-guggulsterone. Several clinical studies have shown gugulipid has an ability to lower both cholesterol and triglyceride levels. Typically cholesterol levels will drop 14%-27% in a 4 to 12 week period while triglyceride levels will drop from 22%-30%.

The mechanism of action for gugulipid's cholesterol lowering action is its ability to increase the liver's metabolism of LDL-cholesterol; guggulsterone increases the uptake of LDL-cholesterol from the blood by the liver.

The dosage of gugulipid is based on its guggulsterone content. The standard dosage is 25 mg of guggulsterone 3 times daily.

Safety studies in rats, rabbits, and monkeys have demonstrated gugulipid to be nontoxic. It is also considered safe to use in pregnancy.

Hawthorn (*Crataegus oxyacantha; C. monogyna*)

Possible applications:

        Atherosclerosis
        Cardiac Arrhythmia
        Congestive Heart Failure
        Hypertension
        Peripheral Vascular Disease
        Vascular Fragility

Hawthorn extracts are widely used by physicians in Europe for their effect on the cardiovascular system. Studies have demonstrated hawthorn extracts are effective in reducing angina attacks, as well lowering blood pressure and serum cholesterol levels.

The beneficial effects of hawthorn extracts in the treatment of angina are a result of improvement in the blood and oxygen supply to the heart by dilating the coronary vessels, as well as improvement of the metabolic processes in the heart.

Various flavonoid components in hawthorn have been shown to inhibit constriction of vessels in a manner similar to the calcium-channel blockers. However, this is only part of the total picture. Hawthorn extracts also incease energy production within the heart due to the ability of flavonoids to improve the utilization of oxygen by the heart. The net result is improved heart function and an increase in the force of contraction. This action is in stark contrast to beta-blockers and calcium-channel blockers, which actually reduce heart function. The effects of hawthorn also make it beneficial in cases of congestive heart failure and rhythm disturbances. In addition, the procyanidins of hawthorn have been shown to decrease cholesterol levels and the size of cholesterol-containing plaques in the arteries.

The mild blood pressure lowering effects of hawthorn extracts have been demonstrated in many experimental and clinical studies. Its action in lowering blood pressure is quite unique in that it does so through a combination of many diverse actions. Specifically, it dilates the larger blood vessels, inhibits angiotensin-converting enzyme (ACE) similar to the drug captopril, increases the functional capacity of the heart, and possesses mild diuretic activity. The blood pressure lowering effects of hawthorn extracts generally require up to two weeks before appearing. This time is necessary in order for adequate tissue concentrations of the flavonoids to be achieved.

The dosage of hawthorn depends on the type of preparation and source material. Standardized extracts are the preferred form for medicinal purposes. The dosage for hawthorn extracts standardized to contain 1.8% vitexin-4[1]-rhamnoside or 10% procyanidins is 120-240 mg three times daily; for extracts standardized to contain 18% procyanidolic oligomers, the dosage is 240 to 480 mg daily.

Hawthorn extracts are without known side effects and are extremely well tolerated.

Licorice (*Glycyrrhiza glabra*)

    Possible applications:

        Acquired Immunodeficiency Syndrome
        Aphthous Stomatitis
        Eczema
        Heartburn
        Hepatitis

Inflammation
Menopausal Symptoms
Peptic Ulcer
Periodontal Disease

Licorice root is one of the most extensively investigated botanical medicines. Licorice components are known to exhibit many pharmacological actions, including: the healing of peptic ulcers; estrogenic activity; aldosterone-like action; anti-inflammatory (cortisol-like action); anti-allergic; antihepatotoxic; antineoplastic; expectorant; and antitussive activities. Although the majority of these effects are attributed to the glycyrrhizinic acid component of licorice, other components, particularly flavonoids, also play a major role in the pharmacological action of licorice.

Because of the aldosterone-like action of glycyrrhetinic acid, licorice root ingestion can cause sodium retention and high blood pressure. The sensitivity to this side effect is individualized. Prevention of the pseudo-aldosteronism may be possible by following a high-potassium, low-sodium diet. Although no formal trial of either of these guidelines has been performed, patients who normally consume high-potassium foods and restrict sodium intake, even those with hypertension and angina, have been reported to be free from the aldosterone-like side effects of glycyrrhizin.

In treating peptic ulcer, deglycyrrhizinated licorice (DGL) is preferred as it produces equally effective results compared to glycyrrhetinic acid, but is free from any side effects.

Three times a day dosages are:

Powdered root: 1-2 g
Fluid extract (1:1): 2-4 ml
Solid (dry powdered) extract (4:1): 250 to 500 mg
Deglycyrrhizinated licorice: 380-760 mg 20 minutes before meals

Panax ginseng (Chinese or Korean Ginseng)

Possible applications:

Anxiety
Cancer
Fatigue
Immunodepression
Menopausal Symptoms

Chinese or Korean ginseng is a small perennial plant which originally grew wild in the damp woodlands of northern China, Manchuria, and Korea. Ginseng is, without question, the most famous medicinal plant of China, where it has been generally used alone or in combination with other herbs for its revitalizing properties, especially after a long illness. It is regarded as being more potent than Siberian ginseng (see below).

The mental and physical anti-fatigue effects of ginseng have been demonstrated in both animal studies and double-blind clinical trials in humans. From a practical standpoint, ginseng's antifatigue properties may be useful whenever fatigue or lack of energy is apparent. Athletes, in particular, may derive some benefit from ginseng use.

The dosage of ginseng is related to the ginsenoside content. The use of standardized ginseng preparations is recommended to insure sufficient ginsenoside content, consistent therapeutic results, and reduced risk of toxicity. The typical dose (taken one to three times daily) for general tonic effects should contain a saponin content of at least 10 mg of ginsenoside Rg1 with a ratio Rg1 to Rb1 of 1:2. The standard dose for high quality ginseng root is in the range of 4 to 6 grams daily.

As each individual's response to ginseng is unique, care must be taken to observe possible ginseng toxicity (*see below*). It is best to begin at lower doses and increase gradually. The Russian approach for long-term administration is to use ginseng cyclically for a period of 15 to 20 days followed by a two-week interval without any ginseng.

The following side effects can appear with ginseng toxicity: anxiety, irritability, nervousness, insomnia, hypertension, breast pain, and menstrual changes. Upon the appearance of any of these side effects, dosage should be reduced or the product should be discontinued.

Procyanidolic Oligomers

Possible applications:

> Atherosclerosis
> Diabetes Mellitus
> Peripheral Vascular Disease
> Retinopathy
> Vascular Fragility
> Visual Dysfunction
> Wound Healing

Procyanidolic oligomers (PCOs), also known as leukocyanidins or pycnogenols, are complexes of flavonoids (polyphenols). Most commercial preparations use PCOs extracted from grape seed skin (*Vitis vinifera*), although PCOs can also be extracted from other sources - such as the bark of Landes' pine, the bracts of the lime tree, and the leaves of the hazel-nut tree.

PCOs have very strong 'vitamin P' activity. Among their effects is an ability to increase intracellular vitamin C levels, decrease capillary permeability and fragility, scavenge oxidants and free radicals, and a unique ability to bind to collagen structures directly, as well as inhibit destruction of collagen.

Collagen, the most abundant protein of the body, is responsible for maintaining the integrity of 'ground substance', as well as the integrity of tendons, ligaments, and cartilage. Collagen also is the support structure of the dermis and blood vessels. Leukocyanidins and other flavonoids are remarkable in their effect in supporting collagen structures and preventing collagen destruction. They affect collagen metabolism in several ways:

> 1. They have the unique ability to crosslink collagen fibers, resulting in reinforcement of the natural crosslinking of collagen that forms the so-called collagen matrix of connective tissue (ground substance, cartilage, tendon, etc.).
> 2. They prevent free radical damage with their potent antioxidant and free radical scavenging action.

3. They inhibit enzymatic cleavage of collagen by enzymes secreted by white blood cells during inflammation, and microbes during infection.

4. They prevent the release and synthesis of compounds that promote inflammation, such as histamine, serine proteases, prostaglandins, and leukotrienes.

These effects on collagen are put to good use in the treatment of capillary fragility, easy bruising, and varicose veins.

The standard dosage of PCOs are 150 to 300 mg per day.

Detailed toxicology studies, as well as empirical use, have shown grape seed extract to be without toxicity and well-tolerated.

Sarsaparilla (*Smilax sarsaparilla*)

Possible application:

Psoriasis

Sarsaparilla species have been used all over the world in many different cultures for the same conditions, namely gout, arthritis, fevers, digestive disorders, skin disease, and cancer. Sarsaparilla contains saponins or steroid-like molecules which bind to gut endotoxins. This effect may support the plant's historical use as a 'blood purifier' and tonic in human health conditions associated with high endotoxin levels, most notably psoriasis, eczema, arthritis, and ulcerative colitis.

In the U.S., sarsaparilla has been widely touted as a 'sexual rejuvenator' with some commercial suppliers even claiming that it is a rich source of human testosterone. In fact, while sarsaparilla may have tonic effects, there is no testosterone in the plant and it is unlikely that the steroid-like substances in sarsaparilla are absorbed in any great degree. It is also unlikely sarsaparilla has any significant anabolic effects, as there is no evidence to support the claim that it increases muscle mass in any historical text, as well as from clinical or experimental studies.

The confusion arises because the sarsaparilla saponin, sarsapagenin, can be synthetically transformed in the laboratory to testosterone. However, it is highly unlikely that this reaction could take place in the human body.

The three times a day dosage for sarsaparilla is as follows:

Dried root: 1-4 g
Fluid extract (1:1): 1-4 ml
Solid (dry, powdered) extract (4:1): 250 mg

No notable side effects have been reported due to sarsaparilla root ingestion.

Saw Palmetto (*Serenoa repens*)

Possible application:

Benign Prostatic Hyperplasia

Saw palmetto is a small scrubby palm tree native to the West Indies and the Atlantic coast of North America from South Carolina to Florida. It bears berries that have a long folk history of use as an aphrodisiac and sexual rejuvenator. These berries also have been used for centuries in treating conditions of the prostate. Numerous clinical studies on the fat-soluble extract of saw palmetto berries have shown it to greatly improve the signs and symptoms benign prostatic hyperplasia (BPH).

The therapeutic effect of the saw palmetto extract in BPH appears to be due to its inhibition of dihydrotestosterone, the compound that causes the prostate cells to multiply excessively. However, the saw palmetto extract also inhibits the binding of dihydrotestosterone at cellular binding sites and exerts a mild anti-inflammatory effect within the prostate.

The standard dosage of the fat-soluble saw palmetto extract standardized to contain 85% to 95% fatty acids and sterols is 160 mg twice daily.

No significant side effects have ever been reported in the clinical trials of the extract or with saw palmetto berry ingestion. Detailed toxicology studies on the extract have been carried out on mice, rats, and dogs and indicate that the extract has no toxic effects.

Siberian Ginseng (*Eleutherococcus senticosus*)

Possible applications:

> Fatigue
> Immunodepression

Siberian ginseng is a shrub that grows abundantly in parts of the Soviet Far East, Korea, China, and Japan. Siberian ginseng root extract has been administered to more than 2,100 healthy human subjects in clinical trials for the purpose of evaluating its 'adaptogenic' effects. These studies indicated Siberian ginseng: (1) increases the ability of humans to withstand many adverse physical conditions (i.e., heat, noise, motion, work load increase, exercise, and decompression); (2) increases mental alertness and work output; and (3) improves the quality of work under stressful conditions and athletic performance.

Siberian ginseng extract also has been administered to more than 2,200 human subjects in clinical trials for the purpose of evaluating its 'adaptogenic' effects in disease states. A variety of illnesses were included in these studies including angina, hypertension, hypotension, acute pyelonephritis, various types of neuroses, acute craniocerebral trauma, rheumatic heart disease, chronic bronchitis, and cancer. Siberian ginseng displayed good adaptogenic activity in these diseases as well.

The standard dosage of the fluid extract used in the majority of studies ranged from 2.0 to 4.0 ml (up to 16.0 ml), one to three times a day, for periods up to 60 consecutive days. The dosage using an extract standardized to contain greater than 1% eleutheroside E would be 100 to 200 mg three times daily. With long-term use there is usually a two to three week interval between 60 day courses.

Toxicity studies in animals have demonstrated that Siberian ginseng extracts are virtually nontoxic. In human studies, it was demonstrated that Siberian ginseng extracts are well tolerated and side effects are infrequent. However, side effects, including insomnia, irritability, melancholy, and anxiety, are often reported at higher dosages. In individuals with rheumatic heart disease, symptoms such as pericardial pain, headaches, and elevations in blood pressure have been reported.

Silymarin

Possible applications:

> Alcoholic Liver Disease
> Atherosclerosis
> Gallbladder Disease
> Hepatitis
> Immunodepression
> Psoriasis

Silybum marianum or milk thistle is a stout, annual or biennial plant, found in dry rocky soils in southern and western Europe and some parts of the United States. The seeds, fruit, and leaves are used for medicinal purposes.

An extract of milk thistle, silymarin is composed of three flavonoid molecules. In numerous clinical studies, silymarin has been shown to have positive effects in treating virtually every type of liver disease, including cirrhosis, hepatitis, and chemical or alcohol-induced fatty liver.

Silymarin's ability to prevent liver destruction and enhance liver function is due largely to silymarin's inhibition of the factors that are responsible for liver damage coupled with its ability to stimulate the growth of new liver cells to replace old damaged cells. Silymarin prevents free radical damage by acting as an antioxidant. Silymarin is many times more potent in antioxidant activity than vitamin E.

Many American are taking silymarin products to aid detoxification of harmful chemicals from the environment. Silymarin has been shown to increase the glutathione (GSH) content of the liver by more than 35% in healthy subjects. Since glutathione is responsible for detoxifying a wide range of toxic chemicals, silymarin not only protects the liver from damage, but also increases the capacity for detoxification reactions for many substances including pesticides and heavy metals (e.g., lead, mercury, cadmium, arsenic, etc.).

The standard dose of milk thistle is based on its silymarin content (70 to 210 mg three times daily). For this reason, standardized extracts are preferred.

Silymarin preparations are widely used medications in Europe, where a considerable body of evidence points to very low toxicity. When used at high doses for short periods of time, silymarin given by various routes to mice, rats, rabbits, and dogs has shown no toxic effects.

As silymarin possesses an ability to increase bile flow, it may produce a looser stool. If higher doses are used, it may be appropriate to use bile-sequestering fiber compounds (e.g., guar gum, pectin, psyllium, oat bran, etc.) to prevent mucosal irritation and loose stools.

St. John's wort (*Hypericum perforatum*)

Possible applications:

> Acquired Immunodeficiency Syndrome
> Anxiety
> Depression

St. Johns Wort or hypericum is a shrubby perennial plant native to many parts of the world including Europe and the United States. A tremendous amount of excitement about St. John's wort occurred after researchers demonstrated in a preliminary study that the St. John's wort components, hypericin and pseudohypericin, inhibit a variety of retroviruses including the retrovirus associated with AIDS (the human immunodeficiency virus or HIV). More research is needed to determine if St. John's wort is an appropriate recommendation in AIDS patients based on its antiviral activity, but there is clinical research showing St. John's wort to be useful in relieving depression, a common finding in AIDS patients. Hypericin also has been shown to inhibit the Epstein-Barr virus.

Recent studies have demonstrated the standardized extract of St. John's Wort can significantly improve symptoms of anxiety, depression, and feelings of worthlessness. In fact, the effectiveness of the St. John's wort extract in relieving depression has been shown to be greater than that produced by standard drugs including amitriptyline and imiprimine. While these drugs are associated with significant side effects (most often drowsiness, dry mouth, constipation, and impaired urination), St. John's wort extract at the usually prescribed level of intake is not associated with any significant side effect. However, as St. John's wort can cause severe photosensitivity in animals grazing extensively on the plant, and there is some evidence that St. John's wort at high levels can produce photosensitivity in humans, individuals taking larger amounts of St. John's wort extracts (or hypericin) should avoid exposure to strong sunlight. In addition to improving mood, the extract has been shown to greatly improve sleep quality.

The dosage of St. John's wort extract used in the studies in depression has typically been 300 mg of the extract (0.125% hypericin content) three times daily.

Tea tree oil

Possible applications:

> Acne Vulgaris
> Candidiasis
> Infection
> Wound healing

Tea tree (*Melaleuca alternifolia*) is a small tree native to only one area of the world - the northeast coastal region of New South Wales, Australia. The leaves are the portion of the plant that is used medicinally. The leaves are the source of a valuable therapeutic oil - tea tree oil. The medical world's first mention of tea tree appeared in the Medical Journal of Australia in 1930. A surgeon in Sydney reported some impressive results a solution of tea tree oil for cleaning surgical wounds.

Tea tree oil possesses significant antiseptic properties and is regarded by many as the ideal skin disinfectant as it is active against a wide range of organisms, possesses good penetration, and is non-irritating to the skin. Tea tree oil has been used in the following conditions: acne, apthous stomatitis (canker sores), athlete's foot, boils, burns, carbuncles, corns, empyema, gingivitis, herpes, impetigo, infections of the nail bed, insect bites, lice, mouth ulcers, psoriasis, root canal treatment, ringworm, sinus infections, sore throat, skin and vaginal infections, tinea, thrush, and tonsilitis.

A variety of tea tree oil based products exist on the marketplace including toothpastes, shampoos and conditioners, creams, hand and body lotions, soaps, gels, liniments, and nail polish removers. Apply as instructed on the product label.

Valerian (*Valeriana officinalis*)

Possible applications:

Infection
Insomnia

Valerian is a perennial plant native to North America and Europe that has been widely used in folk medicine as a sedative. Recent scientific studies have substantiated valerian's ability to improve sleep quality and relieve insomnia.

In a large double-blind study involving 128 subjects, an aqueous extract of valerian root improved the subjective ratings for sleep quality and sleep latency (the time required to get to sleep) but left no 'hangover' the next morning.

In a follow-up study, valerian extract significantly reduced sleep latency and improved sleep quality in sufferers of insomnia under laboratory conditions suggesting that it was as effective in reducing sleep latency as small doses of benzodiazepines. The difference, however, is that synthetic compounds also increase morning sleepiness, while valerian reduces morning sleepiness.

As a mild sedative, valerian may be taken at the following dosage 30 to 45 minutes before retiring:

Dried root (or as tea): 1-2 grams
Tincture (1:5): 4-6 ml
Fluid extract (1:1): 1-2 ml
Solid (dry powdered) extract (1.0-1.5% valtrate or 0.8% valeric acid): 150-300 mg.

Valerian is generally regarded as safe and is approved for food use by the U.S. Food and Drug Administration. If morning sleepiness occurs, reduce the dosage. If the initial dosage is ineffective, eliminate those factors that disrupt sleep, such as caffeine and alcohol, before considering a dosage increase.

ACNE VULGARIS

Chaste berry:

The chaste tree (*Vitex agnus castus*) is native to the Mediterranean. Its berries that have long been used for female complaints. As its name signifies, chaste berries were used in suppressing the libido.

Administration may be beneficial, especially for women.

> **Review Article:** Several uncontrolled studies have shown an extract of the berries of *Vitex agnus castus* can improve acne vulgaris and other acne-form skin conditions by normalizing sexual hormone levels including follicle stimulating hormone and leutinizing hormone. *Vitex agnus castus* appears to exert its effects on the pituitary and hypothalamus (*Ammon VW. [Akne vulgaris und agnus castus (Agnolyt®)]. Z Allgemeinmed 51:1645-8, 1975) (in German).*

Gugulipid:

Gugulipid is the standardized extract produced from the oleoresin of *Commiphora mukul*. (See: '*ATHEROSCLEROSIS*').

Administration may be beneficial.

> **Experimental Study:** 30 pts. with severe to moderate acne were treated with gugulipid (500 mg three times daily) for six weeks. Excellent, good and moderate response was seen in 9 (30%), 14 (47%) and 7 (23%) pts., respectively. Only 3 (10%) of the pts. reported relapse when examined at a 3 month follow-up visit (*Dogra J et al. Oral gugulipid in acne vulgaris management. Ind J Dermatol Venereol Leprol 56(1):381-3, 1990*).

Tea tree oil:

The essential oil extracted from the Australian tea tree (*Melaleuca alternifolia*) contains a mixture of plant terpenes with proven antimicrobial wound healing action. (*See: 'WOUND HEALING'*)

Topical application may be beneficial.

> **Experimental Single-blind Study:** 124 pts. with mild to moderate acne randomly received either a 5% gel of tea tree oil or 5% benzoyl peroxide lotion to be applied topically daily. Subject gps. were similar for age, sex, and severity of acne. After 3 mo., both treatments produced a significant improvement in mean number of both non-inflamed and inflamed lesions - only with non-inflamed lesions was benzoyl peroxide found to be more effective. There were fewer reports of side effects (dryness, pruritis,

stinging, burning, and skin redness) with tea tree oil (44% vs. 79%) (*Bassett IB et al. A comparative study of tea-tree oil versus benzoyl peroxide in the treatment of acne. Med J Aust 153:455-8, 1990*).

ACQUIRED IMMUNODEFICIENCY SYNDROME (A.I.D.S.)

See Also: IMMUNODEPRESSION
INFECTION

Aloe vera:

Acemannan, a water-soluble, long-chain polydispersed beta-(1,4)-linked mannan polymer interspersed with O-acetyl groups found in *Aloe vera*, is a potent immunostimulant. Approximately 1/2 to 1 liter of *Aloe vera* juice is required to provide 800-1,600 mg of acemannan.

Administration may be beneficial.

Negative Experimental Double-blind Study: 62 male pts. with advanced HIV disease having CD4 counts of 50 to 300/mm3 (x2) within 1 month of entry and had received ≥ 6 months of antiretrovirals, at a stable dose for the month prior to entry received either acemannan (400 mg 4 X d) or placebo. CD4 counts were done every 4 weeks for 48 weeks. P24 antigen was measured at entry and every 12 weeks thereafter. Quantitative viral cultures were similarly done in a subset of patients. AZT pharmacokinetics were assessed at baseline, 4 and 24 weeks. CD4's were 165/mm^3 and 144/mm^3 in the placebo and acemannan gps., respectively; 90% were on AZT at entry (30% were later switched to ddI). 10 pts. in each gp. discontinued study therapy prematurely, none due to serious adverse reactions. 7 pts. in the acemannan and 5 in the placebo gp., respectively, developed AIDS-defining illnesses. There was no difference between gps. in CD4's at 48 weeks. Among AZT treated pts., median rate of CD4 change (delta CD4) over the initial 16 weeks was -121 and -120 cells/year in the acemannan and placebo gp., respectively (p=0.45); delta CD4 from week 16 to 48 was 0 and -65 cells/year in the acemannan and placebo groups (p=0.04), respectively. There was no statistical difference between groups with regard to adverse events, p24 antigen, quantitative virology or pharmacokinetics. At the dose tested, acemannan is well tolerated and has no pharmacokinetic interaction with AZT. Although the rate of decline of helper cell count from 16 to 48 weeks favored the acemannan gp., there was no difference between groups in helper cell count at 48 weeks. Acemannan showed no significant effect on p24 antigen and quantitative virology (*Singer J. A randomized placebo-controlled trial of oral acemannan as an adjunctive to anti-retroviral therapy in advanced HIV disease. Int Conf AIDS 9(1):494[abstract no. PO-B28-2153], 1993*).

Experimental Study: A 6th year analysis was done on 5 survivors of a 1986 open-label clinical pilot to evaluate the potential efficacy of oral acemannan (ACM) in the treatment of symptomatic HIV-1 infected patients. In addition to existing medication, patients consumed each day a beverage which contained 500-800 mg acemannan. CD4 and CD8 levels and clinical status of these 5 patients and clinical deterioration of 10 deceased study patients closely paralleled their compliance for the daily intake of ACM. Deceased patients had lived 18-24 months after voluntarily ceasing the ACM intake. The survival of these 5 patients may be due to the expansion of cytotoxic CD8 lymphocyte population through complex leukocyte interactions essential for host defense. The induction of cytokines synthesis, as well as expansion of the CD8 population with maintenance of CD4 levels, may provide a rational basis for long-term survival of these 5 HIV-1 infected patients (*McDaniel HR, Rosenberg LJ, McAnalley BH. CD4 and CD8 lymphocyte levels in acemannan (ACM)-treated HIV-1 infected long-term survivors. Int Conf AIDS 9(1):498[abstract no. PO-B29-2179], 1993*).

Experimental Study: 14 HIV pts. prescribed oral acemmanan (800 mg/day) demonstrated significant increases in circulating monocytes/macrophages. In particular, there were significant increases in the number of large circulating monocytes indicating improvement in phagocytizing, processing, and presenting cells in the blood (*McDaniel HR et al. An increase in circulating monocyte/macrophages (MM) is induced by oral acemannan (ACE-M) in HIV-1 patients. Am J Clin Pathol 94:516-7, 1990*).

Experimental Study: 15 AIDS pts. receiving an oral dose of acemannan (800 mg/day) demonstrated significant improvement in the average scores of Modified Walter Reed Clinical (MWR) scoring, absolute T-4, absolute T-8, and p24 core antigen levels. Respectively, pretreatment values of 6.5, 322/mm3, 469/mm3, and 5 out of 15 positive improved to the following values at the end of 900 days: MWR 2.0, absolute T-4 324, absolute T-8 660, and positive p24 core antigen values in 4 out of 12. Two patients died of AIDS; another committed suicide. It has been suggested that prognostic criteria to determine the most responsive patients are those with an absolute T-4 count greater than 150/mm3 and p24 levels less than 300 (*McDaniel HR et al. Extended survival and prognostic criteria for acemannan (ACE-M) treated HIV-1 patients. Antiviral Res 13(Suppl.1):117, 1990*).

Acemannan may potentiate the antiviral drug azidothymidine (AZT). Researchers believe that the use of acemannan may reduce the amount of AZT required by as much as 90%. As AZT is very expensive and its use is often associated with serious side effects, confirmation of the efficacy of acemannan in clinical settings would be an important therapeutic advance.

In vitro study: Acemannan demonstrated significant antiviral activity against several viruses including the human immunodeficiency virus type 1 (HIV-1), influenza virus, and measles virus. Although acemmanan demonstrated some direct antiviral activity against HIV-1 by inhibiting glycosylation of viral glycoproteins, its main promise in treating AIDS and HIV is to enhance the action of AZT. When acemannan is combined with suboptimal noncytotoxic concentrations of AZT or acyclovir it acts synergistically to inhibit the replication of HIV and herpes simplex type 1 (HSV-1) (*Kahlon JB et al. In vitro evaluation of the synergistic antiviral effects of acemannan in combination with azidothymidine and acyclovir. Mol Biother 3:214-23, 1991*).

See also:

In vitro study: *Kahlon JB et al. Inhibition of AIDS virus replication by aceman-nan in vitro. Mol Biother 3:127-35, 1991*

In vitro study: *Kemp MC. In-vitro evaluation of the antiviral effects of aceman-nan on the replication and pathogenesis of HIV-1 and other enveloped viruses: Modification of the processing of glycoprotein precursors. Antiviral Res 13(Suppl 1):83, 1990*

Bloodroot (*Sanguinaria canadensis*) and
Celandine (*Chelidonium majus*):

Bloodroot and celandine contain alkaloids with *in vitro* anti-HIV activity (*Kakiuchi N et al. Effect of benzo[c]phenanthridine alkaloids on reverse transciptase and their binding proper-ties to nucleic acids. Planta Med 53(1):22-7, 1987*).

Administration may be beneficial.

Experimental Study: 13 pts. with HIV infection were evaluated after receiving a product (Retro-ZIP®) containing freeze-dried celandine and bloodroot. Improvements were noted in persistent generalized lymphadenopathy and CD8 values (*D'Adamo P. Chelidonium and Sanguinaria alkaloids as anti-HIV therapy. J Nat Med 3:31-4; 1992*).

Ukrain, a semi-synthetic thiophosphoric acid compound of chelidonine, an alkaloid of *Chelidonium majus*, given in injectable form may also be effective, especially in the treat-ment of Kaposi's sarcoma.

Experimental Study: Several HIV positive individuals with biopsy proven Kaposi's sarcoma (KS) were given 10 mg IV every other day for a total of 10 injections. Total CD4+ cells improved and clinically the KS lesions were noted to be diminished in size, thickness and color; no new lesions were noted (*Martinez G et al. Effect of the alka-loid derivative Ukrain in AIDS patients with Kaposi's sarcoma. Int Congress AIDS 9(1):401[abstract no. PO-B12-1596], 1993*).

Garlic (*Allium sativum*):

Administration may enhance immune function. (*See: 'IMMUNODEPRESSION'*)

Experimental Study: 7 AIDS pts. received an aged processed extract (SGP, Waku-naga) 5 g/d for 6 wks. and 10 g/d for another 6 weeks. At baseline, natural killer cell activity in all 7 was >2 S.D. below the mean for normal controls. After 6 wks., 6/7 pts. had normal NK activity; after 12 wks., all 7 had normal activity. After 12 wks., the helper/suppressor ratio normalized in 3/7 pts., improved in 2, worsened in 1 and was unchanged in 1. During the study period diarrhea (Cryptosporidia), genital herpes, can-didiasis of the oropharynx and esophagus, and pansinusitis with recurrent fever im-proved. The pt. with pansinusitus had not responded to antibiotics for over a year. In 1 pt., the platelet count increased from 103,000 to 280,000 mm^3 in 4 months (*Abdullah TH, Kirkpatrick DV, Carter J. Enhancement of natural killer cell activity in AIDS with garlic. Dtsch Zschr Onkol 21:52-3, 1989*).

Administration may be effective against a number of opportunistic microbes that are associ-ated with AIDS, including:

Candida albicans:　(See: '*CANDIDIASIS*')

Cryptococcus:

> *Hunan Medical College of China. Garlic in cryptococcal meningitis: A preliminary report of 21 cases. Chin Med J 93:123, 1980*

> *Frontling RA, Bulmer GS. In vitro effect of aqueous extract of garlic on the growth and viability of Cryptococcus neoformans. Mycopathologia 70:397-405, 1978*

Herpesvirus hominis type I:

> *Tsai Y et al. Antiviral properties of garlic: In vitro effects on influenza B, herpes simplex I, and coxsackie viruses. Planta Medica 5:460-1, 1985*

Mycobacteria:

> *Delaha EC, Garagusi VL. Inhibition of mycobacteria by garlic extract (Allium sativum). Antimicrob Agents Chemother 27(4):485-6, 1985*

> *Rao RR et al. Inhibition of Mycobacterium tuberculosis by garlic extract. Nature 157, 1946*

Glycyrrhizin:

Licorice root (*Glycyrrhiza glabra*) contains about 6-14% glycyrrhizin, the glycone of glycyrrhetinic acid. Glycyrrhetinic acid exhibits profound pharmacological activity including antiviral, immune-enhancing, and anti-inflammatory properties.

> WARNING: If ingested regularly, licorice root (>3 g/d for more than 6 weeks) or glycyrrhizin (>100 mg/d) may cause sodium and water retention, hypertension, hypokalemia, and suppression of the renin-aldosterone system through a pseudo-aldosterone action of glycyrrhetinic acid. Monitoring of BP and electrolytes and increasing potassium intake is suggested　(*Farese RV et al. Licorice-induced hypermineralocorticoidism. N Engl J Med 325(17):1223-7, 1991; MacKenzie MA et al. The influence of glycyrrhetinic acid on plasma cortisol and cortisone in healthy young volunteers. J Clin Endocrinol Metab 70:1637-43, 1990*).

> > There is a great individual variation in the susceptibility to the symptom-producing effects of glycyrrhizin. Adverse effects are rarely observed at levels below 100 mg/day while they are quite common at levels above 400 mg/day (*Stormer FC, Reistad R, Alexander J. Glycyrrhizic acid in liquorice - Evaluation of health hazard. Fd Chem Toxicol 31(4):303-12, 1993*).

> > Prevention of the side effects of glycyrrhizin may be possible by following a high-potassium, low-sodium diet. Although no formal trial of either of these guidelines has been performed, patients who normally consume high-potassium foods and restrict sodium intake, even those with hypertension and angina, have been reported to be free from the aldosterone-like side effects of

glycyrrhizin (*Baron J et al. Metabolic studies, aldosterone secretion rate and plasma renin after carbonoxolone sodium as biogastrone. Br Med J 2:793-5, 1969*).

Administration may be beneficial.

Note: Intravenous administration may not be necessary as glycyrrhizin is easily absorbed orally and well-tolerated.

Experimental Double-blind Study: The clinical effectiveness of glycyrrhizin (GL) by long-term oral administration to 16 asymptomatic HIV-1 carrier (AC) pts. with hemophilia was studied. Pts. received daily doses of 150-225mg of GL for 3 to 7 years. CD4+ and CD8+ T lymphocyte numbers, p24, p17 and Nef antibody levels, GL and glycyrrhetinic acid (GA) levels in sera were monitored. Neither progression of immunologic abnormalities nor development to AIDS has been seen. Orally administered GL was converted into GA which was detected in sera, without manifesting any side effect, while untreated patients showed decreases in CD4+ and CD8+ cell counts and antibody levels. Two of them developed AIDS (*Ikegami N et al. Prophylactic effect of long-term oral administration of glycyrrhizin on AIDS development of asymptomatic patients. Int Conf AIDS 9(1):234[abstract no. PO-A25-0596], 1993*).

- with Cysteine and Glycine:

An intravenous glycyrrhizin-containing product, Stronger Neominophagen C (SNMC), consisting of 0.2% glycyrrhizin, 0.1% cysteine and 2.0% glycine in physiological saline solution, is used in Japan primarily for the treatment of hepatitis. The other components, glycine and cysteine, appear to modulate glycyrrhizin's actions. Glycine has been shown to prevent the aldosterone effects of glycyrrhizin, while cysteine aids in detoxification via increased glutathione synthesis and cystine conjugation. (*See: 'HEPATITIS'*)

Experimental Study: 42 hemophiliacs with HIV infection were treated with high-dose glycyrrhizin, Stronger Neo-Minophagen C (SNMC). The dose was 100-200 ml of SNMC in 21 patients and 400-800 ml in the other 21. The patients were divided into an asymptomatic carrier (AC) gp. and AIDS related-complex (ARC)/AIDS group. SNMC was administered intravenously daily for the first 3 weeks, and every second day for the following 8 weeks to the 42 HIV-infected hemophilia patients, in accordance with the protocol proposed by the Japanese National Research Committee. The CD4/CD8 ratio and CD4 positive lymphocyte counts did not change during the treatment period. However, significant improvement was noted in some cases. A slight increase in mitogenic responsiveness to phytohemagglutinin, Concanavalin A and pokeweed mitogen was noted in most patients of both groups, especially significant improvement was seen in the AC gp. administered over 400 ml of SNMC. Furthermore, complete improvement was noted in liver dysfunction, which has been thought to be one of the major problems for hemophiliacs treated with blood products. Thus, prophylactic administration of high-dose SNMC to HIV positive hemophiliacs who have impaired immunological ability and liver dysfunction was considered to be effective in preventing the development from AC/ARC to AIDS (*Mori K et al. Effects of glycyrrhizin*

(SNMC: Stronger Neo-Minophagen C) in hemophilia patients with HIV-1 infection. Tohoku J Exp Med 162(2):183-93, 1990).

Experimental Controlled Study: 10 HIV positive pts. without AIDS took 150-225 mg glycyrrhizin daily. After 1-2 yrs., none developed symptoms associated with AIDS or AIDS-related complex (ARC), while 1/10 pts. of a matched control gp. developed ARC and 2 progressed to AIDS and subsequently died *(Ikegami N et al. Clinical evaluation of glycyrrhizin on HIV-infected asymptomatic Hemophiliac patients in Japan. Fifth International Conference on AIDS. Abstract W.B.P. 298, June 1989 cited in AIDS Treatment News, No. 103, May 18, 1990).*

Experimental Study: 9 asymptomatic HIV-positive pts. received 200-800 mg glycyrrhizin IV daily. After 8 wks., the gp. had increased helper T cells, improved helper/suppressor ratios and improved liver function *(Mori K et al. The present status in prophylaxis and treatment of HIV infected patients with hemophilia in Japan. Rinsho Byhori 37(11):1200-08, 1989).*

Experimental Study: 6 AIDS pts. received 400-1600 mg glycyrrhizin IV daily. After 30 days, 5/6 showed a reduction or disappearance of the 'P24 antigen' which indicates active disease *(Hattori T et al. Preliminary evidence for inhibitory effect of glycyrrhizin on HIV replication in patients with AIDS. Antiviral Res 11:(5-6), 255-61, 1989).*

St. John's Wort (*Hypericum perforatum*):

Hypericin, a constituent, exerts anti-HIV activity. Although it can occasionally cause photosensitivity, it must interact with light in order to inactivate the HIV virus. Extracts standardized for hypericin may be the most beneficial.

> *Note: Its benefits at the usual doses appear to be due to an antidepressant effect rather than to its anti-viral effect (Bergner P. Hypericum and A.I.D.S. Med Herbalism 2(1) January, 1990).*

Administration may be beneficial.

Clinical Observation: 65/112 pts. who received Hypericum, including some who were asymptomatic at the start, reported some benefits including improved outlook, more energy, less fatigue, and feeling better. Two pts. reported photosensitivity, and a few others reported rashes and drowsiness   *(James JS. AIDS Treatment News. Issue #74, February 24, 1989).*

Clinical Observation: Hypericum administration appears to make most AIDS pts. feel better, including those who are seriously ill   *(James JS. AIDS Treatment News. Issue #91, November 17, 1989).*

Animal and In vitro Experimental Study: Mice were infected with retroviruses (leukemia viruses). A single dose of hypericin and pseudohypericin, constituents of hypericum, administered within a day of infection, completely inhibited the establishment of the virus in the hosts, while treatments given over a period of time successfully inhibited the spread of the virus in previously infected mice. There was no significant toxicity at the effective doses. In addition, preliminary investigation demonstrated that one of the compounds reduced the spread of HIV virus *in vitro* (*Meruelo et al. Therapeutic agents with dramatic antiretroviral activity and little toxicity at effective doses; aromatic polycyclic diones hypericin and pseudohypericin. Proc Natl Acad Sci U S A 85:5230-4, 1988*).

See also:

> **In vitro Study:** *Degar S et al. Inactivation of the human immunodeficiency virus by hypericin: Evidence for photochemical alterations of p24 and a block in uncoating. AIDS Res Human Retrovir 8:1929-36, 1992*

> **In vitro Study:** *Hudson JB et al. Antiviral activities of hypericin. Antiviral Res 15:101-12, 1991*

> **In vitro Study:** *Lopez-Bazzochi I et al. Antiviral activity of photoactive plant pigment hypericin. Photochem Photobiol 54:95-8, 1991*

Trichosanthin:

Trichosanthin (Compound Q) and a related compound (GLQ223) are plant proteins purified from the roots of *Trichosanthes kirilowi*.

Administration may be beneficial.

> **Experimental Study:** 20 pts. with AIDS (n=5), AIDS-related complex (ARC) (n=10), or asymptomatic HIV infection (HIV+) (n=5) were given 20 mcg/kg-3 trichosanthin (TCS) once every four weeks for up to 12 weeks. With the concurrent administration of ibuprofen and/or acetaminophen, the drug was moderately well tolerated, with most pts. experiencing mild arthralgia, hives, and malaise. 4/20 showed progressive reductions in viral activity (p-24 antigen and beta-2-macroglobulin levels decreased). 10 ARC and HIV+ pts. improved immunological status. No subject with oral candidiasis experienced improvement. "In the short term, TCS seems to have the ability to reduce viral activity and improve certain symptoms in healthy ARC patients and HIV+ asymptomatics although it may not be able to restore immune competence in persons with advanced AIDS or poor prognosis ARC. Additionally, the drug may pose a special risk for patients with HIV-related dementia" (*Mayer RA et al. Trichosanthin treatment of HIV-induced immune dysregulation. Eur J Clin Invest 22:113-22, 1992*).

See Also:

> **Experimental Study:** *Kahn J et al. The safety and pharmacokinetics of GLQ223 in subjects with AIDS and AIDS related complex: a phase 1 study. AIDS 4:197-204, 1990*

> **In vitro Study:** *McGrath M et al. Effect of GLQ223 on HIV replication in human monocyte/macrophages chronically infected in vitro with HIV. Aids Res Retrovir 6(8):1039-43, 1990*

In vitro Study: *McGrath M et al. GLQ223: Inhibitor of HIV replication in acutely and chronically infected cells of lymphocytes and mononuclear phagocyte lineage. Proc Natl Acad Sci 86:2844-8, 1989*

ALCOHOL CRAVING

Kudzu (*Peuraria thunbergiana*):

A perennial vine, native to eastern Asia.

Chinese herbal physicians have traditionally treated alcoholism and drunkenness with a tea made from the roots, seeds, or flowers.

Administration of the extract may reduce alcohol craving.

> **Animal Experimental Study:** Syrian Golden hamsters prefer and consume large amts. of ethanol in a 2-bottle free-choice regimen. As drugs that suppress ethanol intake in alcohol-dependent humans also reduce ethanol intake in this animal model, the model has high predictive validity. A crude extract of *Radix puerariae* suppressed (>50%) free-choice ethanol intake in the experimental animals. There was no significant change in body weight or in food or water intake (*Keung WM, Vallee BL. Daidzin and daidzein suppress free-choice ethanol intake by Syrian golden hamsters. Proc Natl Acad Sci U S A 90(21):10008-12, 1993*).

Administration of daidzin, an isoflavone isolated from Kudzu and shown to be a selective inhibitor of mitochondial aldehyde dehydrogenase, may reduce alcohol craving (*Keung WM, Vallee BL. Daidzin: a potent, selective inhibitor of human mitochondrial aldehyde dehydrogenase. Proc Natl Acad Sci U S A 90(4):1247-51, 1993*).

> **Animal Experimental Study:** Syrian Golden hamsters prefer and consume large amts. of ethanol in a 2-bottle free-choice regimen. As drugs that suppress ethanol intake in alcohol-dependent humans also reduce ethanol intake in this animal model, the model has high predictive validity. Daidzin and daidzein, two major constitutents of *Radix puerariae*, suppressed free-choice alcohol intake by more than 50%. There was no significant change in body weight or in food or water intake (*Keung WM, Vallee BL. Daidzin and daidzein suppress free-choice ethanol intake by Syrian golden hamsters. Proc Natl Acad Sci U S A 90(21):10008-12, 1993*).

ALCOHOLIC LIVER DISEASE

See Also: HEPATITIS

Berberine:

Berberine is an alkaloid found in goldenseal (*Hydrastis canadensis*), barberry root bark (*Berberis vulgaris*), and Oregon grape root (*Berberis aquifolium*).

> *Note: The dosage of crude herb or extract should approximate the dosage of berberine.*

Administration may be beneficial in cirrhosis.

Experimental Controlled Study: Berberine (600-800 mg/day) was shown to correct the hypertyraminemia of patients with liver cirrhosis. Berberine prevents the elevation of serum tyramine following oral tyrosine load by inhibiting the enzyme tyrosine decarboxylase found in bacteria in the large intestine. The accumulation of tyramine and its derivatives in cirrhosis causes lowering of peripheral resistance, with resultant high cardiac output, reduction in renal function, and cerebral dysfunction (*Watanabe A et al. Berberine therapy of hypertyraminemia in patients with liver cirrhosis. Acta Med Okayama 36:277-81, 1982*).

Catechin:

Catechin is a flavonoid that is found in high concentrations in *Acacia catechu* (black catechu, black cutch) and *Uncaria gambier* (pale catechu, gambier).

Administration of isolated catechin or plant extracts concentrated for catechin may be beneficial.

WARNING: Catechin can induce autoimmune hemolysis. Use with caution.

Negative Experimental Double-blind Study: 3-palmitoyl-(+)-catechin at a dose of 1500 mg daily for 3 months failed to demonstrate statistically significant clinical, biochemical or histological benefit in pts. with biopsy-proven alcoholic liver disease (*World MJ et al. Palmitoyl-catechin for alcoholic liver disease: results of a three-month clinical trial. Alcohol Alcohol 22(4):331-40, 1987*).

Negative Experimental Double-blind Study: The effects of catechin 1.5-2.0 g/d versus placebo over the course of one year was studied in pts. with toxic alcoholic precirrhotic liver disease. Catechin produced significant improvement in subjective symptoms like asthenia and anorexia, and in serum aspartate-transaminase (GOT) levels. However, it is possible that the improvement was in part due to abstinence from alcohol. Results showed a more favorable, but not significantly better, response in pts. receiving catechin versus placebo (*Abonyi M, Kisfaludy S, Szalay F. Therapeutic effect of (+)-cyanidanol-3 in toxic alcoholic liver disease and in chronic active hepatitis. Acta Physiol Hung 64(3-4):455-60, 1984*).

Negative Experimental Double-blind Study: While a prospective randomized double-blind trial of (+)-cyanidanol-3 at a dose of 2 g daily for 6 mo. vs. placebo failed to demonstrate statistically significant clinical, biochemical or histological benefit in pts. with biopsy-proven alcoholic liver disease, the gp. receiving the active drug tended to drink more both before and during the trial and their mean serum AST and GGT levels were higher on admission to the trial yet, after the 4th wk. of treatment, the mean serum levels of these enzymes remained consistently lower in this gp. compared to controls. It is suggested that further clinical trials should employ higher dosages which would be more in keeping with those found beneficial in animal studies (*World M et al. (+)-cyanidanol-3 for alcoholic liver disease: Results of a six month clinical trial. Alcohol Alcoholism 19:23-9, 1984*).

Experimental Double-blind Study: 39 pts. with pre-cirrhotic alcohol-related liver disease were given either catechin (2 g/d) or placebo over a three month period. 41% (16/39) abstained from alcohol and showed significant improvements (p) in mean values for serum aspartate transaminase, serum gamma glutamyl transpeptidase, and mean corpuscular volume. 10 of the 16 showed overall histological improvement on liver biopsy. 59% continued to drink, though significantly reducing their mean daily alcohol intake. No significant changes occurred in this group in mean serum enzyme values, though the mean value for mean corpuscular volume improved significantly and 16 of the 23 showed overall histological improvement. Changes occurred irrespective of treatment with catechin (*Colman JC et al. Treatment of alcohol-related liver disease with (+)-cyanidanol-3: a randomised double-blind trial. Gut 21(11):965-9, 1980*).

Centella asiatica:

Administration of *Centella asiatica* (Gotu kola) extracts containing the total triterpenoid fraction (TTFCA) may be beneficial in cirrhosis.

Experimental Study: Histological improvement was noted in in 5 of 6 pts. with alcohol-related cirrhosis treated with a daily dose of 90 to 150 mg TTFCA (*Darnis F et al. [Use of a titrated extract of Centella asiatica in chronic hepatic disorders]. Sem Hop Paris 55(37-38):1749-50, 1979*) (*In French*).

Silymarin:

The flavonoid complex of milk thistle (*Silybum marianum*).

Administration may reduce mortality from cirrhosis.

Experimental Double-blind Study: 87 cirrhotics (46 with alcoholic cirrhosis) received silymarin (Legalon®) 140 mg 3 times daily, while 83 cirrhotics (45 with alcoholic cirrhosis) received a placebo. The mean observation period was 41 months. There were 14 dropouts in the treatment gp. and 10 dropouts in the controls. In the treatment gp., there were 24 deaths with 18 related to liver disease while, in the controls, there were 37 deaths with 31 related to liver disease. The 4-yr. survival rate was 58±9% in the treatment gp. compared to 39±9% in the controls. Analysis of subgroups indicated that treatment was effective in pts. with alcoholic cirrhosis (p=0.01) *(Ferenci P et al. Randomized controlled trial of Silymarin treatment in patients with cirrhosis of the liver. J Hepatology 9:105-13, 1989).*

Administration may improve immune function in immunocompromised patients.

Experimental Double-blind Study: The effects of the hepatoprotective, antioxidant drug silymarin (Legalon®) on some cellular immune parameters of pts. with histologically proven chronic alcoholic liver disease were studied in a six month double-blind study. The lectin-induced proliferative activity of the lymphocytes was enhanced, the originally low T cell percentage and the originally high CD8+ cell percentage was normalized, the antibody-dependent and natural cytotoxicity of the lymphocytes decreased during silymarin therapy. All these changes were significant, while in the placebo group no significant changes occurred, except for a moderate elevation of the T cell percentage. The immunomodulatory activity of silymarin might be involved in the hepatoprotective action of the drug and improves the depressed immunoreactivity of the pts. *(Deak G et al. [Immunomodulator effect of silymarin therapy in chronic alcoholic liver diseases.] Orv Hetil 131(24):1291-2, 1295-6, 1990) (in Hungarian).*

- with Phosphatidylcholine:

Administration may be more effective when complexed with phosphatidylcholine. *(See: 'GALLBLADDER DISEASE'; 'HEPATITIS')*

Experimental Study: A phase-II trial was performed to evaluate the dose-response relationship of IdB 1016, a complex of silybin and phosphatidylcholine, in pts. with chronic hepatitis of either viral or alcoholic etiology. 20 pts. received 80 mg b.i.d., 20 pts received 120 mg twice daily, and 20 pts. received 120 mg 3 times daily for two weeks. At all tested doses, IdB treatment produced a remarkable and statistically significant decrease of mean serum aspartate aminotransferase (p<0.001) and of total bilirubin (p<0.05-0.001). When used at the dose of 240 or 360 mg per day, it also resulted in a remarkable and statistically significant decrease of alanine aminotransferase (p<0.01-0.001) and gamma-glutamyl transpeptidase (p<0.01-0.001). The results indicate that even short-term treatment of viral or alcohol-induced hepatitis with IdB 1016 is effective at a daily dose of 160 mg per day, but there are significant advantages at 240 mg, and still greater benefits at 360 mg per day *(Vailati A et al. Randomized open study of the dose-effect relationship of a short course of IdB 1016 in patients with viral or alcoholic hepatitis. Fitoterapia 44(3):219-28, 1993).*

ALLERGY
(ALTERED REACTIVITY)

See Also: BRONCHIAL ASTHMA
ECZEMA

Feverfew (*Tanacetum parthenium*):

Feverfew, which has confirmed clinical benefit in the treatment of migraine headaches, may also be effective in other allergic and inflammatory conditions.

> *Note: The effectiveness of feverfew is dependent upon adequate levels of parthenolide, the active ingredient. The preparations used in the clinical trials in migraine headaches had a parthenolide content of 0.4-0.66%.*

> **Animal Ex vivo Study:** Extracts of fresh feverfew caused a dose- and time-dependent, irreversible inhibition of the contractile response of rabbit aortic rings to all receptor-acting agonists tested. The presence of potentially SH reacting parthenolide and other sesquiterpene alpha-methylenebutyrolactones in these extracts, and the close parellelism of pure parthenolide, suggest that the inhibitory effects are due to these compounds. Extracts of the dry leaves were not inhibitory and actually caused potent and sustained contractions of aortic smooth muscle; these extracts were found to be devoid or parthenolide or butyrolactones (*Barsby RWJ, Salan U, Knight BW, Hoult JRS. Feverfew and vascular smooth muscle: Extracts from fresh and dried plants show opposing pharmacological profiles, dependent upon sesquiterpene lactone content. Planta Medica 59:20-5, 1993*).

> **Chemical Analysis:** The parthenolide content of over 35 different commercial preparations of feverfew was determined by bioassay, 2 HPLC methods, and NMR. The results indicate a wide variation in the amounts of parthenolide in commercial preparations. The majority of products contained no parthenolide or only traces (*Heptinstall S et al. Parthenolide content and bioactivity of feverfew (Tanacetum parthenium (L.) Schultz-Bip.). Estimation of commercial and authenticated feverfew products. J Pharm Pharmacol 44:391-5, 1992*).

In vitro Study: An extract of feverfew produces a dose-dependent inhibition of histamine release from mast cells (*Hayes NA and Foreman JC. The activity of compounds extracted from feverfew on histamine release from rat mast cells. J Pharm Pharmacol 39:466-7, 1987*).

See Also:

Heptinstall S et al. Extracts of feverfew inhibit granule secretion in blood platelets and polymorphonuclear leukocytes. Lancet i:1071-4, 1985

Makheja AM, Bailey JM. A platelet phospholipase inhibitor from the medicinal herb feverfew (Tanacetum parthenium). Prostagland Leukotri Med 8:653-60, 1982

Garlic (*Allium sativum*) or
Onion (*Allium cepa*):

Regular consumption of garlic or onion may be beneficial.

Experimental Double-blind Study: An alcohol/onion extract (5% ethanol) was injected simultaneously with 20 IU and 200 IU rabbit anti-human-IgE intradermally in 12 adult volunteers (6 atopics, 6 non-atopics). Diameters of wheals and flares were measured 10 min after and compared with control sites challenged with 20 IU and 200 IU anti-IgE in a 5% ethanol solution. The skin sites were then treated epidermally with 45% alcohol/onion extract and 45% ethanol under occlusion. Diameters of late cutaneous reactions were measured hourly. Edema formation was clinically estimated according to an arbitrary scale and skin thickness measured with a caliper. In the onion-treated skin sites, the wheal areas were significantly reduced (20 IU: control 108 mm^2; onion 69 mm^2; 200 IU anti-IgE: control: 152 mm^2, onion 138 mm^2). The edema formation during the late phase skin reaction was significantly markedly depressed at 2,4,6 and 8 hours. The extent of late skin reactions was slightly, but not significantly, reduced (*Dorsch W, Ring J. Suppression of immediate and late anti-IgE-induced skin reactions by topically applied alcohol/onion extract. Allergy 39(1):43-9, 1984*).

Ginkgo biloba:

Ginkgo biloba contains several unique terpene molecules known collectively as ginkgolides that antagonize platelet activating factor (PAF), a key chemical mediator in asthma, inflammatory, and allergies. PAF plays a central role in many inflammatory and allergic processes including neutrophil activation, increasing vascular permeability, smooth muscle contraction including bronchoconstriction, and reduction in coronary blood flow. Ginkgolides compete with PAF for binding sites and inhibit the various events induced by PAF. Mixtures of ginkgolides (BN 52063) as well as the *Ginkgo biloba* extract standardized to contain 24% ginkgoflavonglycosides have shown clinical effects.

Experimental Study: Clinical and histopathologic responses to intradermal PAF were evaluated in 12 pts. before and after administration of 120 mg BN 52063. Without BN 52063 pretreatment, PAF produced an immediate acute wheal and flare reaction. The reaction was characterized by a predominantly neutrophilic response, which was seen at 30 min. and was maximal at 4 hours. Eosinophils were observed in the infiltrate as early as 30 min. after injection, and were maximal by 12 hours. BN 52063 antagonized the acute flare response to intradermal PAF-acether but had little effect on cellular recruitment at the site of injection (*Markey AC et al. Platelet activating factor-induced clinical and histopathologic responses in atopic skin and their modification by the platelet activating factor antagonist BN52063. J Am Acad Dermatol 23(2):263-8, 1990*).

Experimental Study: 6 healthy males given a single 15-ml oral dose of Tanakan, a standardized *Ginkgo biloba* extract, demonstrated a reduction in platelet aggregation induced by PAF and adenosine diphosphate (ADP), collagen or PAF-acether (*Guinot P et al. Tanakan inhibits platelet-activating-factor-induced platelet aggregation in healthy male volunteers. Haemostasis 19(4):219-23, 1989*).

Case Report: BN 52063, 240 mg daily for three weeks, produced dramatic improvement in an adult with systemic mastocytosis inducing erythema on the face and trunk with recurrent facial flushing, conjunctivitis, palpitation, dizziness, abdominal pain, diarrhea, nausea, and severe hypotension (*Guinot P et al. Treatment of adult systemic mastocytosis with a PAF-acether antagonist BN52063. Lancet ii:114, 1988*).

Experimental Double-Blind Study: Wheal and flare responses to 400 ng PAF, examined 2 h after ingestion of BN 52063 (80 mg and 120 mg), were inhibited in a dose-related manner. After 120 mg the flare area was reduced by a mean 62.4% and the wheal volume by a mean 60%. Both doses of BN 52063 significantly inhibited PAF-induced platelet aggregation in platelet-rich plasma (*Chung KF et al. Effect of a ginkgolide mixture (BN 52063) in antagonising skin and platelet responses to platelet activating factor in man. Lancet i:48-51, 1987*).

Experimental Study: At a oral dose of 80 mg, BN 52063 inhibited the inflammatory response to a subcutaneous injection of PAF (400 ng). A late cutaneous response was not observed in any of the subjects. BN 52063 was also demonstrated to be well tolerated at doses of 20, 40, 80 and 120 mg with no significant side effects (*Guinot P et al. Inhibition of PAF-acether induced wheal and flare reaction in man by a specific PAF antagonist. Prostaglandins 32(1):160-3, 1986*).

See Also:

> **Review Article:** *Koltai M et al. Platelet activating factor (PAF). A review of its effects, antagonists and possible future clinical implications (Part I). Drugs 42(1):9-29, 1991; Koltai M et al. PAF. A review of its effects, antagonists and possible future clinical implications (Part II). Drugs 42(2):174-204, 1991*

> **Review Article:** *Braquet P Hosford D. Ethnopharmacology and the development of natural PAF antagonists as therapeutic agents. J Ethnopharmacol 32:135-9, 1991*

> **Review Article:** *Braquet P. The ginkgolides: Potent platelet-activating factor antagonists isolated from Ginkgo biloba: Chemistry, pharmacology and clinical applications. Drugs Future 12:643-9, 1987*

Stinging Nettles (*Urtica dioica*) :

A perennial plant found commonly throughout Europe.

Administration of freeze-dried preparations of stinging nettles (*Urtica dioica*) may be effective in allergic rhinitis.

> **Experimental Double-Blind Study:** 69 pts. with allergic rhinitis were randomly given either a freeze-dried preparation of *Urtica dioica* or placebo. In the treatment gp., 58% rated it moderately effective, compared to only 37% in the placebo group. A one-week trial period taking two 300 mg capsules of freeze-dried *Urtica dioica* appears to be

sufficient to identify those individuals who will respond favorably (*Mittman P. Randomized, double-blind study of freeze-dried Urtica dioica in the treatment of allergic rhinitis. Planta Med 56:44-7, 1990*).

ANXIETY

See Also: DEPRESSION

Ashwagandha (*Withania somnifera*):

Ashwagandha is referred to as 'Indian ginseng' as it appears to exert many of the same 'adaptogenic' activities of *Panax ginseng*. Ashwagandha has been used in Ayurvedic medicine for more than 2,500 years.

In vivo and in vitro Study: A methanolic extract of *W. somnifera* root inhibited the specific binding of GABA and TBPS and enhanced the binding of flunitrazepam to their receptor sites. Additional studies indicated the W. somnifera extract contains an ingredient which has a GABA-mimetic activity (*Mehta AK, et al. Pharmacological effects of Withania somnifera root extract on GABA receptor complex. Ind J Med Res 94(B):312-5, 1991*).

Experimental Controlled Study: A formulation containing primarily Ashwagandha was used in the treatment of 34 diagnosed cases of anxiety neurosis. After 12 weeks of therapy, a significant reduction in 5-hydroxytryptophan levels was observed. Circulating monamine oxidase and GABA showed an increasing trend along with decreased glutamic acid levels after treatment. Psychological complaints were considerably decreased after 12 weeks (*Upadhaya L et al. Role of an indigenous drug Geriforte on blood levels of biogenic amines and its significance in the treatment of anxiety neurosis. Acta Nerv Super 32(1):1-5, 1990*)

See Also:

In vitro Study: *Ghosal S et al. Immunomodulatory and CNS effects of sitoindosides IX and X, two new glycowithanolides from Withania somnifera. Phytother Res 3(5):201-6, 1989*

In vitro Study: *Bhattacharya SK et al. Anti-stress activity of sitoindosides VII and VIII, new acylsterylglycosides from Withania somnifera. Phytother Res 1(1):32-7, 1987*

Kava (*Piper mythysticum*):

Kava was historically consumed during Polynesian religious rites for its ability to relax and soothe the mind. Kava was also used for its medicinal effects including as a sedative.

Experimental Double-Blind Study: 58 pts. received either kava extract (100 mg three times daily) or placebo over a four week period. The Hamilton-Anxiety-Scale overall score of anxiety and other anxiety scales revealed a significant reduction in the group receiving the kava extract. No adverse effects were noted (*Kinzler E, Kromer J and*

51

Lehmann E. Effect of a special kava extract in patients with anxiety-, tension- and excitation states of non-psychotic genesis. Double blind study with placebos over 4 weeks. Arzneim Forsch 41(6):584-8, 1991).

Lemongrass (*Cymbopogon citratus*):

Lemongrass tea is used in Brazilian folk medicine in anxiety.

Negative Experimental Double-Blind Study: Eighteen subjects with high scores of trait-anxiety were submitted to an anxiety-inducing test following taking lemongrass or placebo. Their anxiety levels were similar, indicating the plant has no clinical anxiolytic properties. In another part of the study, 50 patients were given either lemongrass or placebo and analyzed for various parameters which may indicate a hypnotic effect (i.e., sleep induction, sleep quality, dream recall and reawakening. There were no differences between those receiving the lemongrass compared to those receiving placebo (*Leite JR et al. Pharmacology of lemongrass (Cymbopogon citratus Stapf). III. Assessment of eventual toxic, hypnotic and anxiolytic effects on humans. J Ethnopharmacol 17(1):75-83, 1986*).

Panax Ginseng:

Panax ginseng root may be effective when anxiety is due to stress.

Animal Experimental Study: The anxiolytic activity of *Panax ginseng* root was investigated in rats and mice using a number of experimental paradigms of anxiety and compared with diazepam. The effects produced by ginseng were comparable to those induced by diazepam *(Bhattacharya SK and Mitra SK. Anxiolytic activity of Panax ginseng roots: an experimental study. J Ethnopharmacol 34:87-92, 1991)*

Animal Experimental Study: A *Panax ginseng* root extract containing 15% ginsenosides demonstrated an anti-stress effect in mice after subchronic administration *(Della Loggia R et al. Anti-stress activity of a ginseng extract: A subchronic study in mice Planta Med 57(Suppl.2):A6-7, 1991).*

Experimental Double-Blind Study: Nurses who had switched from day to night duty rated themselves for competence, mood, and general well-being, and were given an objective test of psychophysical performance, blood counts, and blood chemistry. The group administered ginseng demonstrated higher scores in competence, mood parameters, and objective psychophysical performance when compared with those receiving a placebo (*Hallstrom C et al. Effect of ginseng on the performance of nurses on night duty. Comp Med East West 6:277-82, 1982).*

Animal Experimental Study: *Panax ginseng* increased tolerance to stress *(Fulder SJ. Ginseng and the hypothalamic-pituitary control of stress. Am J Chin Med 9:112-8, 1981).*

- -

COMBINATION TREATMENT

<u>Suanzaorentang</u>:

Suanzaorentang is an ancient Chinese remedy composed of five herbs: zizyphi seed (*Zizyphus jujuba*), poria (*Poria cocos*), ligustrum root (*Ligustrum lucidum*), bunge root (*Anemarrhea asphodeloides*) and licorice root (*Glycyrrhiza glabra*). Pharmacological studies have shown two components (zizyphi and ligustrum) exert anti-anxiety effects, however, these effects are not nearly as strong as that of Suazaorentang.

Experimental Double-blind Study: Suanzaorentang (250 mg 3 times daily) and diazepam (2 mg 3 times daily) had almost the same anxiolytic effect in patients with anxiety, weakness, irritability, and insomnia. However, Suanzaorentang, but not diazepam, improved psychomotor performance during the daytime. No side effects were observed during the treatment with Suanzaorentang (*Suanzaorentang versus diazepam: a controlled double-blind study in anxiety. <u>Int J Clin Pharmacol Ther Toxicol</u> 24(12)646-50, 1986*).

Experimental Double-Blind Crossover Study: In 60 patients with cardiac symptoms of anxiety such as palpitations, chest pain, and shortness of breath, Suanzaorentang demonstrated significant anxiolytic effects as well as an ability to reduce the elevated plasma norepinephrine and blood lactic acid levels (*Hsieh MT and Chen HC. Suanzaorentang in cardiac patients with anxiety. <u>Eur J Clin Pharmacol</u> 30:481-4, 1986*).

APHTHOUS STOMATITIS
(CANKER SORES)

<u>Deglycyrrhizinated Licorice:</u>

Administration as a mouthwash or chewable tablet may be beneficial.

Experimental Study: 20 pts. were instructed to use a solution of deglycyrrhizinated licorice as a mouthwash (200 mg powdered DGL dissolved in 200 ml warm water) 4 times daily. 15/20 (75%) experienced 50-75% improvement within 1 day, followed by complete healing of the ulcers by the third day (*Das SK, Gulati AK, Singh VP. Degly-cyrrhizinated liquorice in aphthous ulcers. <u>J Assoc Physicians India</u> 37(10):647, 1989*).

- -

COMBINATION TREATMENT

'<u>LongoVital</u>':

A commercial product based on dried and ground herbs from pumpkin seeds, arnica flowers, rosemary leaves, paprika and milfoil flower along with vitamins A, B_1, B_2, B_3, B_5, B_6, C, D and E).

Administration may be beneficial.

Experimental Double-blind Crossover Study: 29 otherwise healthy pts., mean age 36, with an estimated ave. number of recurrences the previous yr. of 12.8 (range 3-30), randomly received either LongoVital (LV) 3 tabs with breakfast or placebo. The number of recurrences was significantly reduced on LV the latter 4 of the 6 mo. trial period (p<0.01), and 31% of pts. were totally free of recurrences at the 360 day follow-up. Subjective overall evaluations were significantly in favor of LV. There were no side effects (*Pedersen A et al. LongoVital in the prevention of recurrent aphthous ulceration. <u>J Oral Pathol Med</u> 19(8):371-5, 1990*).

Efficacy may be due to improvement in immune function.

Experimental Double-blind Crossover Study: 31 otherwise healthy pts. were studied while participating in a randomized double-blind crossover study of LongoVital (LV). 14 had LV during the first 6 mo. (GrA) and 17 during the latter 6 mo. (GrB). OKT4+ percentages increased significantly during the LV period in both gps. (p<0.05). OKT8+ percentages increased in both gps.; however, only significantly in GrA (p<0.05). Results suggest that LV acts as an immunostimulant in pts. with recurrnet aphthous ulcerations and that the increase in T-lymphocyte subsets may account for its benefits in LV prevention (*Pedersen A, Klausen B, Hougen HP, et al. [Immunomodulating effect*

*of LongoVital in patients with recurrent aphthous stomatitis.] <u>Ugeskr Laeger</u>
153(37):2561-4, 1991).*

See Also:

*Johansen K. [LongoVital and aphthous stomatitis.] Letter. <u>Ugeskr Laeger</u>
153(47):3335, 1991 (in Danish)*

ATHEROSCLEROSIS
(including CORONARY HEART DISEASE)

**See Also: CARDIAC ARRHYTHMIA
CEREBROVASCULAR DISEASE
PERIPHERAL VASCULAR DISEASE**

KEY: A = *concerns angina pectoris*
C = *concerns total cholesterol*
F = *concerns fibrinolysis*
G = *concerns atherogenesis*
H = *concerns HDL cholesterol*
L = *concerns LDL cholesterol*
M = *concerns CVD mortality and MI*
P = *concerns platelet adhesiveness and/or aggregation*
R = *concerns plaque regression*
T = *concerns triglycerides*

- -

Alfalfa (*Medicago sativa*):
(C,G,H,L)

Rich in saponins which are capable of binding to cholesterol and bile salts in the gut to prevent absorption. In addition, the interaction of other components with bile acids may be equally important (*Story JA, LePage SL, Petro MS, et al. Interactions of alfalfa plant and sprout saponins with cholesterol in vitro and in cholesterol-fed rats. Am J Clin Nutr 39:917-29, 1984*).

Animal Experimental Study (C,H,L): Following 3 wks. on a diet enriched with 10 tsp. alfalfa seed powder daily, blood cholesterol levels declined as much as 20% and HDL/LDL ratios improved by up to 40% (*Malinow MR, McLaughlin P, Stafford C, et al. Comparative effects of alfalfa saponins and alfalfa fiber on cholesterol absorption in rats. Am J Clin Nutr 32(9):1810-12, 1979*).

See Also:

Animal Experimental Study (C): *Malinow MR, McLaughlin P, Papworth L, et al. Effect of alfalfa saponins on intestinal cholesterol absorption in rats. Am J Clin Nutr 30(12):2061-7, 1977*

Administration may cause regression and dissolution of plaque.

Animal Experimental Study (G): A semipurified high-cholesterol diet was fed to cynomolgus monkeys. After 6 mo., a gp. of them were killed for evaluation of the extent of atherosclerosis. Although their cholesterol intake was as high as in the usual Western diet, the remaining monkeys who were placed on a semipurified diet showed a reduction in the extent of aortic and coronary atherosclerosis as well as reduction in cholesterolemia and plasma phospholipid levels, and normalization in the distribution of plasma lipoproteins, but only if their diet was enriched with 50 gm alfalfa meal daily *(Malinow MR et al. Effect of alfalfa meal on shrinkage (regression) of atherosclerotic plaques during cholesterol feeding in monkeys. Atherosclerosis 30(1):27-43,1978).*

Artichoke (*Cynara scolymus*) extracts:
(C,T)

Artichoke contains caffeylquinic acid compounds. The most widely studied component is cynarin (1,5-dicaffeyl ester of quinic acid) even though cynarin is found at minimal concentrations in artichoke and artichoke extracts. Although most of the clinical research has focused on cynarin, there is experimental evidence that the monocaffeylquinic acids are more potent and artichoke extracts standardized for caffeylquinic acids (e.g., 35%) may produce better clinical results than cynarin in lowering triglyceride and cholesterol levels *(Lietti A. Choleretic and cholesterol lowering properties of two artichoke extracts. Fitoterapia 48(4):153-8, 1977).*

Administration may may help normalize lipid metabolism.

Negative Experimental Study (C,T): 17 pts. with Type IIa or Type IIb hyperlipoproteinemia given 250 mg or 750 mg of cynarin demonstrated no significant change in cholesterol or triglyceride levels within 3 months *(Heckers H et al. Inefficiency of cynarin as a therapeutic regimen in familial Type II hyperlipoproteinaemia. Atheroscler 26:249-53, 1977).*

Experimental Double-Blind Study (C,T): 30 pts. given 500 mg of cynarin per day for 50 days demonstrated significant reductions in the levels of total cholesterol (avg. reduction 20%), triglyceride (avg. reduction 15%), and pre-beta-lipoprotein (avg. reduction 20%) compared to a matched placebo group *(Montini M et al. Controlled trial of cynarin in the treatment of the hyperlipidemic syndrome. Observations in 60 cases. Arzneim Forsch 25(8):1311-4, 1975) (in German).*

See Also:

Experimental Study (C,T): *Mars G, Brambilla G. Wirkung von 1,5-dicaffeyl-chinasaure (cynarin) auf die hypertriglyceridamie im fortgeschritten. Med Welt 25:1572-4, 1975 (in German).*

Experimental Study (C,T): *Pristautz H. Cynarin in der modernen hyperlipamie-behandlung. Weiner Med Wschr 69:705-8, 1975 (in German).*

Berberine:
(M)

Berberine is an alkaloid extracted from the roots and bark of various plants such as golden-seal (*Hydrastis canadensis*), barberry root bark (*Berberis vulgaris*), and Oregon grape root (*Berberis aquifolium*).

Administration may protect against coronary artery ischemia and reperfusion injury. (*See: 'CARDIAC ARRHYTHMIA'*)

> **Animal Experimental Study (M):** In anesthetized rats, tetrahydroberberine reduced infarct size in the ischemic and reperfused myocardium following coronary artery ligation and markedly decreased the incidences of ventricular tachycardia and ventricular fibrillation during the reperfusion period. Also, following pretreatment with tetrahydroberberine, the malondialdehyde content and xanthine oxidase activity were decreased ($p<0.01$; $p<0.05$) (*Zhou J, Xuan B, Li DX. Effects of tetrahydroberberine on ischemic and reperfused myocardium in rats. Chung Kuo Yao Li Hsueh Pao 14(2):130-3, 1993*).

See Also:

> **Animal Experimental Study (M):** *Huang Z, Chen S, Zhang G, et al. Protective effects of berberine and phentolamine on myocardial reoxygenation damage. Chin Med Sci J 7(4):221-5, 1992*

> **Animal Experimental Study (M):** *Huang WM, Yan H, Jin JM, et al. Beneficial effects of berberine on hemodynamics during acute ischemic left ventricular failure in dogs. Chin Med J (Engl) 105(12):1014-9, 1992*

Bilberry (*Vaccinium myrtillus*):
(P)

Bilberry, or European blueberry, is a shrubby perennial plant that grows in the woods and forest meadows of Europe.

The standard dose for bilberry extracts is based on its anthocyanoside content, as calculated by its anthocyanidin percentage. The dosage for a bilberry extract standardized for an anthocyanidin content of 25% is 80 to 160 mg three times daily.

Administration may reduce platelet aggregation (*Buliero G. The inhibitory effects of anthocyanosides on human platelet aggregation. Fitoterapia 60:69, 1989*), probably due to increased release of prostacyclin - which has potent blood vessel dilating and platelet anti-aggregatory activities (*Morrazzoni P, Magistretti MJ. Effects of anthocyanosides on prostacyclin activity in arterial tissue. Fitoterapia 57:11, 1986*).

Bromelain:
(A,F,G,P,R)

Bromelain is a mixture of sulfur-containing proteolytic enzymes or proteases obtained from the stem of the pineapple plant (*Ananas comosus*). The fibrinolytic activities of bromelain may be useful in many cardiovascular diseases. (*See: 'THROMBOPHLEBITIS'*)

The standard dosage of bromelain (1,800-2,000 m.c.u.) is 125-450 mg 3 times daily on an empty stomach.

Administration may be beneficial.

Review Article (F,P): The combination of fibrinolytic and antithrombotic properties of bromelain appear to be effective, and 2 large scale tests on heart pts. have shown a practically complete elimination of thrombosis *(Felton GE. Fibrinolytic and antithrombotic action of bromelain may eliminate thrombosis in heart patients. Med Hypotheses 6(11):1123-33, 1980).*

Review Article: The cardiovascular applications of bromelain are presented including results from several uncontrolled trials in angina, hypertension, and thrombophlebitis. Bromelain inhibits platelet aggregation, exerts anti-anginal activity, promotes fibrinolysis, and relaxes vasoconstriction. These actions make it particularly useful in angina and thrombophlebitis *(Taussig S and Nieper H. Bromelain: Its use in prevention and treatment of cardiovascular disease present status. J Int Assoc Prev Med 6:139-51, 1979).*

Experimental Study (A): 14 pts. with angina pectoris received 1000-1400 mg daily with disappearance of symptoms in all pts. within 4 - 90 days depending upon the severity of the coronary sclerosis. Symptoms recurred when bromelain was discontinued *(Nieper HA. Effect of bromelain on coronary heart disease and angina pectoris. Acta Med Empirica 5:274-5, 1978; Nieper HA. Wirkung von Bromelain auf koronare Herzkrankheit un Angina Pectoris. Erfahungsheilkunde 5:274-5, 1978.).*

Animal Experimental Study (R): Bromelain broke down arteriosclerotic plaque in rabbit aorta both *in vivo* and *in vitro* *(Chen JR. In vivo and in vitro studies of the effect of bromelain on cholesterol-protein binding. Dissert Abstr B 1975 35 (2 Pt) 6013, Ord. No. 75-13, 735).*

Experimental Study (P): 2 tablets reduced platelet aggregability in 2 hours in 8/9 pts. with hyper-aggregable platelets and 8/11 pts. with normal platelet sensitivity *(Heinicke RM, Van der Wal L, Yokoyama MM. Effect of bromelain (Ananase) on human platelet aggregation. Experientia 28:844-5, 1972).*

See Also:

> **Review Article:** *Taussig S, Batkin S. Bromelain, the enzyme complex of pineapple (Ananas comosus) and its clinical application. An update. J Ethnopharmacol 22:191-203, 1988.*

Curcumin:
(C,P)

Curcumin is the yellow pigment of turmeric *(Curcuma longa).*

Administration may be beneficial.

Animal Experimental Study (C): Rats fed a diet containing as low as 0.1% curcumin and cholesterol, the levels of cholesterol fell to one-half of those rats fed cholesterol and no curcumin. This data indicates that even at small doses, curcumin may be effective (*Rao DS et al. Effect of curcumin on serum and liver cholesterol levels in the rat. J Nutri 100:1307-16, 1970*).

Animal Experimental Study (C): Curcumin's cholesterol-lowering actions include interfering with intestinal cholesterol-uptake; increasing the conversion of cholesterol into bile acids by increasing the activity of hepatic cholesterol-7-alpha-hydroxylase, the rate-limiting enzyme of bile acid synthesis; and increasing the excretion of bile acids (*Srinivasan K, Samaiah K. The effect of spices on cholesterol 7 alpha-hydroxylase activity and on serum and hepatic cholesterol levels in the rat. Int J Vitam Nutr Res 61:364-9, 1991*).

In vitro Study (P): Curcumin inhibits platelet aggregation by inhibiting the formation of thromboxanes, a promoter of aggregation, while simultaneously increasing prostacyclin, an inhibitor of aggregation (*Srivastava R et al. Effect of curcumin on platelet aggregation and vascular prostacyclin synthesis. Arzneim Forsch 36:715-7, 1986*).

See Also:

   Srivastava R et al. Anti-thrombotic effect of curcumin. Throm Res 40:413-7, 1985

Eggplant (*Solanum melongena*):
(G)

Administration may inhibit the development of atheromatous plaques.

   Animal Experimental Study (G): Animals fed violet eggplant were protected from developing atheromatous plaques (*Mitschek GH [Histological studies on cholesterol-induced atheromatosis in rabbits in mean- and long-term tests.] Exp Pathol (Jena) 10(3-4):156-66, 1975*) (*in German*).

Fenugreek (*Trigonella foenum-graecum*):
(C,H,L,T)

Fenugreek seeds or debitterized fenugreek seed powder may lower blood lipids. (*See: 'DIABETES MELLITUS'*)

Experimental Study (C,H,L,T): Ingestion of experimental diets containing 100 g of debitterized fenugreek powder for 20 days resulted in significant reduction in the serum total cholesterol (-24%), LDL and VLDL cholesterol (-32%), and triglyceride (-37%) levels. Although HDL cholesterol levels were not altered, the ratio of HDL to LDL and VLDL was significantly increased by 42% (*Sharma RD et al. Hypolipidemic effect of fenugreek seeds, a clinical study. Phytother Res 5:145-7, 1991*).

Experimental Double-blind Study (C,H.L,T): Isocaloric diets with and without fenugreek were each given randomly for 10 days to type I diabetics. Defatted fenugreek seed powder (100 g), divided into two equal doses, was incorporated into the diet and served during lunch and dinner. Serum total cholesterol, LDL and VLDL cholesterol and triglycerides were significantly reduced. The HDL cholesterol fraction, however, remained unchanged (*Sharma RD et al. Effect of fenugreek seeds on blood glucose and serum lipids in type I diabetes. Eur J Clin Nutr 44(4):301-6, 1990*).

Experimental Study (T): Fenugreek seeds given at a dose of 25 g/d for 3 weeks to type II diabetics led to a reduction in serum cholesterol levels (*Sharma RD. Effect of fenugreek seeds and leaves on blood glucose and serum insulin responses in human subjects. Nutr Res 6:1353-64, 1986*).

Animal Experimental Study (C,H,T): Administration of the defatted seed (in daily doses of 1.5-2 g/kg) to both normal and diabetic dogs reduced fasting and after-meal blood levels of total cholesterol and triglycerides, while increasing HDL-cholesterol levels (*Ribes G et al. Antidiabetic effects of subfractions from fenugreek seeds in diabetic dogs. Proc Soc Exp Biol Med 182(2):159-66, 1986*).

Gamma-oryzanol:
(C,H,L,T)

A mixture of ferulic acid derivatives found in rice bran.

Administration may be beneficial.

Experimental Study (C,H,L,T): 67 pts. with type IIA (n=35), type IIB (n=19), or type IV (n=13) hyperlipoproteinemia received 300 mg/d of gamma-oryzanol for 3 months. Mean plasma cholesterol in type IIA and IIB pts. decreased significantly from the second month (-8% and -12%, respectively) due to a fall in LDL-cholesterol levels. Mean plasma triglyceride levels of all pts. decreased significantly (-14%) by the third month. HDL-cholesterol increased significantly after 3 mo. in the type IIB subjects (*Yoshino G et al. Effects of gamma-oryzanol on hyperlipidemic subjects. Curr Ther Res 45:543-52, 1989*).

Garlic (*Allium sativum*) or
Onion (*Allium cepa*):
(C,F,G,H,L,M,P,T)

The beneficial effects of garlic and onions are thought to be due to a variety of sulfur-containing compounds, especially allicin. Commercial garlic preparations concentrated for alliin appear to be the most effective and because alliin is relatively 'odorless' until it is converted to allicin in the body, these preparations are more socially acceptable. The compound alliin is converted to allicin by the enzyme alliinase which is activated when garlic is crushed. The dosage of the commercial product should provide a daily dose of 8 mg alliin or a total allicin potential of 4,000 mcg.

Meta-analytic Study (C): Based on a meta-analysis of 5 randomized, placebo-controlled studies of pts. with initial cholesterol levels greater than 200 mg/dL (5.17 mmol/L), it was conservatively estimated that garlic, in an amount approximating 1/2 clove per day, decreases total serum cholesterol levels by about 9% (23 mg/dL; 0.59 mmol/L) ($p < 0.001$) (*Warshafsky S, Kamer RS, Sivak SL. Effect of garlic on total serum cholesterol. Ann Intern Med 119:599-605, 1993*).

Experimental Double-blind Study (C,L): 42 healthy human volunteers with a serum total cholesterol level greater than 220 mg/dl received either 900 mg/day of a standardized dried garlic preparation (Kwai®) containing 1.3% alliin or placebo. After twelve weeks, total cholesterol dropped by 6% and LDL dropped 11% in the group receiving the garlic. The placebo group had no change (*Jain AK et al. Can garlic reduce levels of serum lipids? A controlled clinical study. Am J Med 94:632-5, 1993*).

Experimental Double-blind Study (H,T): 24 human volunteers with low HDL levels were given either 900 mg/day of dried garlic preparation (Sapec®; Kwai®) containing 1.3% alliin or placebo for 6 weeks. When these volunteers were fed a standardized test meal contining 100 g of butter, the gp. receiving the garlic had a reduced postprandial increase of triglycerides. Compared to the placebo gp., the uptake of triglycerides in the garlic gp. were up to 35% lower (*Rotzch W et al. [Postprandial lipaemia under treatment with Allium sativum. Controlled double-blind study in healthy volunteers with reduced HDL₂- cholesterol levels.] Arzneim Forsch 42(10):1223-7, 1992*) (*in German*).

Experimental Placebo-controlled Study (C,T): 261 pts. with total cholesterol and/or triglycerides >200 mg/dl (mostly hyperlipoproteinemia types IIa/IIb) randomly received tablets containing 800 mg garlic powder (standardized to 1.3% alliin content) daily or placebo. After 16 wks., mean serum cholesterol levels decreased in the experimental gp. from 266 to 235 mg/dl (12%), and mean triglyceride levels decreased from 226 to 188 mg/dl (17%). Pts. with initial total cholesterol levels of 250-300 mg/dl showed the best results (*Mader FH. Treatment of hyperlipidemia with garlic-powder tablets. Arzneim Forsch 40:1111-6, 1990*).

Review Article (C,F,P): Claims for beneficial effects on cholesterol levels, fibrinolytic activity and platelet aggregation have been made for fresh garlic and onions or their extracts and to commerically available preparations. These claims have been confirmed for fresh garlic, but only at very high dosages. For onions and commercially available supplements, contradictory results have been reported. All published trials show severe methodological shortcomings; some were not randomized and/or not blinded, and in only one-third of studies >25 pts. participated in each treatment group. In no trial was prognostic comparability of the treatment and the control gps. ascertained. Thus, there is inadequate scientific justification for garlic or onion supplementation (*Kleijnen J et al. Garlic, onions and cardiovascular risk factors: A review of the evidence from human experiments with emphasis on commercially available preparations. Br J Clin Pharmacol 28(5):535-44, 1989*).

Experimental Double-blind Crossover Study (C,H,T): 30 pts. with primary hyperlipidemia randomly received 2 garlic capsules of a spray-dried preparation (350 mg/cap) for 2 mo. or placebo for 2 mo. in either order. Results showed some trends for reduction of serum cholesterol and triglycerides and elevation of HDL cholesterol (*Plengvidhya C et al. Effects of spray dried garlic preparation on primary hyperlipoproteinaemia. J Med Assoc Thai 71(5):248-52, 1988*).

Review Article (M): The action of both garlic and onion on blood coagulability is more clearly defined than their effect on the other risk factors. While many of the studies have serious methodological shortcomings, there is some evidence to suggest that use of certain formulations of garlic and/or onion is accompanied by favorable effects on risk factors in normal subjects and in patients. The possibility of toxicity resulting from acute and chronic ingestion of large amounts is unresolved. Accordingly, further clinical and epidemiological studies are required before the role of these plants in the prevention and control of cardiovascular disorders is understood and can be realized (*Kendler BS. Garlic (Allium sativum) and onion (Allium cepa): A review of their relationship to cardiovascular disease. Prev Med 16(5):670-85, 1987*).

Review Article (C,F,P): The results of numerous studies are reviewed that show that garlic can bring about normalization of plasma lipids, enhancement of fibrinolytic activity and inhibition of platelet aggregation (*Ernst E. Cardiovascular effects of garlic (Allium sativum): A review. Pharmatherapeutica 5(2):83-9, 1987*).

Experimental Study (C,H,L,T): Subjects with moderately high cholesterol levels added 4 capsules (1 ml/cap) daily of Kyolic® liquid garlic to their usual diet. Blood fat levels rose for the first few months; then, in most pts., lipid levels dropped. After 6 mo., total cholesterol levels were an ave. of 44 mg/dl lower than at the start of the study. High-density lipoproteins rose, while LDL, VLDL and triglycerides fell (*Lau BH et al. Effect of an odor-modified garlic preparation on blood lipids. Nutr Res 7:139-49, 1987*).

Experimental Double-blind Crossover Study (C,H,P): 20 normal volunteers were randomly divided into 2 gps., each of which rotated for 4-wk. periods through 2 different sequences during which they received 18 mg of garlic oil (extracted from 9 gms of fresh garlic) and placebo laced with garlic oil. During garlic administration, the amt. of platelet aggregation decreased ($p<0.005$), total serum cholesterol decreased ($p<0.011$) and serum high density lipoprotein levels rose ($p<0.001$). There was also a significant rise in arachidonic acid in RBC phospholipids, suggesting that garlic may reduce the conversion of arachidonic acid to thromboxane A_2 (*Barrie, SA et al. Effects of garlic oil on platelet aggregation, serum lipids and blood pressure in humans. J Orthomol Med 2(1):15-21, 1987*).

Negative Experimental Double-blind Study (H,L,T): A simple dried garlic preparation did not produce any effects on HDL or LDL cholesterol and triglycerides (*Luley C et al. Lack of efficacy of dried garlic in patients with hyperlipoproteinemia. Arzneim Forsch 36(4):766-8, 1986*).

Note: The negative results may have been due to the lack of potency of this non-standardized preparation.

Experimental Controlled Study (C,T): 10 hypercholesterolemic pts. were treated with 600 mg garlic powder daily (equivalent to 1800 mg fresh garlic) and showed a 10% mean decrease in cholesterol levels and a significant decrease in plasma viscosity, levels of triglycerides and low density lipoproteins compared to controls (*Ernst E et al. Garlic and blood lipids. Br Med J 291:139, 1985*).

Increasing the garlic content of the diet may be beneficial.

Experimental Studies (C,H,T): 1.) 20 healthy volunteers were fed garlic for 6 mo. and then followed for another 2 mo. without garlic. Garlic significantly lowered serum cholesterol and triglycerides while raising high density lipoproteins. 2.) 62 pts. with CHD and elevated serum cholesterol were randomly divided so that one gp. received garlic for 10 mo. while the other gp. served as a control. Garlic decreased serum cholesterol ($p<0.05$), triglycerides ($p<0.05$) and low-density lipoprotein ($p<0.05$) while increasing the high-density fraction ($p<0.001$) (*Bordia A. Effect of garlic on blood lipids in patients with coronary heart disease. Am J Clin Nutr 34:2100-3, 1981*).

Animal Experimental Study (C,G): Garlic fed to rabbits on a high cholesterol diet prevented a rise in blood cholesterol and inhibited development of atherosclerosis in the aorta (*Jain RC. Effect of alcoholic extraction on garlic in atherosclerosis. Am J Clin Nutr 31:1982-3, 1978*).

Animal Experimental Study (G): The administration of garlic and onion prevented the formation of experimental AS in rabbits (*Bordia A et al. Effect of essential oil of onion and garlic on experimental atherosclerosis in rabbits. Atherosclerosis 26:379-82, 1977*).

Onion may produce similar benefit to garlic in lowering cholesterol levels.

Experimental Study (C): Crude onion oil was given to 34 pts. with moderate hypertension or hypercholesterolemia, or both at a dose of 1 tbsp. 2-3 times daily. In 13 of 20 pts. with hypertension, there was a clear blood pressure reduction of an average 25 mm Hg for the systolic and/or 15 mm Hg for the diastolic. In 9 of 18 pts with hypercholesterolemia, total cholesterol levels fell between 7% and 33% (*Louria DB et al. Onion extract in treatment of hypertension and hyperlipidemia: A preliminary communication. Curr Ther Res 37(1):127-31, 1985*).

Both onions and garlic inhibit platelet aggregation by blocking thromboxane synthesis for several hours (*Makheja AN et al. Inhibition of platelet aggregation and thromboxane synthesis by onion and garlic. Letter. Lancet i:781, 1979*).

Experimental Double-blind Crossover Study (F,P): When 12 healthy human volunteers received 900 mg/day of a dried garlic preparation (Sapec®; Kwai®) containing 1.3% alliin significant increases in fibrinolytic activity and tissue plasminogen activator activity were noted along with reduced platelet aggregation (*Legnani C et al. Effects of dried garlic preparation on fibrinolysis and platelet aggregation in healthy subjects. Arzneim Forsch 43(1):119-21, 1993*).

Experimental Double-blind Study (P): 120 pts. with increased platelet aggregation were given either 900 mg/day of a dried garlic preparation containing 1.3% alliin or a placebo for 4 weeks. In the garlic group, spontaneous platelet aggregation disappeared, the microcirculation of the skin increased by 47.6%, plasma viscosity decreased by 3.2%, diastolic blood pressure dropped from an average of 74 to 67 and fasting blood glucose concentration dropped from an average of 89.4 to 79 (*Kiesewetter H, Jung F, Pindur G, et al. Effect of garlic on thrombocyte aggregation, microcirculation, and other risk factors. Int J Clin Pharmacol Ther Toxicol 29(4):151-5, 1991*).

In vitro Experimental Study (P): Aqueous extracts of onion and garlic inhibited platelet aggregation induced by several aggregation agents, including arachidonate, in a dose-dependent manner (*Srivastava KC. Aqueous extracts of onion, garlic and ginger inhibit platelet aggregation and alter arachidonic acid metabolism. Biomed Biochim Acta 43(8/9):S335-S346, 1984*).

Experimental Study (P): 100-150 mg./kg. fresh garlic completely inhibited platelet aggregation to 5-hydroxytryptamine for 1-2 1/2 hours after ingestion (*Boullin DJ. Garlic as a platelet inhibitor. Lancet i:776-7, 1981*).

Experimental Study (P): 6 healthy subjects took 25 mg. of garlic oil daily. After 5 days, platelet aggregation induced by 3 different aggregating agents was inhibited (*Bordia A. Effect of garlic on human platelet aggregation in vitro. Atherosclerosis 30:355-60, 1978*).

See Also:

> *Vanderhoek JY et al. Inhibition of fatty acid oxygenases by onion and garlic oils. Biochem Pharm 29:3169, 1980*

> *Baghurst KI et al. Onions and platelet aggregation. Lancet January 8, 1977*

Administration may increase fibrinolytic activity.

Experimental Study (F): Onion increased fibrinolytic activity (*Baghurst KI et al. Onions and platelet aggregation. Lancet January 8, 1977*).

Experimental Study (F): When garlic (equivalent to the essential oil of garlic extracted from 1 gm of raw garlic per kgm of body weight) was given within 24 hrs. after a MI, fibrinolytic activity increased 63% after 10 days and 95% after 20 days. When given to normals, fibrinolytic activity rose 130% (*Bordia AK et al. Effect of garlic oil on fibrinolytic activity in patients with CHD. Atherosclerosis 28:155-9, 1977*).

Administration of garlic may reduce lipoprotein (LDL) oxidation, a process that is believed to play an important role in the development of atherosclerosis.

Experimental Double-blind Crossover Study: 10 healthy human volunteers given 600 mg/day of a dried garlic preparation (Kwai®) containing 1.3% alliin and a placebo, in random order, for two weeks had a 34% lower susceptibility to lipoprotein oxidation when receiving garlic compared to when receiving placebo (p) (*Phelps S, Harris WS. Garlic supplementation and lipoprotein oxidation susceptibility. Lipids 28:475-7, 1993*).

Ginger (*Zingiber officinale*):
(C,P)

Administration may inhibit platelet aggregation.

Review Article (P): Ginger is a potent inhibitor of thromboxane synthetase as is aspirin and other inhibitors of platelet aggregation. In contrast to other platelet aggregation inhibitors, however, it raises levels of prostacyclin without a concomitant rise in inflammatory prostaglandins; thus it should cause substantially fewer side-effects (*Backon J. Ginger: Inhibition of thromboxane synthetase and stimulation of prostacyclin: Relevance for medicine and psychiatry. Med Hypotheses 20:271, 1986*).

In vitro Study (P): Ginger inhibited platelet aggregation *in vitro* more than either onion or garlic (*Srivastava KC. Effects of aqueous extracts of onion, garlic and ginger on platelet aggregation and metabolism of arachidonic acid in the blood vascular system: In vitro study. Prostaglandins Med 13:227, 1984*).

In vitro Study (P): Platelet-rich plasma was preincubated for 1-60 min. with an ethanol extract of ground ginger. The extract completely inhibited arachidonate-induced platelet aggregation, whereas the ethanol vehicle was without effect (*Dorso CR et al. Chinese food and platelets. Letter N Engl J Med 303:756-7, 1980*).

Administration may reduce cholesterol levels.

Animal Experimental Study (C): *Gujaral S et al. Effect of ginger (Zinger officinale roscoe) oleoresin on serum and hepatic cholesterol levels in cholesterol fed rats. Nutr Rep Int 17:183-9, 1978*

Ginkgo biloba:
(F,P)

The 24% ginkgoflavonglycosides extract may be effective in reducing fibrinogen levels and plasma viscosity. (*See: 'CEREBROVASCULAR DISEASE'; 'PERIPHERAL VASCULAR DISEASE'*)

Experimental Study (F,P): 20 pts. with a long history of elevated fibrinogen levels and plasma viscosity were given 240 mg per day of *Ginkgo biloba* extract for 12 weeks. At the end of the study significant improvements were noted (*Witte S et al. [Improvement of hemorrheological parameters by Ginkgo biloba extract.] Fortsch Med 13:247-50, 1992*) (*in German*).

See Also:

> *Koltringer P et al. [Hemorheologic effects of ginkgo biloba extract EGb 761. Dose- dependent effect of EGb 761 on microcirculation and viscoelasticity of blood]. Fortschr Med 111(10):170-2, 1993 (in German)*

Gugulipid (*Commiphora mukul*):
(C,H,L,P,T)

Gugulipid refers to the extract of the oleoresin (gum guggul or guggulu) of the mukul myrrh tree standardized for guggulsterones. It is the preferred form. While the crude oleoresin (gum guggul), alcohol extract, and petroleum ether extract all exert lipid-lowering and anti-inflammatory action, they are associated with side effects (skin rashes, diarrhea, etc.) at doses required to produce a clinical effect. No side effects are noted with gugulipid. The dosage of gugulipid depends on the guggulsterone content, 25 mg of guggulsterones three times per day is the effective dose (*Gugulipid. Drugs of the Future 13(7):618-9, 1988; Dev S. Chemistry of Commiphora mukul and development of a hypolipidemic drug. Econ Med Plant Res 5:47-82, 1991; Satyavati GV. Gum guggul (Commiphora mukul) - The success story of an ancient insight leading to a modern discovery. Ind J Med Res 87:327-35, 1988*).

Administration may improve the lipid profile.

Experimental Double-blind Crossover Study (C,H,L,T): 125 pts. received gugulipid while 108 received clofibrate. With gugulipid, the ave. decrease in serum cholesterol and triglycerides was 11% and 16.8%, respectively; with clofibrate, the ave. decrease was 10% and 21.6%, respectively. The lipid lowering effect of both drugs became evident 3-4 wks. after starting administration and was unrelated to age, sex or concomitant drug intake. Hypercholesterolemic pts. responded better to gugulipid than hypertriglyeridemic pts. - who responded better to clofibrate. In mixed hyperlipidemic pts., the response to both drugs was comparable. HDL cholesterol increased in 60% of the pts. who responded to gugulipid, while clofibrate had no effect. LDL cholesterol significantly decreased in responders to each drug (*Nityanand S et al. Clinical trials with Gugulipid: A new hypolipidemic agent. J Assoc Phys India 37(5):323-8, 1989*).

Experimental Placebo-controlled Study (C): 205 pts received gugulipid (a standardized extract of gum guggul containing 25 mg of guggulosterones per capsule) 500 mg 3 times daily or placebo. Total cholesterol was significantly lowered in 70-80% of patients. One pt. had GI symptoms which did not necessitate withdrawal of the drug (*Nityanand S et al. Clinical trials with Gugulipid: A new hypolipidemic agent. J Assoc Phys India 37(5):323-8, 1989*).

Experimental Placebo-controlled Study (C,H,L,T): 40 pts. aged 40-60 with hyperlipidemia type IIa or IIb randomly received either purified gum guggul 2.25 g twice daily or placebo. Serum cholesterol decreased by 7.8%, 15.78% and 21.75% at the end of the 4th, 8th, and 16th wk., respectively, while serum triglyceride levels decreased by 6.7%, 17.1% and 27.1% over the same time period. HDL cholesterol gradually increased; by the end of the 16th wk., it had increased approx. 35.8%. VLDL and LDL cholesterol significantly decreased during the study. There were no reported side effects (*Verma SK, Bordia A. Effect of Commiphora mukul (gum guggul) in patients of hyperlipidemia with special reference to HDL-cholesterol. Indian J Med Res 87:356-60, 1988*).

See Also:

> **Animal Experimental Study (L):** *Singh V et al. Stimulation of low density lipoprotein receptor activity in liver membrane in guggulsterone treated rats. Pharmacol Res 22(1):37-44, 1990*

Administration may inhibit platelet aggregation (*Mester L et al. Inhibition of platelet aggregation by "gugglu" steroids. Planta Med 37(43):367-9, 1979*).

Hawthorn (*Crataegus* spp.):
(A)

Extracts of hawthorn berries, leaves, or flowering tops are widely used by physicians in Asia and Europe for their cardiotonic effects. The beneficial effects of hawthorn extracts are due to the presence of procyanidin flavonoids. (*See: 'Procyanidolic Oligomers' below*.)

Standardized extracts, similar to those used in the clinical studies cited below are the preferred form. The dosage for hawthorn extracts standardized to contain 1.8% vitexin-4[1] - rhamnoside or 10% procyanidins is 120-240 mg three times daily; for extracts standardized to contain 18% procyanidolic oligomers, the dosage is 240-480 mg daily. (*See: 'CARDIAC ARRHYTHMIA'; 'CONGESTIVE HEART FAILURE'; 'HYPERTENSION'*)

Administration may improve myocardial function.

In vitro Study: The water-soluble fraction of Crataegus exerted a cardioprotective effect through a mechanism other than increasing coronary blood flow (*Nasa Y et al.*

Protective effect of Crataegus extract on the cardiac mechanical dysfunction in isolated perfused working rat heart. Arzneim Forsch 43(9):945-9, 1993).

Experimental Double-blind Study (A): 46 pts. with angina were given either a tablet containing *Crataegus pinnatifida* leaves 100 mg or placebo for 4 weeks. The overall effectiveness of Crataegus was 84.8% compared to 37% for the placebo group (p). 46.4% of pts. on Crataegus demonstrated improved ECG readings compared to 3.3% in the placebo group *(Weng WL et al. Therapeutic effect of Crataegus pinnatifida on 46 cases of angina pectoris — a double blind study. J Tradit Chin Med 4(4):293-4, 1984).*

Animal Experimental Study (A): Crude extract from the leaf of *Crataegus pinnatifida* simulataneously decreased oxygen consumption and improved oxygen utilization and heart function when given to dogs *(Lianda L et al. Studies on hawthorn and its active principle. I. Effect on myocardial ischemia and hemodynamics in dogs. J Trad Chin Med 4(4):283-8, 1984).*

Review Article: Preparations of Crataegus are used in minor forms of heart disease including angina, minor forms of congestive heart failure, and cardiac arrythmia. From experiments with animals, preparations of Crataegus exhibited the following effects: increased coronary blood flow, decreased arterial blood pressure, increased peripheral blood flow, decreased heart rate, and improved contractility of the heart muscle. Crataegus preparations are extremely well-tolerated. The acute oral toxicity (LD50) of Crataegus preparations and constituents was found to be in the range of 6 g/kg *(Ammon HPT, Handel M. [Crataegus, toxicology and pharmacology, Part I: Toxicity]. Planta Med 43(2):105-20, 1981; Part II: Pharmacodynamics. Planta Med 43(3):209-39, 1981; Part III: Pharmacodynamics and pharmacokinetics. Planta Med 43(4):313-22, 1981) (in German).*

Animal Experimental Study (A): Oral and intravenous administration of Crataegus procyanidins led to a significant rise in blood flow through the myocardium for several hours depending on the dose. The highest increase reached an average value to +70% of resting flow *(Roddewigg C, Hensel H. [Reaction of local myocardial blood flow in non-anesthetized dogs and anesthetized cats to oral and parenteral application of a Crataegus fraction (Oligomere procyanidines). Arzneim Forsch 27(7):1407-9, 1977) (in German).*

See Also:

Experimental Double-blind Study (A): *Iwamoto M, Sato T, Ishizaki T. [The clinical effect of Crataegutt® in heart disease of ischemic or hypertensive origin. A multicenter double-blind study]. Planta Med 42(1):1-16, 1981 (in German)*

Animal Experimental Study (A): *Roddewig VC, Hensel H. Reaction of local myocardial blood flow in non-anesthetized dogs and anesthetized cats to oral and parenteral application of a crataegus fraction (oligomere procyanidins). Arzneim Forsch 27:1407-10, 1977 (in German)*

Animal Experimental Study (A): *Mavers VWH, Hensel H. Changes in local myocardial blood flow following oral administration to a crataegus extract to non-anesthetized dogs. Arzniem Forsch 24:783-5, 1974*

Experimental Double-blind Study (A): *Massoni G. [On the use of hawthorn extract (Crataegus) in the treatment of certain ischemic myocardial diseases in old age]. G Gerontol 16(9):979-84, 1968 (in Italian)*

Experimental Double-blind Study (A): *Hammerl H, et al. [Clinico-experimental metabolic studies using a Crataegus extract]. Arzneim Forsch 21(7):261-4, 1967 (in German)*

Animal Experimental Study (A): *Rewerski VW et al. Some pharmacological properties of oligomeric procyanidin isolated from hawthorn (Crataegus oxyacantha). Arzniem Forsch 17:490-1, 1967 (in German)*

Khella (*Ammi Visnaga*):
(A,C)

Khella is an ancient medicinal plant native to the Mediterranean region where it has been used in the treatment of angina and other heart ailments since the time of the pharaohs. Several of its components have demonstrated effects in dilating the coronary arteries. Its mechanism of action appears to be very similar to the calcium-channel blocking drugs.

Most clinical studies used preparations contain 70 to 80% khellin and 20 to 30% visnagin. At higher doses, 120-160 mg per day, these preparations were associated with mild side effects such as insomnia, anorexia, nausea, and dizziness in some cases. Although most clinical studies used high dosages, several studies show that as little as 30 mg of khellin per day appears to offer as good as results with fewer side effects. Rather than using isolated khellin, khella extracts standardized for khellin content (typically 12%) can be used.

Administration of the extracts may reduce angina.

Experimental Double-blind Study (A): Of the 41 pts. with angina given 1 tablet of Khelltron (khellin 20 mg, sestron monocitrate 40 mg, thiamine hydrochloride 3 mg) 3 times daily, definite improvements was noted in 27. However, it had to be discontinued in 8 of these because of toxic effects (*Hejtmancik MR et al. Clinical effects of Khelltron in angina pectoris. Texas State J Med 49:679-82, 1953*).

Experimental Study (A): 42 pts. treated with khellin: 30 (71%) had a favorable response, 3 had an unfavorable response, and 6 remained unchanged. The incidence of side effects, mainly nausea and vomiting was 62% (*Conn JJ et al. Treatment of angina pectoris with khellin. Part I. Ann Int Med 36:1173-8, 1952*).

Experimental Double-blind Study (A): Of 32 pts. receiving an average of 160 mg of pure khellin daily, 26 experienced a decrease in frequency and severity of anginal pains, a drop in nitroglycerin requirements and an increase in exercise tolerance. Improvement was considered marked in 11 pts., moderate in 11 and slight in 4, the remaining 6 showed no improvement. In contrast, only 1 pt. in the placebo group a drop in nitroglycerin and no pts. demonstrated improved exercise tolerance. 5 additional pts. with severe and often intractable angina also noted marked or moderate improvements. "The high proportion of favorable results, together with the striking degree of improvement frequently observed, has led us to the conclusion that khellin, properly used, is a safe and effective drug for the treatment of angina pectoris" (*Osher HL et al. Khellin in the treatment of angina pectoris. N Engl J Med 244:315-21, 1951*).

Experimental Study (A): Of 250 pts treated with khellin (average dose 120 mg/day), 225 (90%) were considered to be improved — 140 (56%) markedly and 85 (34%) moderately (*Anrep GV et al. Coronary vasodilator action of khellin. Am Heart J 37:531-42, 1949*).

See Also:

Experimental Study (A): *Conn JJ et al. Treatment of angina pectoris with khellin. Part II. Ann Int Med 38:23-7, 1953*

Experimental Study (A): *Armburst CA et al. Treatment of angina pectoris with preparations of khellin (Ammi visnaga). Am J Med Sci 220:127-32, 1950*

Administration of the extracts may lower cholesterol.

Animal Experimental Study (C): Khellin and a related compound, methoxsalen caused a marked reduction in LDL and total cholesterol when fed to rats even at low doses (0.23 mg/100 g b.wt./day). No toxic side effects were noted (*Naser HE, Gaffar EA, Mahmoud SS. Hypocholesterolemic effect of khellin and methoxsalen in male albino rats. Arzneim Forsch 42(2):140-2, 1992*).

Malabar Tamarind (*Garcinia camboga*):
(*C,T*)

The Malabar tamarind or Brindall berry is a yellowish fruit that is about the size of an orange, with a thin skin, and deep furrows similar to an acorn squash. It is native to South India where it is dried and used extensively in curries. It has also been historically used in the Ayurvedic treatment of obesity. (*See: 'OBESITY'*)

The dried fruit contains about 30% (-)-hydroxycitric acid (HCA). Citrin®, a commercial preparation, contains about 50% HCA.

The recommended dosage of HCA is 500 mg 3 times daily with meals.

HCA inhibits lipogenesis by interfering with adenosine triphosphate (ATP) citrate lyase. As a result it reduces the level of acetyl coenzyme A, the extramitochondrial precursor of fatty acid synthesis.

HCA may lower cholesterol and triglyceride levels.

In vitro Study (C): HCA-incubated liver cells demonstrated significant inhibition of cholesterol synthesis (*Berkhout TA, et al. The effect of HCA on the activity of the low-density-lipoprotein receptor and 3-hydroxy-3-methylglutaryl-CoA reductase levels in the human hepatoma cell line Hep G2. Biochem J 15;272(1):181-6, 1990*).

Animal Experimental Study (T): HCA produced a significant reduction in food intake, body weight, and serum triglyceride levels in rats compared to a control gp. (*Rao RN, Sakariah KK. Lipid-lowering and antiobesity effect of (-)-hydroxycitric acid. Nutr Res 8:209-12, 1988*).

Animal Experimental Study (T): Zucker obese rats fed HCA demonstrated a significantly decreased rate of fatty acid synthesis and level of serum triglycerides compared to their lean litter mates (*Sullivan AC, Triscari J, Spiegel JE. Metabolic regulation as a control for lipid disorders. II. Influence of (-)-hydroxycitrate on genetically and experimentally induced hypertriglyceridemia in the rat. Am J Clin Nutr 30(5):777-84, 1977*).

Animal Experimental Study (C,T): In all models, the mature rat, the goldthioglucose-induced obese mouse, and the ventromedial hypothalmic lesioned obese rat, food intake and body weight gain were reduced signficantly by the chronic oral administration of HCA. Body composition analyses of mature rats treated with HCA demonstrated a significant depression of body lipid levels and an unaltered body protein content (*Sullivan C, Triscari J. Metabolic regulation as a control for lipid disorders. I. Influence of (-)-hydroxycitrate on experimentally induced obesity in the rodent. Am J Clin Nutr 30(5):767-76, 1977*).

Animal Experimental Study (C,T): *In vivo* hepatic rates of fatty acid and cholesterol synthesis determined in meal-fed normolipidemic rats were suppressed significantly by the oral administration of HCA for 6 hr, when control animals exhibited maximal rates of lipid synthesis; serum triglyceride and cholesterol levels were significantly reduced by HCA. In two hypertriglyceridemic models-the genetically obese Zucker rat and the fructose-treated rat-elevated triglyceride levels were due, in part, to enhance hepatic rates of fatty acid synthesis. HCA significantly reduced the hypertriglyceridemia and hyperlipogensis in both models (*Hamilton JG, Sullivan AC, Kritchevsky D. Hypolipidemic activity of (-)-hydroxycitrate. Lipids 12(1):1-9, 1977*).

In vitro Study (C,T): HCA reduced equivalently the biosynthesis of triglycerides, phospholipids, cholesterol, diglycerides, cholesteryl esters, and free fatty acids in isolated liver cells (*Hamilton JG, Sullivan AC, Kritchevsky D. Hypolipidemic activity of (-)-hydroxycitrate. Lipids 12(1):1-9, 1977*).

Procyanidolic Oligomers:
(A,C,P,R)

Also known as leukocyanidins or pycnogenols, procyanidolic oligomers are complexs of flavonoids (polyphenols).

Administration of procyanidin-rich extracts may lower cholesterol levels, reduce plaque size, and inhibit platelet aggregation. They may also reduce angina (*see: 'Hawthorn' above*).

Animal Experimental Study (C,R): Rabbits fed with normal and cholesterol-rich diets were fed 50 mg/kg of procyanidolic oligomers (PCOs) or placebo. After 10 weeks, the cholesterol content of the blood and excised aortic-media were significantly lower in the animals fed PCOs (*Wegrowski J, Robert AM, Moczar M. The effect of procyanidolic oligomers on the composition of normal and hypercholesterolemic rabbit aortas. Biochem Pharm 33:3491-7, 1984*).

See Also:

In vitro Study (P): *Chang WC, Hsu FL. Inhibition of platelet aggregation and arachidonate metabolism in platelets by procyanidins. Prostagland Leukotri Essent Fatty Acids 38:181-8, 1989.*

Silymarin:
(C,H)

Silymarin, the flavonoid complex from milk thistle (*Silybum marianum*) may be effective for type II hyperlipidemia or hyperlipidemias secondary to liver disease. (*See: 'HEPATITIS'*).

Experimental Placebo-controlled Study (C,H): Blood lipid, lipoprotein and apolipoprotein concentrations, as well as liver and renal function parameters were measured during a 7-month open clinical study on 14 type-II hyperlipidaemic outpatients with silymarin (Legalon). After determining baseline values, pts. were treated with 420 mg silymarin daily for three months. After a two-month placebo period, the treatment was repeated with silymarin for a further month. In respect to the serum lipid and lipoprotein concentrations, there were no remarkable changes except that the total cholesterol and HDL-cholesterol levels slightly decreased. At the 12th week, in all cases, the apolipoprotein levels were somewhat decreased compared to the baseline values. By the significant decrease of both apo A-I and A-II values, a decrease of the total structural protein amount of HDL, and thus a relative increase in the proportion of cholesterol in HDL fraction, was suggested. There were minor changes in serum protein concentration and liver function tests, but all values remained within the normal range. All of the renal function parameters remained unchanged during both treatments and the placebo periods (*Somogyi A et al. Short term treatment of type II hyperlipoproteinaemia with silymarin. Acta Med Hung 46(4):289-95, 1989*).

COMBINATION TREATMENT

Abana:
(A)

Abana is an Ayurvedic herbomineral medicinal preparation. A 400 mg capsule of Abana contains: 30 mg *Terminalia arjuna*; 20 mg *Withania somnifera*; 20 mg *Tinospora cordifolia*; 10 mg *Boerhaavia diffusa*, and 10 mg *Nardostachys jatamansi*.

Administration may reduce angina.

Experimental Double-blind Study (A): 25 pts. with ischemic heart disease (IHD) and 25 pts. with IHD and mild hypertension (HTN) received either Abana or a placebo. The effect of Abana was evaluated by means of LV apex cardiogram (ACG), phonocardiogram and carotid pulse tracing and ECG before and at the end of 8 weeks of treatment. As compared to placebo, Abana significantly reduced the frequency and severity of anginal episodes, as judged by clinical improvement and nitrate consumption. Significant improvement in ventricular function was observed as reflected by a decrease in ACG A amplitude and A wave duration, along with a significant increase in LV ejection fraction and VCF. The decrease in double and triple products reflected decreased MVO_2. A significant fall in diastolic blood pressure was noted in pts. with mild hypertension. Abana seems to reduce preload and afterload and improve diastolic function and pump function, which may be responsible for the beneficial effects of Abana in ischemic heart disease (*Antani JA et al. Effect of Abana on ventricular function in ischemic heart disease. Jpn Heart J 31(6):829-35, 1990*).

BENIGN PROSTATIC HYPERPLASIA

<u>*Pygeum africanum*</u>:

A tropical African evergreen tree.

Administration of extracts of the bark (standardized to contain 14% beta-sitosterol and 0.5% n-docosanol) may be beneficial at a dosage of 50-100 mg twice daily.

Experimental Study: 18 pts. with benign prostatic hypertrophy or chronic prostatitis and, simultaneously, sexual disturbances, received an extract of *Pygeum africanum* (Tadenan®, Roussel-Pharma) 200 mg daily. After 60 days, the extract had improved all the urinary parameters that were investigated. Also, sexual behavior was reported to be improved despite a lack of change in the levels of sex hormones or in nocturnal penile tumescence and rigidity. No side effects were observed (*Carani C, Salvioli V, Scuteri A, et al. [Urological and sexual evaluation of treatment of benign prostatic disease using Pygeum africanum at high doses.] <u>Arch Ital Urol Nefrol Androl</u> 63(3):341-5, 1991*) (*in Italian*).

Experimental Double-blind Study: 263 pts. received *Pygeum africanum* extract 50 mg twice daily or placebo. After 60 days, the experimental treatment led to a marked subjective improvement. A comparison of quantitative parameters (residual urine, uroflowmetry and diurnal and nocturnal pollakiuria) showed a significant difference between gps. with respect to therapeutic response. Micturition improved in 66% of treated pts. compared to 31% of controls (p<0.001). 5 pts. had GI side effects, and 2 of them discontinued treatment because of these side effects (*Barlet A et al. [Efficacy of Pygeum africanum extract in the medical therapy of urination disorders due to benign prostatic hyperplasia: evaluation of objective and subjective parameters. A placebo-controlled double-blind multicenter study.] <u>Wien Klin Wochenschr</u> 102(22):667-73, 1990*) (*in German*).

Experimental Double-blind Study: 120 pts. randomly received either an extract of *Pygeum africanum* or placebo. While 50% of pts. in the placebo gp. improved, pts. in the treatment gp. showed significantly greater improvements in nocturnal frequency, difficulty in starting micturition, and incomplete emptying of the bladder (*Dufour B et al. [Controlled study of the effects of Pygeum africanum extract on the functional symptoms of prostatic adenoma.] <u>Ann Urol (Paris)</u> 18(3):193-95, 1984*) (*in French*).

Experimental Study: In an open trial, thirty patients with BPH given 100 mg/day of the standardized Pygeum extract for 75 days demonstrated significant improvements in subjective and objective parameters: maximum flow rate increased from 5.43 ml/sec to 8.20 ml sec and the residual urine content dropped from 76 ml to 33 ml (*Zurita IE et* *al. Treatment of prostatic hypertrophy with Pygeum africanum extract. Rev Bras Med 41:364-6, 1984).*

Experimental Double-blind Study: Both pts. and physicians rated the placebo and Pygeum extract to be effective in improving subjective symptoms of daytime frequency, nocturia, weak stream, after dribbling, hesitation, and interruption of flow. Urodynamic variables (flow, frequency, and histogram) also clearly demonstrated the superiority of Pygeum over placebo (*Donkervoort T et al. A clinical and urodynamic study of Tadenan® in the treatment of benign prostatic hypertrophy. Urol 8:218-25, 1977).*

See Also:

> **Experimental Controlled Study:** *Bassi P et al. [Standardized extract of Pygeum africanum in the treatment of benign prostatic hypertrophy. Controlled clinical study versus placebo.] Minerva Urol Nefrol 39(1):45-50, 1987 (in Italian)*

> **Experimental Double-blind Study:** *Colpi G, Farina U. Study of the activity of chloroformic extract of Pygeum africanum bark in the treatment of urethral obstructive syndrome caused by non-cancerous prostapathy. Urologia 43:441-8, 1976*

> **Experimental Double-blind Study:** *Del Valio B. The use of a new drug in the treatment of chronic prostatitis. Minerva Urol 26:81-94, 1974 (in Italian)*

> **Experimental Double-blind Study:** *Doremieux J et al. Prostatic hypertrophy, clinical effects and histological changes produced by a lipid complex extracted from Pygeum africanum. J Med Strasbourg 4:253-7, 1973*

> **Experimental Double-blind Study:** *Maver A. Medical therapy of the fibrousademateuse hypertrophy of the prostate with a new vegetal substance. Minerva Med 63:2126-36, 1972*

> **Experimental Double-blind Study:** *Bongi G. Tadenan in the treatment of prostatic adenoma. Minerva Urol 24:129-39, 1972 (in Italian)*

> **Animal Experimental Study:** *Thieblot L et al. [Preventive and curative action of a bark extract from an African plant, Pygeum africanum, on experimental prostatic adenoma in rats.] Therapie 26(3):575-80, 1971 (in French)*

Saw Palmetto (*Serenoa repens*):

The liposterolic extract of the saw palmetto berry standardized to contain 85-95% fatty acids and sterols may be effective at a dosage of 160 mg twice daily.

Benign hyperplasia is believed to involve the accumulation of dihydrotestosterone within the prostate.

The standardized liposterolic extract of Serenoa (LSE) inhibits inhibits the binding of a ligand to the cytosolic and nuclear androgen receptors of the prostate, and inhibits the activities of both 5-alpha-reductase and 3-ketosteroid reductase (*Carilla E et al. Binding of Per-*

mixon, a new treatment for prostatic benign hyperplasia, to the cytosolic androgen receptor in the rat prostate. J Steroid Biochem 20(1):521-23, 1984; Sultan C et al. Inhibition of androgen metabolism and binding by a liposterolic extract of "Serenoa repens B" in human foreskin fibroblasts. J Steroid Biochem 20(1):515-19, 1984).

Administration of the liposterolic extract may be beneficial.

Experimental Study: In a multicenter study, the effect of the liposterolic extract of *Serenoa repens* (Permixon) was evaluated. Symptom score and quantitative indicators of urinary flow, postmicturition residues, prostate volume and other parameters of the urodynamic examination provided evidence of the effectiveness of the preparation *(Hanus M, Matouskova M. [Alternative therapy of benign prostatic hypertrophy—Permixon (Capistan)]. Rozhl Chir 72(2):75-9, 1993) (in Czech).*

Experimental Double-blind Study: 40 pts. with moderate BPH were given either LSE at a dose of 160 mg twice daily or placebo for three months. Significant improvements were noted in the treatment gp. in the number of daytime voiding, nocturia, incomplete voiding, dysuria, and urine retention. Transrectal and superpubic ultrasound indicated the residual urine content dropped from 110 ml at the beginning of the study to 45 ml at the end. There was no significant change in the size of the prostate in either gp. *(Mattei FM et al. Serenoa repens extract in the medical treatment of benign prostatic hypertrophy. Urologia 55:547-52, 1988).*

Negative Experimental Double-blind Study: LSE (160 mg twice daily) or placebo was given. In both gps. there was a significant improvement in flow rate and subjective symptoms with no significant difference between gps. *(Reece Smith H et al. The value of Permixon® in benign prostatic hypertrophy. Br J Urol 58(1):36-40, 1986).*

Experimental Double-blind Study: In a study of 168 pts., after 60-90 days, pts. receiving LSE demonstrated significant improvements compared to controls in dysuria, urinary frequency and residual urine *(Cukier A et al. Permixon versus placebo. C R Ther Pharmacol Clin 4(25):15-21, 1985).*

Experimental Double-blind Study: In a study of 30 pts., after 31-90 days, pts. receiving LSE demonstrated significant improvements compared to controls in urinary frqeuency and urine flow measurements *(Tamca A et al. [Treatment of obstructive symptomatology caused by prostatic adenoma with an extract of Serenoa repens. Double-blind clinical study vs. placebo.] Minerva Urol Nefrol 37(1):87-91, 1985) (in Italian).*

Experimental Double-blind Study: After 45 days, ingestion of LSE resulted in >45% reduction in episodes of nocturia, a >45% increase in urinary flow rate, and a 42% decrease in post-micturition residue in treated pts.; those on placebo showed no significant improvements and post-micturition residue worsened. Of the 50 treated pts. completing the study, 14/50 had greatly improved, 31/50 had improved, and 5/50 were unchanged or worse; of the controls, none had greatly improved, 16/44 had improvement, and 28/44 were unchanged or worse *(Champault G et al. A double-blind trial of an extract of the plant Serenoa repens in benign prostatic hyperplasia. Br J Clin Pharmacol 18:461-2, 1984).*

Experimental Double-blind Study: 110 pts. with prostatic adenoma requiring medical treatment due to symptoms but not surgery received either LSE or placebo. After 1 mo., PA 109 appeared significantly more effective than placebo, especially in the objective criteria (nocturnal pollakiuria, urinary output, postmictional residue) ($p < 10^{-9}$). This efficacy was confirmed in a supplementary study of 47 pts. with a mean follow-up of 14.6 months. There were no adverse side-effects (*Champault G et al. [Medical treatment of prostatic adenoma. Controlled trial: PA 109 vs. placebo in 110 patients.] Ann Urol (Paris) 18(6):407-10, 1984*) (*in French*).

Experimental Double-blind Study: 22 pts. received LSE (320 mg/d) or placebo. After 60 days, there were significant differences for volume voided, maximum and mean urine flow, dysuria and nocturia. There were no side effects (*Boccafoschi S, Annoscia S. Comparison of Serenoa repens extract with placebo by controlled clinical trial in patients with prostatic adenomatosis. Urologia 50:1257-68, 1983*).

Experimental Double-blind Study: 30 pts. received LSE (320 mg/d) or placebo. After 30 days, there were significant differences in the number of voidings, strangury, maximum and mean flow, and residual urine (*Emili E et al. Clinical trial of a new drug for treating hypertrophy of the prostate (Permixon). Urologia 50:1042-8, 1983*).

See Also:

> **Clinical Observations:** *Ollé Carreras J. [Our experience with an hexane extract of Serenoa repens in the treatment of benign prostatic hypertrophy.] Arch Esp Urol 40(5):310-3, 1987 (in Spanish)*

Saw Palmetto vs. *Pygeum africanum*:

Experimental Study: 30 pts. were given extracts of either *Pygeum africanum* or Saw Palmetto. After 30 days, pts. treated with Saw Palmetto demonstrated a greater reduction of symptoms and a greater increase of micturitional rate than those on *Pygeum africanum*. While Saw Palmetto did not induce side effects, *Pygeum africanum* caused gastric symptoms in 13% of pts. (*Duvia R et al. Advances in the phytotherapy of prostatic hypertrophy. Med Praxis 4:143-8, 1983*).

Saw Palmetto vs. *Pygeum africanum* with or without amino acids:

Experimental Double-blind Study: 100 pts. with grade I - II prostatic adenoma received either *Pygeum africanum, Serenoa repens, Pygeum africanum* combined with amino acids or placebo. Based on both objective and subjective evaluations, the results with both *Pygeum africanum* and *Serenoa repens* were good, the results with the combination of *Pygeum africanum* and amino acids were excellent, and the results with placebo were poor (*Menendez Fernandez H et al. [Use of amino acids as a combination in the treatment of prostatic hypertrophy. Arch Esp Urol 41(7):495-9, 1988 (in Spanish)*).

Urtica dioica (Stinging Nettles):

In studies on the interaction of an extract of *Urtica dioica* root with the sexual hormone binding globulin of the blood plasma and with the androgen receptor of the prostatic cytosol, it was found that the extract influences the binding of 5-alpha-dihydrotesterone with the binding proteins (*Schmidt K. [Effect of radix urticae extract and its several secondary extracts on blood SHBG in benign prostate hyperplasia.] Fortschr Med 101(15):713-16, 1983; Tosch M, Müssigang H. Medikamentöse Behandlung der benignen Prostatahyperplasie. Euromed 6, 1983*).

Administration of the extract may be beneficial.

Experimental Study: The effects of fluid of the roots of *Urtica dioica* and *Urtica urens* on 67 men of over 60 years of age, suffering from BPH, were studied. Functional symptoms such as nocturia were alleviated, particularly in less severe cases, and no side effects were reported (*Belaiche P, Lievoux O. Clinical studies on the palliative treatment of prostatic adenoma with extract of Urtica root. Phytother Res 5:267-9, 1991*).

Experimental Study: 30 pts. with prostatic hyperplasia stages I and II received capsules containing 300 mg of Bazoton®(Kanoldt), an extract of *Urtica dioica* root. After an ave. of 3.5 mo., there was a significant decrease in the volume of residual urine There was also a significant increase in mean urinary flow which increased in 50% of the cases. Pts. reported marked subjective relief (*Romics I. Observations with Bazoton in the management of prostatic hyperplasia. Int Urol Nephrol 19(3):293-7, 1987*).

Experimental Double-blind Study: 50 pts. in phases I or II received capsules containing either an extract of *Urtica dioica* root or placebo. After 9 wks., both gps. noted improvement in subjective symptoms. However, there were significant objective differences as there was a significant improvement of the micturition volume and maximum urinary flow as well as a highly significant (p=0.0005) decrease in the sex hormone binding globulin in the treatment group. Improvement of ave. flow in the treatment gp. was not significant. Length of treatment and treatment dosage may not have been optimal for this gp. of pts. (*Vontobel HP et al. [Results of a double-blind study on the effectiveness of ERU (extractum radicis Urticae) capsules in conservative treatment of benign prostatic hyperplasia.] Urologe [A] 24(1):49-51, 1985*) (*in German*).

Experimental Study: 4550 pts. received Bazoton®(Kanoldt), an extract of *Urtica dioica* root. 83.2% of pts. with stage I, and 80.4% of pts. with stage II, prostatic hypertrophy noted subjective benefit (*Tosch M, Müssigang H. Medikamentöse Behandlung der benignen Prostatahyperplasie. Euromed 6, 1983*).

Experimental Study: 30 pts. with prostatic adenomas received Prostatin®, an extract of *Urtica dioica* root. In almost all cases, there was a clear decrease in residual urine as seen in sonograms performed before and after its administration. Micturation frequency decreased by 24.4% during the day and by 52.6% at night. 3 pts. had side effects (*Barsom S, Bettermann AA. Prostatic adenoma: Conservative therapy with Urtica extract. ZFA (Stuttgart) 55(33):1947-50, 1979*).

See Also:

> **Experimental Study:** *Maar K. [Regression of the symptoms of prostatic adenomas Results of 7 months' conservative treatment using ERU capsules.] Fortschr Med 10591):18-20, 1987* (*in German*)

Experimental Study: *Stahl HP. [Therapy of prostatic nocturia with standardized extractum radix urticae.] ZFA (Stuttgart) 60(3):128-32, 1984 (in German)*

Case Report: *Djulepa J. [Conservative therapy of prostatic hyperplasia with urinary retention.] Med Welt 34(48):1377-9, 1983 (in German)*

Experimental Study: *Ziegler H. [Cytomorphologic studies of benign prostatic hyperplasia treated with extract radicis urticae (ERU). Preliminary results.] Fortschr Med 100(39):1832-4, 1982 (in German)*

Experimental Study: *Hallwachs O. [Urination disorders caused by prostatic hyperplasia. Effect of Baxoton, Harzol and Prosta-capsules.] MMW 123(44):1675-6, 1981 (in German)*

– –

COMBINATION TREATMENT

Flower Pollen:

Administration of a standardized extract of flower pollen may be beneficial.

Experimental Double-blind Study: 60 pts. with outflow obstruction due to BPH received either pollen extract (Cernilton®, A.B. Cernelle, Sweden) or placebo. After 6 mo., there was a statistically significant subjective improvement with the extract (69% of pts.) compared with placebo (30%). There was a significant decrease in residual urine and in the antero-posterior diameter of the prostate on ultrasound in the pts. treated with pollen extract. However, differences in respect to flow rate and voided volume were not statistically significant (*Buck AC et al. Treatment of outflow tract obstruction due to benign prostatic hyperplasia with the pollen extract, Cernilton®. A double-blind, placebo-controlled study. Br J Urol 66(4):398-404, 1990*).

Experimental Double-blind Study: 192 pts. received either Cernilton® or a mixture of L-glutamic acid, L-alanine and glycine (Paraprost®). After 4 wks., moderate or greater improvement was seen more often in the Cernilton® gp. as was the frequency of improvement in protracted micturition. The Cernilton® gp. showed a significant improvement in residual urinary volume, ave. flow rate, maximum flow rate, prostatic weight and phased change of residual urinary volume and it reported no side effects. Cernilton® was judged more than moderately effective in 49.1% of pts. while Paraprost® was judged more than moderately effective in 46.3% of patients. There was no significant difference in outcome between the 2 gps. (*Maekawa M et al. [Clinical evaluation of Cernilton on benign prostatic hypertrophy - - a multiple center double-blind study with Paraprost.] Hinyokika Kiyo 36(4):495-516, 1990*) (*in Japanese*).

Experimental Study: 20 pts. received pollen extract (Cernilton®) 6 tabs daily. After an ave. of 13.2 wks., sense of residual urine improved in 92%, retardation improved in 86%, night frequency improved in 85%, strain on urination improved in 56%, protraction improved in 53% and the force of the urinary stream improved in 53%. There was overall subjective efficacy in 80% of pts., and overall objective efficacy in 54% of patients. Night frequency, residual urine volume and tidal urine volume significantly improved. No side effects were observed (*Hayashi J et al. [Clinical evaluation of*

Cernilton® *in benign prostatic hypertrophy.] Hinyokika Kiyo 32(1):135-41, 1986) (in Japanese).*

Experimental Study: 30 pts. received pollen extract (Cernilton®) 2 tablets 3 times daily. After at least 12 wks., the overall subjective efficacy was 80%, and the overall subjective efficacy was 43%. No serious side effects were observed   (*Horii A et al. [Clinical evaluation of Cernilton®*   *in the treatment of benign prostatic hypertrophy.] Hinyokika Kiyo 31(4):739-46, 1985) (in Japanese).*

Experimental Study: 22 pts. with stage I or II BPH whose ave. age was 67 yrs. received pollen extract (Cernilton®). After at least 4 wks., there was an excellent improvement in subjective symptoms and the improvement rate for dysuria was over 85%. 18/22 pts. were rated as moderately improved or better, 2 were slightly improved and 2 remained unaltered. Objective symptoms such as residual urine volume and urinary flow rate were improved in 3 pts., although shrinkage of the prostate was not observed. There were no side effects   (*Ueda K et al. [Clinical evaluation of Cernilton on benign prostatic hyperplasia.] Hinyokika Kiyo 31(1):187-91, 1985) (in Japanese).*

BRONCHIAL ASTHMA

See Also: ALLERGY

Aloe vera:

Administration may be effective for patients who are not dependent upon corticosteroids.

Experimental Study: The oral administration of an extract of *Aloe vera* for six months was shown to produce good results in the treatment of asthma in some individuals of various ages. The extract was produced from the supernatant of fresh leaves stored in the dark at 4°C for 7 days. Subjecting the leaves with dark and cold results in an increase in the polysaccharide fraction. One gram of the crude extract obtained from leaves stored in cold and dark produced 400 mg of neutral polysaccharide compared to only 30 mg produced from leaves not subjected to cold or dark. The dosage was 5 ml of a 20% solution of the Aloe extract in saline twice daily for 24 weeks; 11 of 27 pts. (40%) without corticosteroid dependence felt very much better at the study's conclusion. The mechanism of action is thought to be via restoration of protective mechanisms followed by augmentation of the immune system (*Shida T et al. Effect of Aloe extract on peripheral phagocytosis in adult bronchial asthma. Planta Med 51:273-5, 1985*).

Coleus forskohlii:

The root of *Coleus forskohlii*, an herb used in Ayurvedic medicine, contains a diterpene molecule known as forskolin which is a powerful activator of adenylate cyclase in various tissues leading to an elevation of cAMP. In the bronchial tissues this increase causes bronchodilation.

The forskolin content of Coleus root is typically 0.2-0.3%, therefore the forskolin content of some Coleus products may not be sufficient to produce a pharmacological effect. It is best to use standardized extracts which have concentrated the forskolin content. The dosage of the extract should provide a daily intake of 5-10 mg of forskolin, although oral administration of 50 mg/kg of an ethanol extract of Coleus was as effective as 10 mg/kg of pure forskolin in reducing blood pressure in rats. Evidently the activity of the extract is higher than would be expected from its forskolin content. If this ratio holds true for humans, a daily intake as little as 0.5-1 mg of forskolin provided in a Coleus extract may be sufficient.

Oral administration of Coleus extracts may promote bronchodilation.

Experimental Double-blind Crossover Study: The airway and tremor response and cardiovascular and hypokalemic effects of single doses of inhalative fenoterol dry powder capsules (0.4 mg) were compared with the fenoterol metered dose inhaler (0.4 mg) and colforsin (forskolin) dry powder capsules (10.0 mg) in 16 patients with asthma.

Subjects were investigated in a randomized, double-blind, placebo-controlled, four-period, crossover trial for a 120 minute period. All active drugs caused a significant increase in specific airway conductance; the order of potency (mean SEM maximum increase from baseline) was fenoterol metered dose inhaler (0.51 sec-1 x kPa-1), fenoterol dry powder capsules (0.49), and colforsin dry powder capsules (0.30). A marked increase in finger tremor amplitude resulted after fenoterol metered dose inhaler only (62.93%) in contrast to fenoterol dry powder capsules (15.84%) and colforsin dry powder capsules (12.87%) (*Bauer K et al. Pharmacodynamic effects of inhaled dry powder formulations of fenoterol and colforsin in asthma. Clin Pharmacol Ther 53(1):76-83, 1993*).

Forskolin administered by a metered dose inhaler may be beneficial.

Experimental Double-blind Crossover Study: The bronchodilating effect (after 5 min.) of forskolin was as good as following fenoterol in 12 healthy volunteers (nonsmokers) as determined by whole body plethysmography. At the beginning (after 3 and 5 min.) the protective effect of forskolin against inhaled acetylcholine was as good as following fenoterol while later on (after 15 and 30 min.) fenoterol resulted in a stronger action. Both drugs were administered by metered dose inhalers (*Kaik G, Witte PU. [Protective effect of forskolin in acetylcholine provocation in healthy probands. Comparison of 2 doses with fenoterol and placebo]. Wien Med Wochenschr 136(23-24):637-41, 1986*) (*in German*).

See Also:

> *Lichey I et al. Effect of forskolin on methacholine-induced bronchoconstriction in extrinsic asthmatics [letter]. Lancet ii(8395):167, 1984*

Ephedra or Ma Huang (*Ephedra sinica*):

> WARNING: The FDA advisory review panel on nonprescription drugs recommended that ephedrine not be taken by patients with heart disease, high blood pressure, thyroid disease, diabetes, or difficulty in urination due to enlargement of the prostate gland. Nor should ephedrine be used in patients on antihypertensive or antidepressant drugs. Ephedra preparations can produce the same side effects that ephedrine can (i.e., increased blood pressure and heart rate, insomnia, and anxiety) but, according to the American Pharmaceutical Association, "There is far more discussion of ephedrine tachyphylaxis (rapid decrease in effectiveness) or tolerance than is evidenced as a significant problem in the scientific literature" (*American Pharmaceutical Association. Handbook of Nonprescription Drugs, 8th ed. American Pharmaceutical Association, Washington, DC, 1986:183*).

Administration may promote bronchodilation.

Experimental Double-blind Study: 16 asthmatic children between the ages of 7 and 13 years were studied for 8 weeks to evaluate efficacy, toxicity, and development of tolerance to the combination of ephedrine sulfate and theophylline. Results of the study indicated ephedrine is a potent bronchodilator that, in appropriate doses, can be administered safely along with therapeutic doses of theophylline without the fear of progressive tolerance or toxicity. Comparison of data from weeks 1 and 8 showed no evidence of the development of tolerance (*Tinkelman DG, Avner SE. Ephedrine therapy in asthmatic children. JAMA 237:553-7, 1977*).

Galphimia glauca:

Galphimia glauca is native to Central and South America where it is used by traditional healers in hayfever and asthma.

Administration may be effective (*Dorsch W, Wagner H. New antiasthmatic drugs from traditional medicine. Int Arch Allergy Appl Immunol 94:262-5, 1991*).

Animal Experimental Study: A methanolic extract from *Galphimia glauca* at a dose of 320 mg/kg given orally inhibited acute bronchial reactions to allergen and platelet-activating factor in inhalation challenges, but not to histamine or acetylcholine. Gallic acid and flavonoids, including quercetin, were identified as active compounds (*Dorsch W, Bittinger M, Kaas A, et al. Antiasthmatic effects of Galphimia glauca, gallic acid, and related compounds prevent allergen- and platelet-activating factor-induced bronchial obstruction as well as bronchial hyperreactivity in guinea pigs. Int Arch Allergy Immunol 97:1-7, 1992*).

See Also:

> **Animal Experimental Study:** *Neszmelyi A, Kreher B, Muller A, et al. Tetragalloylguinic acid, the major antiasthmatic principle of Galphimia glauca. Planta Med 59(2):164-7, 1993*

Ginkgo biloba:

Ginkgo biloba contains several unique terpene molecules known collectively as ginkgolides that antagonize platelet activating factor (PAF), a key chemical mediator in asthma, inflammation, and allergies (*See: 'ALLERGY'*). Ginkgolides compete with PAF for binding sites and inhibit the various events induced by PAF.

Administration may be effective.

> *Note: BN 52063 is a mixture of ginkgolides A, B and C.*

Experimental Study: The effects of orally administered or inhaled BN 52063 on the response to isocapnic hyperventilation with dry cold air (ISH study) and exercise (EIA study) were assessed in a single dose and short term treatment study in 10 patients with exercise induced asthma. ISH challenge was performed twice within 1 h after administration of either placebo, 240 mg BN 52063 orally, or inhalation of 2.4 mg BN 52063. Oral pretreatment with BN 52063 did not result in a reduction of bronchoconstriction; however a significant increase of respiratory function was noted immediately after inhalation of BN 52063. A significant inhibition of PAF induced platelet aggregation (by a factor of 2) occurred after oral administration of BN 52063 following both ISH challenges. No significant inhibition of PAF-induced platelet aggregation was seen after inhalation of BN 52063. In the EIA study the patients were challenged on the third day of treatment with either placebo or 240 mg BN 52063 orally or 5 mg BN 52063 by inhalation. Oral administration of BN 52063 was effective in improving pulmonary function and protecting against EIA; inhalation of BN 52063 was not (*Wilkens JH et* *al. Effects of a PAF-antagonist (BN 52063) on bronchoconstriction and platelet activation during exercise induced asthma. Br J Clin Pharmacol 29(1):85-91, 1990).*

Experimental Double-Blind Study: 8 pts. received 3 days of treatment with BN 52063 (120 mg daily) or placebo, separated by a one week washout. On the third day of treatment, subjects were challenged with nebulized house dust mite or pollen allergen. BN 52063 significantly antagonized early bronchoconstriction and showed a tendency to inhibit residual bronchial hyperreactivity, assessed 6 hours after allergen challenge by a provocation test to acetylcholine. No side effects were reported during active treatment *(Guinot P et al. Effect of BN 52063, a specific PAF-acether antagonist, on bronchial provocation test to allergens in asthmatic patients. A preliminary study. Prostaglandins 34(5):723-31, 1987).*

See Also:

> **Animal Ex vivo Study:** *Puglisi L, Salvadori S, Gabrielli G, Pasargiklian R. Pharmacology of natural compounds. Smooth muscle relaxant activity induced by a Ginkgo biloba L. extract on guinea-pig trachea. Pharmacol Res Commun 20:573-89, 1988*

Khella (*Ammi visnaga*):

Khella is an ancient medicinal plant native to the Mediterranean region where it has been used in the treatment of asthma as well as angina and other heart ailments since the time of the pharaohs. In angina, its mechanism of action appears to be very similar to the calcium-channel blocking drugs. The same would be true in asthma, although other mechanisms may also be important. Khellin, the chief active component of khella served as the prototype to disodium chromoglycate (Intal®).

Most clinical studies in the treatment of angina and asthma used preparations standardized to contain 70 to 80% khellin and 20 to 30% visnagin were used. At doses 120 mg per day, mild side effects such as insomnia, anorexia, nausea, and dizziness were common. Rather than using isolated khellin, khella extracts standardized for khellin content (typically 12%) are preferred by many practitioners.

Administration may be effective.

> **Experimental Study:**   12 pts. received khella. 3 pts. with chronic asthma improved (EFR increased by 64 - 239%) and 2 pts. with emphysema improved (EFR increased by 18% and 26%). The findings in the remaining 7 pts. were inconclusive *(Kennedy MCS, Stock JPP. The bronchodilator action of khellin. Thorax 7:43-65, 1952).*

Lobelia inflata:

Lobelia (Indian tobacco) is an indigenous North American plant that has a long folk-use in the treatment of asthma. Lobeline, an alkaloid, is the major active component.

Administration may be effective.

> **Animal Experimental Study:**   Lobeline has many of the same pharmacological actions as nicotine, but is generally less potent *(Mansuri S, Kelkar V, Jindal M. Some*

pharmacological characteristics of ganglionic activity of lobeline. Arzneim Forsch 23:1271-5, 1973).

Animal Experimental Study: Although lobeline causes bronchoconstriction in dogs and rats, in guinea pigs and (presumably) humans the opposite - bronchodilation - occurs (*Cambar P, Shore S, Aviado D. Bronchopulmonary and gastrointestinal effects of lobeline. Arch Int Pharmacodyn 177:1-27, 1969).*

Review Article: Lobeline causes bronchoconstriction and is a respiratory stimulant *in vitro*, suggesting a cholinergic effect in the respiratory system. However, it also binds to the nicotine acetylcholine receptors in ganglions, thus promoting the release of epinephrine and norepinephrine. Experimentally induced lung edema in rats is responsive to lobeline in many models that are unresponsive to any other medication (*Halmagyi D, Kovacs A, and Neumann P: Adrenocortical pathway of lobeline protection in some forms of experimental lung edema of the rat. Dis Chest 33:285-296, 1958).*

Onion (*Allium cepa*):

Onion exerts antiasthmatic effects in guinea pigs and inhibits leukotriene synthesis and histamine release in human blood cells.

Increasing consumption of onions or the use of onion poultices may be beneficial.

Animal Experimental Study: In a study of the asthmatic reactions of guinea pigs, onion oils counteracted bronchial obstruction caused by the inhalation of platelet-activating factor (PAF) (*Dorsch W, Ettl M, Hein G, et al. Anti-asthmatic effects of onions. Int Arch Allergy Appl Immunol 82:535-6, 1987).*

See Also:

> **Animal Experimental Study:** *Dorsch W et al. Anti-asthmatic effects of onions. Biochem Pharmacol 37(23):4479-86, 1988.*

> **Animal Experimental Study:** *Dorsch W, Weber J. Prevention of allergen-induced bronchial constriction in sensitized guinea pigs by crude alcohol onion extract. Agents Actions 14:626-30, 1984*

Picrorrhiza kurroa:

The root of *Picrorrhiza kurroa* has been used extensively in Ayurvedic medicine in the treatment of hepatic and respiratory diseases.

Administration may be beneficial.

Animal Experimental Study: Extracts of Picrorrhiza prevented allergen, histamine, and platelet-activating factor induced bronchial obstruction in guinea pigs (*Dorsch W, Stuppner H, Wagner H, et al. Antiasthmatic effects of Picrorrhiza kurroa: Androsin prevents allergen- and PAF-induced bronchial obstruction in guinea pigs. Int Arch Allergy Appl Immunol 95:128-33, 1991).*

Negative Experimental Double-blind Study: 72 pts. were given either *Picrorrhiza kurroa* root powder 300 mg or a placebo. After 3 days, there was no significant evidence of reduction in clinical attacks, need for bronchodilator drugs or improvement in lung function   (*Doshi VB et al. Picrorrhiza kurroa in bronchial asthma. J Postgrad Med 29(2):89-95, 1983*).

Tylophora asthmatica:

The leaves of *Tylophora asthmatica* have been used extensively in Ayurvedic medicine in asthma and other respiratory tract disorders.

The mode of action of Tylophora is unknown, but is thought to be due to the alkaloids, especially tylophorine, which have been reported to possess antihistamine and antispasmodic activity as well as inhibition of mast cell degranulation. However, a more central mechanism may be responsible for the clinical effects in asthma.

Animal Experimental Study: Alcoholic and aqueous extracts of Tylophora exerted a direct stimulatory effect on the adrenal cortex and inhibited dexamethasone suppression on adrenal activity   (*Udupa AL, Udupa SL, Guruswamy MN. The possible site of antiasthmatic action of Tylophora asthmatica on pituitary-adrenal axis in albino rats. Planta Med 57:409-13, 1991*).

Animal Experimental Study: Tylophorine inhibited systemic anaphylaxis and inflammatory processes presumably by interfering with the production or degradation of cAMP (*Gopalakrishnan C et al. Effect of tylophorine, a major alkaloid of Tylophora indica, on immunopathological and inflammatory reactions. Ind J Med Res 71:940-8, 1980*).

Animal Experimental Study: Aqueous Tylophora extracts prevented experimentally-induced anaphylaxis presumably by altering immune reactions   (*Haranath PSRK, Shyamalakumari. Experimental study on mode of action of Tylophora asthmatica in bronchial asthma. Ind J Med Res 63:661-70, 1975*).

Administration may be beneficial.

Experimental Double-blind Study: 135 pts. were studied. Those given 200 mg of Tylophora leaves twice daily for 6 days demonstrated improvements in symptoms and respiratory function during the treatment period and for up to 2 weeks after treatment. Symptom score, FEV1, and PEFR were used as parameters. Side effects, like nausea and vomiting, occurred in 9.8% in the Tylophora gp. and 14% in the placebo gp. (*Gupta S et al. Tylophora indica in bronchial asthma — a double blind study. Ind J Med Res 69:981-9, 1979*).

Experimental Double-blind Study: Pts. receiving Tylophora leaves demonstrated improvements in symptoms and respiratory function compared to a placebo and provided similar benefit to a mixture of ephedrine, theophylline, and phenobarbitone   (*Thiruvengadam KV et al. Tylophora indica in bronchial asthma (a controlled comparison with a standard anti-asthmatic drug. J Indian Med Assoc 71(7):172-6, 1978*).

Experimental Double-blind Crossover Study: 103 pts. receiving 40 mg the dry alcoholic extract of *T. indica* daily for only 6 days demonstrated significant improvement in symptoms of asthma compared to a placebo gp. At the end of the first week, 56% had complete to moderate improvement, as compared to 31.6% of the 92 pts. receiving the placebo. At the end of 4 weeks, the respective figures were 32% and 23.8%; at 8 weeks, 23.8% and 8.4%; and at 12 weeks, 14.8% and 7.2%. The incidence of side effects such as nausea, partial diminution of taste for salt, and slight mouth soreness was 16.3% in the Tylophora gp. and 6.6% in the placebo gp. (*Shivpuri DN, Singhal SC, Parkash D. Treatment of asthma with an alcoholic extract of Tylophora indica: A cross-over, double-blind study. Ann Allergy 30:407-12, 1972*).

Experimental Double-Blind Crossover Study: 110 pts. receiving one Tylophora leaf daily for 6 days demonstrated significant relief in asthma and allergic rhinitis. At the end of the first week, 62% had complete to moderate improvement, as compared to 28% in the placebo group. At the end of 4 weeks, the respective figures were 37% and 11%; at 8 weeks, 30% and 7.4%; and at 12 weeks, 16% and O%. Side effects such as sore mouth, loss of taste, and nausea and vomiting occurred in 53% of the Tylophora gp. (*Shivpuri DN, Menon MP, Prakash D. A crossover double-blind study on Tylophora indica in the treatment of asthma and allergic rhinitis. J Allergy 43(3):145-50, 1969*).

CANCER

See Also: IMMUNODEPRESSION

Aloe vera:

Acemannan, a water-soluble, long-chain polydispersed beta-(1,4)-linked mannan polymer interspersed with O-acetyl groups found in _Aloe vera,_ is a potent immunostimulant. Approximately 1/2 to 1 liter of _Aloe vera_ juice is required to provide 800-1,600 mg of acemannan.

While the efficacy of acemannan for the treatment of human malignancies is untested, acemannan has been approved for veterinary use in injectable form for fibrosarcomas and feline leukemia. Feline leukemia, like AIDS, is caused by a retrovirus (Feline leukemia virus or FeLV). The virus is so lethal that once cats develop clinical symptoms they are usually euthanized. Typically over 70% of cats will die within 8 weeks of the onset of clinical signs. Acemannan has shown impressive results. The mechanism is likely related to increased secretion of macrophage secretory products like tumor necrosis factor, interleukin, and interferon leading to increased initiation of immune attack.

> **Animal Experimental Study:** In a study of 44 cats with clinically confirmed feline leukemia, acemannan was injected (2 mg/kg) weekly for 6 weeks and re-examined 6 weeks after termination of treatment. At the end of the 12 week study, 71% of the cats were alive and in good health _(Sheets MA, Unger BA, Giggleman GF Jr, Tizard IR. Studies of the effect of acemannan on retrovirus infections: Clinical stabilization of feline leukemia virus-infected cats. Mol Biother 3(1):41-5, 1991)._

See Also:

> **Animal Experimental Study:** _Peng SY, Norman J, Curtin G, et al. Decreased mortality of Norman murine sarcoma in mice treated with the immunomodulator, acemannan. Mol Biother 3(2):79-87, 1991_

Acemannan may also be effective in animals with spontaneous tumors _(Harris C, Pierce K, King G, et al. Efficacy of acemannan in treatment of canine and feline spontaneous neoplasms. Mol Biother 3(4):207-13, 1991)._

Benzaldehyde:

Benzaldehyde is a volatile oil found in high concentrations in almond oil (95% benzaldehyde). It is also a non-toxic component of amygdalin (laetrile). Recent research suggests that some of laetrile's proposed effects may be due to the benzaldehyde component rather than the cyanide component. A benzaldehyde derivative, 4,6-Benzylidene-D-glucose (BG), which is a component of figs (_Ficus carica_), has demonstrated carcinostatic properties.

Experimental Study: BG was administered IV to 17 pts. with various advanced carcinomas. 58.8% showed a partial antitumor response and there were no adverse side effects. 4/9 pts. with lung cancer showed a partial response; 3/9 showed a minimal response and 2/9 showed progressive disease. 2 pts. with lung metastatic cancer showed a partial response. All the liver metastases in 3 pts. with gastric cancer showed partial responses. 1 pt. with hepatoma showed a partial response, while 1 pt. with pancreatic cancer showed a minimal response as did a pt. with prostatic cancer with multiple bone and lung metastases (*Tatsumura T et al. Antitumor effect of 4,6-benzylidene-D-glucose in clinical studies. Meeting abstract. Proc Annu Meet Am Soc Clin Oncol 6:A559, 1987*).

Experimental Study: 65 pts. with advanced, inoperable carcinomas received IV BG at a daily dose of 720-1800 mg/m^2. The overall objective response was 55%; 7 pts. achieved a complete response, 29 achieved a partial response, 24 remained stable, and 5 showed progressive disease. Prolongation of survival was apparent and toxic reactions were not observed (*Kochi M et al. Antitumor activity of a benzaldehyde derivative. Cancer Treat Rep 69(5):533-7, 1985*).

Berbamine or
Berberine:

Goldenseal (*Hydrastis canadensis*), Oreon grape root (*Berberis aquifolia*) and barberry root bark (*Berberis vulgaris*) may be beneficial due to the presence of berberine and berbamine. Berbamine has been used in China since 1972 in the treatment of leukopenia due to chemotherapy and/or radiation.

Experimental Study: 405 pts. with WBC counts <4000 given 150 mg of berbamine daily (50 mg orally 3 times daily) for 1-4 weeks. Berbamine was viewed as 'significantly effective' if WBC was raised to >4000 after 1 week or increasing WBC >1000 after 2 weeks; 'effectiv' if WBC was raised to >4000 after 2 weeks or increasing WBC >1000 after 4 weeks; and 'ineffective' if there was no change in WBC after 4 weeks of treatment. The overall results for the 405 pts: significantly effective in 163 cases (40.2%), effective in 125 cases (38.8%) and ineffective in 117 cases (29%). The total effective rate was 71%. However, WBC before therapy was related to overall effectiveness. The effective rate was only 54.8% in 31 cases where WBC was <1000 and 82.7% in cases where WBC count was between 3100 and 3800 (*Liu CX et al. Studies on plant resources, pharmacology and clinical treatment with berbamine. Phytother Res 5:228-30, 1991*).

Animal and in Vitro Experimental Studies: Berberine exhibited potent antitumor activity against human and rat malignant brain tumors. Several experimental approaches were used. *In vitro* studies were performed on a series of 6 human malignant brain tumor cell lines and rat 9L brain tumor cells. Berberine used alone at a dose of 150 mcg/ml showed an average cell kill of 91%. This compared quite favorably to 1,3-bis(2-chloro-ethyl)-1-nitrosourea (BCNU), the standard chemotherapeutic agent for brain tumors, which had a cell kill rate of 43%. *In vivo* studies in rats harboring solid 9L brain tumors also showed berberine has antitumor effects. Rats treated with berberine, 10 mg/kg, had a 81% cell kill. This activity was equal to 1/3 the LDV>10 dose of BCNU (4.44 mg/kg). *In vivo* combination treatment with berberine and BCNU exihibited additive cytotoxicity. These results indicate that berberine may prove to be more effective than BCNU or, at the very least, a valuable therapeutic adjunct (*Rong-xun*

Z et al. Laboratory studies of berberine used alone and in combination with 1,3-bis(2-chloroethyl)-1-nitrosourea to treat malignant brain tumors. Chinese Med J 103(8):658-65, 1990).

Animal Experimental Study: Berberine sulfate inhibited the effects of the tumor promoters 12-O-tetradecanoylphorbol-13-acetate and teleocidin. Berberine also markedly inhibited the promoting effect of teleocidin on skin tumor formation in mice initiated with 7,12-dimethyl-benz[a]anthracene *(Nishino H et al. Berberine sulfate inhibits tumor-promoting activity of teleocidin in two-stage carcinogenesis on mouse skin. Oncology 43:131-4, 1986).*

In vitro Study: Berberine exhibited significant activation of macrophages. This activation resulted in macrophages exhibiting potent cytostatic activity against tumor cells *in vitro (Kumazawa Y et al. Activation of peritoneal macrophages by berberine-type alkaloids in terms of induction of cytostatic activity. Int J Immunopharmacol 6(6):587-92, 1984).*

Bromelain:

Bromelain is the proteolytic enzyme complex derived from the stem of the pineapple (*Ananas comosus*).

Administration may be beneficial.

Animal Experimental Study: When added to the diet, bromelain decreased lung metastases of Lewis lung cancer cells implanted subcutaneously in mice. This antimetastatic potential was demonstrated by both the active and inactive bromelain with or without proteolytic, anticoagulant properties *(Batkin S et al. Antimetastatic effect of bromelain with or without its proteolytic and anticoagulant activity. J Cancer Res Clin Oncol 114(5):507-8, 1988).*

In vitro Study: Bromelain induced the differentiation of 3 leukemic cell lines *in vitro*: a myeloid mouse leukemia, a human promyelocytic leukemia, and a human leukemia able to differentiate into the erythroid lineage. These findings may explain the cytostatic potential of bromelain in combination cancer chemotherapy *(Maurer HR, Hozumi M, Honma Y, Okabe-Kado J. Bromelain induces the differentiation of leukemic cells in vitro: An explanation for its cytostatic effects? Planta Med 54(5):377-81, 1988).*

Animal Experimental Study: Feeding 0.3% bromelain to Lewis lung carcinoma-bearing mice decreased the number of metastatic lesions by over 90% *(Batkin S et al. Modulation of pulmonary metastasis (Lewis lung carcinoma) by bromelain, an extract of the pineapple stem (Ananas comosus). Letter. Cancer Invest 6(2):241-2, 1988).*

Experimental Study: Administration of oral bromelain, sometimes given with subtoxic doses of chemotherapeutic drugs such as 5-FU and vincristine, resulted in tumor regressions. Doses <100 mg daily of active bromelain were inadequate; up to 2.4 g/d may be necessary for optimal effects. Not all bromelain preparations were found to be equally beneficial. The therapeutic effect may be due to fribrinolysis 'deshielding' the tumor cell's fibrin coat to provide the immune system with a more ready access to them (*Nieper HA. [Bromelain in der Kontrolle malignen Washstums.] Krebsgeschehen 1:9-15, 1976*) (*in German*).

Animal Experimental Study: When hairless mice were irradiated with UV light, bromelain-feeding enhanced their resistance to the development of skin cancer. Compared to controls, it took twice as long for the bromelain-fed gp. to develop precancerous lesions (*Goldstein N et al. Bromelain as a skin cancer preventive in hairless mice. Hawaii Med J 34:91-4, 1975*).

Experimental Study: 12 pts. with different tumors were treated with 600 mg bromelain daily from 6 mo. to several years. There was resolution of cancerous masses of ovarian carcinoma, and a marked decrease of most breast cancers and metastases (*Gérard G. [Therapeutique anti-cancreuse et bromelaines.] Agressologie 3:261-74, 1972*) (*in French*).

Carnivora®:

Carnivora® is an extract of the pressed juice of the Venus fly trap plant (*Dionaea muscipula*).

Experimental Controlled Study: A total of 44 pts. were studied in a controlled clincal trial with Carnivora®. The patients all had tumors that were too far advanced for surgery, radiotherapy or chemotherapy to have any chance of success. Unequivocal effects on the growth of the tumor (complete or partial remission) were not observed in the 27 pts. receiving Carnivora®. 5 pts. had a number of individual tumor parameters regress, 6 pts. remained unchanged, and the tumor progressed in 16 patients. 10 pts. reported an improved general state of health (*Dietzel VU et al. [Experience with Carnivora.] Fortschr Med 103:760-1, 1985*) (*In German*).

Chaparral (*Larrea tridentata*):

Chaparral is an evergreen desert shrub that is also known as creosote bush. Its main anticancer component is nordihydroguaiaretic acid (NDGA), a potent antioxidant.

WARNING: Administration may cause hepatitis.

Observational Case Studies: Two cases of chaparral-induced toxic hepatitis are reported. One case took three 500 mg capsules of chaparral per day for 6 weeks, the other case took approximately 150 tablets of chaparral over an 11 week period. In both cases, elevated liver enzymes returned to normal after discontinuation of chaparral (*Epidemiologic Notes and Reports. Chaparral-induced toxic hepatitis - California and Texas, 1992. CDC Morbidity and Mortality Weekly Report October 30:812-4, 1992*).

Letter: In response to a press release issued by the FDA on December 10, 1992 warning of hepatitis, the American Herbal Products Association (AHPA) sent a letter on December 11, 1992 to all members that stated support for the FDA's position. However, the AHPA also pointed out that, over the past 20 years, over 200 tons of chaparral have been sold as dietary supplements and these cases appear to be the first associated with consumption of this herb, suggesting the possibility that causes other than chaparral may be involved as the source of these complaints (*American Herbal Products Association, P.O. Box 2410, Austin TX 78768, 1992*).

WARNING: Administration may stimulate tumor growth.

Experimental Study: From November, 1968, through November, 1969, 59 pts. with advanced incurable malignancy were treated with either chaparral tea (36 pts.) at a dose of 2-3 cups daily or with pure NDGA (23 pts.) at daily doses ranging from 250 mg to 3,000 mg. Of the 45 pts. who were evaluable, 4 pts. had significant tumor regression (2 cases of malignant melanoma, one case of choriocarcinoma with metastasis, and one case of lymphosarcoma). While tumor regressions occurred in these few cases, a significant number of of cases appeared to have had tumor stimulation. This result was not entirely surprising as *in vitro* studies with NDGA have shown stimulation of tumor cell growth at lower concentrations and inhibition at higher levels. "Until this phenomena can be clarified, it would seem inadvisable for cancer patients to continue to indiscriminately treat themselves with chaparral tea" (*Smart CR et al. Clinical experience with nordihydroguaiaretic acid - Chaparrel tea in the treatment of cancer. Rocky Mt Med J pp. 39-43, November, 1970*).

Administration may be beneficial.

Animal Experimental Study: Large bowel tumors were chemically induced in rats and the action of nordihydroguaiaretic acid, an inhibitor of lipoxygenase activity of the arachidonic acid cascade, was evaluated. 13/14 rats in the untreated control gp. developed tumors compared to 5/14 treated rats. Although nordihydroguairetic acid treatment does not abolish prostaglandin synthesis, it does reduce the effect of the carcinogen (*Birkenfeld S, Zaltsman YA, Krispin M, et al. Antitumor effects of inhibitors of arachidonic acid cascade on experimentally induced intestinal tumors. Dis Colon Rectum 30(1):43-6, 1987*).

Case Report: An 85 year-old white male refused medical treatment for a documented malignant melanoma of the right check with a large metastasis to the right submandibular area. Over the course of 1 year, the pt. medicated himself with 2-3 cups daily or a tea made from the dried leaves and stems (about 7-8 grams per quart of water) of chaparral. Without any other medical treatment during the year, the facial lesion shrunk from 3 x 4 cm in diameter to 2-3 cm and the submadnibular lesion of 5 x 7 cm in diameter completely disappeared (*Smart CR et al. An interesting observation on nordihydroguaiaretic acid (NSC-4291; NDGA) and a patient with malignant melanoma - a preliminary report. Cancer Chemother Rep 53:147-51, 1969*).

Chlorella:

An algae that grows in fresh water.

Preparations containing the broken cell wall and extracts of *Chlorella pyrenoidosa* may be beneficial.

Experimental Study: Chlorella (Sun Chlorella and Chlorella Wakasa) was added to the diet of 21 pts. being treated for malignant brain tumors. Results indicated chlorella helps maintain immunocompetence and protects against infection. 7 pts. were alive and showing no reappearance of their brain tumor 2 yrs. after treatment (*Merchant RE et al. Dietary Chlorella pyrenoidosa for patients with malignant glioma: Effects on immunocompetence, quality of life, and survival. Phytother Res 4(6):220-31, 1991*).

Coumarin:

Coumarin (1,2-benzopyrone) is a component of several medicinal plants historically used in cancer including dong quai (*Angelica sinensis*), sweet clover (*Meliotus officinalis*) and red clover (*Trifolium pratense*). The latter herb is a component is a popular folk remedy for cancer - the Hoxsey Formula.

> *Note: Coumarin, which possesses no anticoagulant activity, should not be confused with coumadin (warfarin).*

Administration may be beneficial.

Experimental Study: 48 pts. with metastatic hormone-naive (5 stage D1 and 10 stage D2) or hormone-refractory (33 stage D3) prostatic carcinoma were given 3 grams of coumarin daily by mouth and evaluated monthly for toxicity and response by rigid criteria in a multicenter trial. Toxicity was limited to asymptomatic SGOT elevations in 3 pts. and nausea and vomiting in 4 pateints that required cessation of therapy in 2 patients. Although no pts. showed complete response and only 3 pts. showed partial responses, the minimal toxicity of coumarin and the absence of alternative treatment for this cancer suggests a need for further study possibly at a higher dose (*Mohler JL et al. Phase II evaluation of coumarin (1,2-Benzopyrone) in metastatic prostatic carcinoma. Prostate 20:123-31, 1992*).

Experimental Study: In an attempt to define the maximally tolerated dose (MTD) and dose-limiting toxicity (DLT), 54 pts. with advanced malignancies were treated in a phase I trial of coumarin and cimetidine. The dose of coumarin was escalated, with 3 pts treated at each dose level, while the cimetidine dose was held constant at 300 mg four times daily. Pts. received coumarin alone as a single daily dose for 14 days; on day 15, cimetidine was added and both drugs were continued until progression of disease. This trial was initiated with patients receiving coumarin at 400 mg daily and closed at 7 g daily with 4/5 pts. on this dose experiencing nausea and vomiting. Treatment was generally well tolerated over a wide range of coumarin doses. Symptomatic side effects were few, mild, and self limited. Side effects included insomnia, nausea, vomiting, diarrhea, and dizziness. Hepatotoxicity occurred in only one pt. and was manifested by asymptomatic elevations in hepatic transaminases. This may have been a result of the cimetidine. Objective tumor regression was observed in 6 pts. with renal cell carcinoma. Responses occurred at coumarin doses ranging from 600 mg to 5 g daily. Although this study failed to determine the ideal dose of coumarin, it did show it had low toxicity and may offer benefit to some pts. with cancers who are not effectively treated by current medical treatment (*Marshall ME et al. Phase I evaluation of coumarin (1,2-benzopyrone) and cimetidine in patients with advanced malignancies. Mol Biother 3:170-8, 1991*).

Experimental Study: Coumarin exerts a direct effect on tumor cells as well as a profound immunomodulatory effect through activation of monocytes/macrophages. In this study of patients with advanced malignancies, 100 mg of coumarin per day was shown to produce almost immediate increases in the   percentage of monocytes. Evidence of increased monocyte activity was also noted (*Marshall ME et al. Effects of coumarin (1,2-benzopyrone) and cimetidine on peripheral blood lymphocytes, natural killer cells, and monocytes in patients with advanced malignancies. J Biol Resp Mod 8(1):62-9, 1989*).

Experimental Study: 45 pts. with metastatic renal cell carcinoma were treated with coumarin at a low of 100 mg. On day 15 of therapy, cimetidine administration (300 mg four times daily) was added. Both drugs were continued until progression of the disease. Objective responses of greater than or equal to 50% reduction in measurable disease occurred in 33% of the evaluated patients (42). 3 pts. had complete responses, 11 had partial responses, 12 experienced stabilization, and no response was seen in 16 patients. There was no symptomatic, hematologic, or chemical toxicity among the treated patients (*Marshall ME et al. Treatment of metastatic renal cell carcinoma with coumarin (1,2-benzopyrone) and cimetidine: a pilot study. J Clin Oncol 5(6):862-6, 1987*).

See Also:

> *Maucher A et al. Evaluation of the antitumor activity of coumarin in prostate cancer models. J Cancer Res Clin Oncol 119(3):150-4, 1993*

> *Dexeus FH et al. Phase II study of coumarin and cimetidine in patients with metastatic renal carcinoma. J Clin Oncol 8:325-30, 1992*

> *Marshall ME et al. Treatment of advanced malignant melanoma with coumarin and cimetidine: A pilot study. Cancer Chemother Pharmacol 24:65-6, 1989*

> *Berkarda B et al. The effect of coumarine derivatives on the immunological system of man. Agents Actions 13:50-2, 1983*

Curcumin: *See 'Turmeric' below.*

Echinacea:

An extract of the fresh juice of *Echinacea purpurea*, Echinacin®, has been studied as part of a comprehensive 'immunotherapy' protocol in cancer patients. Although given in injectable form in these studies, oral administration may provide similar benefit.

Experimental Study: Outpatients with inoperable metastatic esophageal (n = 6) or colorectal (n = 15) carcinomas receieved immunotherapy consisting of low-dose cyclophosphamide (LDCY) 300 mg/m^2 every 28 days IV, thymostimulin 30 mg/m^2, days 3-10 after low-dose cyclophosphamide i.m. once daily, then twice a week, and Echinacin® 60 mg/m^2 together with thymostimulin IM. All pts. had previous treatment by surgery and/or radio- and chemotherapy. Absolute numbers of CD4 cells increased by 27%, CD8 cells decreased by 16%, NK cells increased by 32%, and NK cell activity increased up to 221%. In 8/15 pts. with colorectal cancer and in 2/6 pts. with esophageal carcinomas, measurable tumors did not enlarge over a period of 3 months. Mean survival time of the pts. with colorectal cancer was 4 months and 3.5 months in the pts. with esophageal tumors (*Lersch C et al. [Simulation of immunocompetent cells in patients with gastrointestinal tumors during an experimental therapy with low dose* *cyclophosphamide, thymostimulin, and Echinacea purpurea extract (Echinacin)]. Tumordiagen Ther 13:115-20, 1992) (In German).*

Experimental Study: Outpatients (n = 15) with metastasizing far advanced colorectal cancers received immunotherapy consisting of low-dose cyclophosphamide (LDCY) 300 mg/m^2 every 28 days IV, thymostimulin 30 mg/m^2, days 3-10 after low-dose cyclophosphamide IM once daily, then twice a week, and Echinacin® 60 mg/m^2 together with thymostimulin IM. All pts. had had previous surgery and/or chemotherapy and had progressive disease upon entering the study. 2 months after onset of therapy, 1 pt. had a partial tumor regression and the disease was stable in 6 other pts. as documented by abdominal ultrasonography, decrease of the tumor markers carcinoembryonic antigen (CEA), CA 19-9, CA 15-3, and/or chest roentgenography, which may also be attributed to the natural course of disease. Mean survival time was 4 months; 2 pts. survived for more than 8 months. Immunotherapy was well tolerated by all pts. without side effects *(Lersch C et al. Nonspecific immunostimulation with low doses of cyclophosphamide (LDCY), thymostimulin, and Echinacea purpurea extracts (echinacin) in patients with far advanced colorectal cancers: preliminary results. Cancer Invest 10(5):343-8, 1992).*

Experimental Study: Outpatients with inoperable far-advanced hepatocellular carcinomas (n = 5) were treated with low-dose cyclophosphamide (LDCY) 300 mg/m^2 IV every 28 days, Echinacin® 60 mg/m^2 IM and thymostimulin 30 mg/m^2 IM days 3-10 after LDCY, then twice a week. Therapy was well tolerated by all pts. and their mean Karnofsky index increased by 10%. A stable disease for more than 8 weeks was documented by abdominal ultrasonography in one patient. Serum levels of Alpha-Fetoprotein (AFP), Carcinoembryonic Antigen (CEA) and Tissue Polypeptide Antigen (TPA) did not increase in 2 patients. Median survival time was 2.5 months. One pt. is still alive after 8 months. Absolute numbers of CD8+ cells significantly (p) decreased for 7% 1 day after LDCY, whereas CD4+ cells increased (p) from day 1-7. Numbers of NK cells increased for 17% (p), their activity for 90% (p). Activities of peripheral polymorphs increased for 27% (p) and of lymphokine activated killer (LAK) cells for 180% (p) *(Lersch C et al. Stimulation of the immune response in outpatients with hepatocellular carcinomas by low doses of cyclophosphamide (LDCY), Echinacea purpurea extracts (Echinacin) and thymostimulin. Arch Geschwulstforsch 60(5):379-83, 1990) (in German).*

In vitro Study: Acidic arabinogalactan, a highly purified polysaccharide from *Echinacea purpurea*, was effective in activating macrophages to cytotoxicity against tumor cells. Furthermore, it induced macrophages to produce tumor necrosis factor, interleukin-1, and interferon-beta 2. It also stimulated macrophages when injected IP, a finding that may have therapeutic implications in the defense against tumors *(Luettig B et al. Macrophage activation by the polysaccharide arabinogalactan isolated from plant cell cultures of Echinacea purpurea. J Natl Cancer Inst 81(9):669-75, 1989).*

Garlic (*Allium sativum*) or
Onion (*Allium cepa*):

Administration may increase natural killer cell activity.

In vitro Study: 3 healthy volunteers ate the equivalent of 2 bulbs (0.5 gm/kg) of garlic daily, while 3 took the equivalent dose in the form of 1800 mg of a cold-aged, odorless garlic capsule (Kyolic®) and 3 served as controls. After 3 wks., natural killer (NK) cells from the subjects ingesting raw garlic killed 140% more lymphoma cells in culture than NK cells from the controls, while NK cells from the subjects ingesting garlic capsules killed 156% more lymphoma cells than controls (*Kandil OM et al. Garlic and the immune system in humans: Its effect on natural killer cells. Fed Proc 46(3):441, 1987*).

Administration may inhibit carcinogenesis.

Animal Experimental Study: In a study of rats fed2% and 4% garlic powder, garlic was found to inhibit the activation of the carcinogenic N-nitroso compounds in both liver and breast tissue (*Lin X, Liu J, Milner J. Dietary garlic powder suhe in vivo formation of DNA adducts induced by N-nitroso compounds in liver and mammary tissues. FASEB J 6:A1392, 1992*).

Animal Experimental Study: Diallyl sulfide demonstrated effective anticancer effects in hamsters (*Nagabhushan M et al. Anticarcinogenic action of diallyl sulfide in hamster buccal pouch and forestomach. Cancer Lett 6:207-16, 1992*).

Review Article: Garlic may be a potent anticarcinogen when consumed regularly prior to cancer-onset or when cancer cell numbers are small. It appears to exert its effects by:

    1) direct action on tumor cell metabolism,

    2) inhibition of the initiation and promotion phase of cancer, and

    3) modulation of the host immune response

(*Lau B et al. Allium sativum (garlic) and cancer prevention. Nutr Res 10:937-48, 1990*).

Animal Experimental Study: The buccal pouches of hamsters who had been exposed to the carcinogen DMBA were painted with garlic extract. Compared to controls, garlic showed an inhibitory effect on DMBA-induced carcinogenesis (*Meng C, Shyu K. Inhibition of experimental carcinogenesis by painting with garlic extract. Nutr Cancer 14:207-17, 1990*).

Animal Experimental Study: The buccal pouches of hampsters were painted 3 times weekly with a cancer-inducing chemical. 20 of the animals also received a 20% onion extract in their drinking water and their buccal pouches were painted 3 times weekly with an onion extract. Another 20 animals also drank the 20% onion extract, but their buccal pouches were only painted with mineral oil, while a third gp. of 20 animals received no extract. Compared to the third gp., onion extract was found to significantly delay tumor formation (*Niukian K et al. Effects of onion extract on the development of hampster buccal pouch carcinomas as expressed in tumor burden. Nutr Cancer 9(2-3):171-6, 1987*).

Animal Experimental Study: Female mice were given oral doses of diallyl sulfide, one of several naturally occurring thioethers in garlic, 3 hrs. before being injected with DMH, a potent colon carcinogen. Mice given diallyl sulfide developed only small-to-microcsopic adenomas, while other animals developed numerous and severe colonic cancers (*Wargovich MJ. Diallyl sulfide, a flavor compound of garlic, inhibits diamethylhydrazine-induced colon cancer. Carcinogenesis 3:487-9, 1987*).

Animal Experimental Study: Garlic oil and onion oil were both effective in decreasing the number and incidence of experimental skin tumors in mice, although garlic was less effective (*Belman S. Onion and garlic oils inhibit tumor promotion. Carcinogenesis 4(8):1063-5, 1983*).

Animal Experimental Study: An aqueous extract of garlic was found to inhibit the growth of Morris hepatomas (*Criss WE et al. Inhibition of tumor growth with low dietary protein and with dietary garlic extracts. Fed Proc 41:281, 1982*).

Animal Experimental Study: Raw garlic was effective in preventing certain experimental tumors in predisposed mice (*Kroning F. Garlic as an inhibitor for spontaneous tumors in mice. Acta Unio Intern Contra Cancrum 20(3):855, 1964*).

See also:

> **Review Article:** *Dorant E et al. Garlic and its significance for the prevention of cancer in humans: a critical review. Br J Cancer 67:424-9, 1993*

> **Review Article:** *Dausch JG, Nixon DW. Garlic: A review of its relationship to malignant disease. Prev Med 19:346-61, 1990*

Gastric Cancer

Experimental Study: Compared to a basal diet, the urinary excretion of N-nitrosoproline in 9 healthy males was much larger when sodium nitrate and proline were added. When garlic was also added, the amt. of N-nitrosoproline was significantly reduced, suggesting that garlic may have a strong blocking effect on the formation of N-nitroso compounds (*Mei X et al. The blocking effect of garlic on the formation of N-nitrosoproline in the human body. Acta Nutr Sin 11(2):144-5, 1989*).

Observational Study: Interviews with 564 pts. with gastric cancer and 1,131 controls in Linqu, a rural county in Shandong Province in northeast China where gastric cancer rates are high revealed a significant reduction in gastric cancer risk with increasing consumption of allium vegetables. Persons in the highest quartile of intake experienced only 40% of the risk of those in the lowest (*You WC et al. Allium vegetables and reduced risk of stomach cancer. J Natl Cancer Inst 81(2):162-4, 1989*).

Observational Study: The residents of Gangshan County, Shandong Province, China regularly eat up to 20 gm garlic daily and have the lowest gastric cancer death rate in the country (3.45/100,000), while the residents of Quixia County rarely eat garlic and have the highest death rate (40/100,000) (*Horwitz N. Garlic as a plat du jour: Chinese study finds it could prevent G.I. cancer. Med Tribune August 12, 1981*).

See Also:

> *Mei X et al. Garlic and gastric cancer - The effect of garlic on nitrite and nitrate in gastric juice. Acta Nutr Sin 4:53-8, 1982*

Administration may reduce the toxicity of cyclophosphamide.

Animal Experimental Study: The intraperitoneal administration of garlic (50 mg/animal, 14 days) along with cyclophosphamide reduced the toxicity of the latter considerably, with an increase in life span of more than 70%. Garlic had no effect on leukopenia, but did reduce SGPT levels and the level of hepatic lipid peroxidation (*Unikrishnan MC et al. Chemoprevention of garlic extract toward cyclophosphamide toxicity in mice. Nutr Cancer 13:201-7, 1990*).

Gossypol:

Gossypol is a component of raw oil from the seeds of the cotton plant (*Gossypium spp.*).

Negative Experimental Study: 34 pts. with advanced cancer were given weekly or daily escalating doses of oral gossypol. There was no evidence of tumor regression in any of the 20 pts. assessed for response (*Stein RC et al. A preliminary clinical study of gossypol in advanced human cancer. Cancer Chemother Pharmacol 30:480-2, 1992*).

Green tea:

Both green tea and black tea are derived from the same plant (*Camellia sinensis*). Green tea is produced by lightly steaming the fresh-cut leaf, while to produce black tea the leaves are allowed to ferment. During fermentation, enzymes present in the tea convert many 'polyphenol' substances that possess outstanding therapeutic action to compounds with much less activity. With green tea, fermentation is not allowed to take place because the steaming process inactivates these enzymes. Green tea is very high in polyphenols with potent antioxidant and anticancer properties and appears to be beneficial, while black tea may be carcinogenic.

Review Article: Studies have demonstrated either a lack of association between tea consumption and cancer incidence at specific organ sites or inconsistent results. On the other hand, many laboratory studies have demonstrated inhibitory effects of tea preparations and tea polyphenols against tumor formation and growth. This inhibitory activity is believed to be mainly due to the antioxidative and possible antiproliferative effects of polyphenolic compounds in green tea. These polyphenolics may also inhibit carcinogenesis by blocking the endogenous formation of N-nitroso compounds, suppressing the activation of carcinogens, and trapping of genotoxic agents. The effect of tea consumption on cancer is likely to depend on the causative factors of the specific cancer. Therefore, a protective effect observed on a certain cancer with a specific population may not be observable with a cancer of a different etiology (*Yang CS, Wang ZY. Tea and cancer. J Natl Cancer Inst 85(13):1038-49, 1993*).

WARNING: Black tea consumption may increase the risk of certain cancers.

Epidemiological Study: The relationship between black tea consumption and cancer risk was analyzed using data from an integrated series of case-control studies conducted in northern Italy between 1983 and 1990. The dataset included 119 histologically confirmed cancers of the oral cavity and pharynx, 294 of the esophagus, 564 of the stomach, 673 of the colon, 406 of the rectum, 258 of the liver, 41 of the gallbladder, 303 of the pancreas, 149 of the larynx, 2,860 of the breast, 567 of the endometrium, 742 of the ovary,

107 of the prostate, 365 of the bladder, 147 of the kidney, 120 of the thyroid, and a total of 6,147 controls admitted to hospital for acute nonneoplastic conditions unrelated to long-term dietary modifications. Multivariate relative risks (RR) for tea consumption were derived after allowance for age, sex, area of residence, education, smoking, and coffee consumption. All the estimates for tea consumption were close to unity, the highest values being 1.4 for rectum, gallbladder, and endometrium. There was no association with cancers of the oral cavity (RR = 0.6), esophagus (RR = 1.0), stomach (RR = 1.0), bladder (RR = 0.8), kidney (RR = 1.1), prostate (RR = 0.9), or any other site considered (*La Vecchia C, et al. Tea consumption and cancer risk. Nutr Cancer 17(1):27-31, 1992*).

Epidemiological Study: In a prospective cohort study, men of Japanese ancestry were clinically examined from 1965 to 1968. For 7,833 of these men, data on black tea consumption habits were recorded. Since 1965, newly diagnosed cancer incidence cases have been identified: 152 colon, 151 lung, 149 prostate, 136 stomach, 76 rectum, 57 bladder, 30 pancreas, 25 liver, 12 kidney and 163 at other (miscellaneous) sites. Compared to almost-never drinkers, men habitually drinking black tea more than once/day had an increased relative risk (RR) for rectal cancer (RR=4.2). This positive association (p = 0.0007) could not be accounted for by age or alcohol intake. We also observed a weaker but significant negative association of black tea intake and prostate cancer incidence (p = 0.020). There were no significant associations between black tea consumption and cancer at any other site (*Heilbrun LK, Nomura A, Stemmermann GN. Black tea consumption and cancer risk: a prospective study. Br J Cancer 54(4):677-83, 1986*).

Green tea consumption with meals may inhibit the formation of nitrosamines.

Note: The popular custom of drinking green tea with meals in Japan and China is believed to be a major reason for the low cancer rates in these countries.

Experimental Study: The effects of 4 fruit juices, processed vegetable juice, orange peel, green tea and low dose vitamin C on endogenous N-nitrosation in 86 subjects from a high-risk area for gastric cancer in Moping County, China were studied using urinary excretion of N-nitrosoproline (NPRO) as an indicator. After ingestion of 300 mg L-proline, urinary excretion of NPRO was significantly increased from a baseline of 2.5 mcg/d to 8.7 mcg/d. Vitamin C (75 mg) administration significantly reduced NPRO formation (62.3%) although NPRO excretion remained significantly higher than the baseline level (4.2 vs 2.2 mcg/d). Intake of fruit juices and green tea extracts (containing 75 mg vitamin C) or of orange peel powder (containing 3 mg vitamin C) together with 300 mg L-proline inhibited NPRO formation effectively to the baseline level or to levels significantly lower than the baseline level (p<0.005). A processed juice of a number of vegetables (300 ml) significantly catalysed endogenous nitrosation (14.7 vs 9.4 mcg/d) (*Xu GP, Song PJ, Reed PI. Effects of fruit juices, processed vegetable juice, orange peel and green tea on endogenous formation of N-nitrosoproline in subjects from a high-risk area for gastric cancer in Moping County, China. Eur J Cancer Prev 2(4):327-35, 1993*).

Review Article: Green tea polyphenol extracts and components exert significant inhibitory effects on the formation of nitrosamines in various animal and human models.

When human volunteers ingested green tea infusions along with 300 mg sodium nitrate and 300 mg proline, nitrosoproline formation is strongly inhibited (*Stich HF. Teas and tea components as inhibitors of carcinogen formation in model systems and man. Prevent Med 21:377-84, 1992*).

Green tea consumption may increase the activity of antioxidant enzymes.

Animal Experimental Study: Following the oral feeding of a polyphenolic fraction isolated from green tea (GTP) in drinking water, an increase in the activities of antioxidant and phase II enzymes in skin, small bowel, liver, and lung of female SKH-1 hairless mice was observed. GTP feeding (0.2%, w/v) to mice for 30 days significantly increased the activities of glutathione peroxidase, catalase, and quinone reductase in small bowel, liver, and lungs, and glutathione S-transferase in small bowel and liver. GTP feeding to mice also resulted in considerable enhancement of glutathione reductase activity in liver. In general, the increase in antioxidant and phase II enzyme activities was more pronounced in lung and small bowel as compared to liver and skin. The significance of these results can be implicated in relation to the cancer chemopreventive effects of GTP against the induction of tumors in various target organs (*Khan SG et al. Enhancement of antioxidant and phase II enzymes by oral feeding of green tea polyphenols in drinking water to SKH-1 hairless mice: possible role in cancer chemoprevention. Cancer Res 52(14):4050-2, 1992*).

Green tea consumption may inhibit mutagenesis and carcinogenesis.

Review Article: The main physiologically active polyphenol in green tea extract is (-)-epigallocatechin gallate (EGCG). Green tea extract has an advantage over EGCG as a cancer chemopreventive agent for humans, as is apparent from the Japanese custom of injesting green tea on a daily basis. Green tea extract similarly inhibited protein kinase C activation by teleocidin, a tumor promoter, as did EGCG. In addition, EGCG and green tea extract showed inhibitory effects on the growth of lung and mammary cancer cell lines with similar potencies. An experiment using the estrogen-dependent MCF-7 cell line showed the mechanisms of action of these compounds to be inhibiting the interaction of estrogen with its receptors. EGCG and compounds in green tea extracts block the interaction of tumor promoters, hormones and growth factors with their receptors: a kind of sealing effect. The sealing effect would account for reversible growth arrest, and may be induced by various kinds of compound (*Komori A et al. Anticarcinogenic activity of green tea polyphenols. Jpn J Clin Oncol 23(3):186-90, 1993*).

See Also:

Animal Experimental Study: *Katiyar SK, Agarwal R, Mukhtar H. Green tea in chemoprevention of cancer. Compr Ther 18(10):3-8, 1992*

In vivo and In vitro Study: *Mukhtar H et al. Tea components: Antimutagenic and anticarcinogenic effects. Prevent Med 21:351-60, 1992*

Animal Experimental Study: *Wang ZY et al. Protection against polycyclic aromatic hydrocarbon-induced skin tumor initiation in mice by green tea polyphenols. Carcinogenesis 10(2):411-5, 1989.*

In vitro Study: *Wang ZY et al. Antimutagenic activity of green tea polyphenols. Mutat Res 223(3):273-85, 1989*

LaPacho (*Tabebuia avellandae*):

LaPacho is a tropical tree native to Brazil. LaPacho is also known as Pau D'Arco, Tahebo, and Ipe Roxo. It has a long history of use by the natives of Brazil. The major active component is lapachol, a substance which has been studied at the U.S. National Cancer Institute.

> *Note: A 1987 analysis of 12 commercially available LaPacho products by the Canadian government showed that only 1 contained lapachol in trace amounts and the other 11 products had none. Since the lapachol content of LaPacho is typically 2-7%, this suggests that many of the products now present on the market are either not truly LaPacho or that processing and transportation have damaged the product. Chemical analysis and standardization for lapachol or napthoquinones by manufacturers is needed (Canadian Health Protection Branch: Herbs and botanical preparations. Information Letter 726, August 13, 1987; Awang DVC. Commercial taheebo lacks active ingredient. Can Pharm J 121:323-6, 1991).*

Experimental Study: Nine pts. with various cancers (e.g., adenocarcinoma of the liver, kidney, breast, and prostate, and squamous cell carcinoma of the palate and uterine cervix) were given pure lapachol at a daily dose of 20-30 mg/kg. The medicine was administered in 250 mg capsules with meals. Lapachol demonstrated an ability to shrink tumors and reduce feelings of pain caused by the tumor in all patients. Three pts. had complete remissions. Nausea and vomiting caused the cessation of treatment in 3 pts.; there were no other significant side effects *(Santana CF et al. [Preliminary observations with the use of lapachol in human patients bearing malignant neoplasms.] Revista do Instituto de Antibioticos 20:61-8, 1980/81) (in Portuguese).*

Animal Experimental Study: A lapachol analog was shown to be effective in increasing the life span by over 80% in mice inoculated with leukemic cells *(Linardi MDC et al. A lapachol derivative active against mouse lymphocyte leukemia P-388. J Med Chem 18(11):1159-62, 1975).*

Negative Experimental Study: The NCI reported that phase I clinical trials on lapachol failed to produce a therapeutic effect largely due to the inability to obtain therapeutic blood levels (>30 mcg/ml) of lapachol without some mild toxic effects such as nausea, vomiting, and anticoagulant effects due to anti-vitamin K activity *(Block JB et al. Early clinical studies with lapachol (NSC-11905). Cancer Chemother Rep 4:27-8, 1974).*

Animal Experimental Study: Lapachol demonstrated highly significant activity against Walker 256 carcinosarcoma when given by intraperitoneal, subcutaneous, intramuscular, and oral routes. The best activity and therapeutic index are shown when the drug was given twice daily by the oral route *(Rao KV et al. Recognition and evaluation of lapachol as an antitumor agent. Canc Res 28:1952-4, 1968).*

See Also:

Rao KV. *Quinone natural products: Streptonigrin (NSC-45383) and lapachol (NSC-11905) structure-activity relationships.* Cancer Chemother Rep *4:11-7, 1974*

Morrison RK *et al. Oral toxicology studies with lapachol.* Toxicol Appl Pharmacol *17:1-11, 1970*

Mistletoe (*Viscum album*):

Mistletoe preparations are widely used in Europe for cancer therapy. These preparations are administered intracutaneously or intravenously as the active components, polypetides (viscotoxins and glycoproteins) known as mistletoe lectins, are not absorbed orally.

Experimental Placebo-Controlled Study: A mistletoe preparation standardized on mistletoe lectin I (Eurixor®) was examined in 40 pts. with advanced carcinoma of the breast. Mistletoe lectin I is a potent inducer of cytokines like interleukin 1, interleukin 6, and tumor necrosis factor. Along with standard chemotherapy (VEC regimen), 21 pts. were assigned to receive mistletoe (treatment group) while 19 pts. were given a placebo (control group). After the fourth cycle of chemotherapy, the treatment group had statistically significantly higher leukocyte levels (p<0.001) compared to the control group. The treatment group had an average white blood cell count of 3,000 while the control group had an average count of 1,000. Futhermore, the parameters of the quality of life and anxiety strain revealed significantly better values in the treatment group than in the control group. These results show that the adjuvant treatment with mistletoe extracts, in this case Eurixor®, is a valuable addition to standard chemotherapy for breast cancer patients (*Heiny BM. [Adjuvant treatment with standardized mistletoe extract reduces leukopenia and improves the quality of life of patients with advanced carcinoma of the breast gettin palliative chemotherapy (VEC regimen)].* Krebsmedizin *12:3-14, 1991) (in German).*

In Vitro and Animal Experimental Study: The effect of Iscador®, a commercial preparation made from *Viscum album*, was studied on several cell lines using *in vitro* tissue culture as well as tumor-bearing animals. Iscador® was found to be cytotoxic to animal tumor cells such as Dalton's lymphoma ascites cells and Ehrlich ascites cells *in vitro* and inhibited the growth of lung fibroblasts, Chinese hamster ovary cells, and human nasopharyngeal carcinoma cells at very low concentrations. Moreover, *in vivo* administration of Iscador® was found to reduce ascites tumors and solid tumors produced by various agents. The effect could be seen when Iscador was given either simultaneously, after tumor development, or when given prophylactically, indicating a mechanism of action very different from other chemotherapuetic drugs (*Kuttan G, Vasudevan DM, Kuttan R. Effect of a preparation from Viscum album on tumor development in vitro and in mice.* J Ethnopharmacol *29:35-41, 1990).*

Experimental Study: Iscador® was shown to have no objective or life-prolonging effects in 14 pts. with stage IV renal adenocarcinoma, a type of cancer that is typically refractive to all types of systemic treatment. However, this study did not seem unreasonable since Iscador® has been reported to produce a highly significant effect as an adjunct treatment on survival compared with historical controls in pts. with breast cancer, gastric cancer, colonic cancer, non small cell lung cancer, bladder cancer, and malignant melanoma irrespective of the tumor type, stage, sex, or other prognostic factor (*Kjaer M. Mistletoe (Iscador) therapy in stage IV renal adenocarcinoma.* Acta Oncol *28(4)489-94, 1988).*

Experimental Study: The immunomodulatory effects of Iscador® were investigated in breast cancer patients. After a single intravenous infusion of Iscador® several immune parameters were examined. After initial decreases during the first 24 hours, significant increases in natural killer and antibody-dependent cell-mediated cytotoxicity activities as well as augmented levels of large granular lymphocytes were observed. Other effects noted were elevations in neutrophil levels, enhanced macrophage phagocytic and cytotoxic activity, and enhanced mitogenic responses to phytohemagluttinin and concanavalin A (*Hajto T. Immunomodulatory effects of Iscador: A Viscum album preparation. Oncology 43(supple 1):51-65, 1986*).

See Also:

> *Oncology Volume 43, Supplement 1, 1986*

> *Rentea R   et al. Biological properties of Iscador: a Viscum album preparation. Lab Invest 44:43-8, 1981*

> *Blocksma N   et al. Cellular and humoral adjuvant activity of a mistletoe extract. Immunobiol 156:309-19, 1979*

Panax ginseng (Chinese or Korean ginseng):

Administration of Chinese or Korean ginseng may inhibit cancer development.

Observational Study: The effects of ginseng consumption on the risk of cancer was investigated by interviewing 905 pairs of cases and controls matched by age, sex, and date of admission to the Korea Cancer Center Hospital in Seoul, Korea. Of the 905 cases, 562 (62%) had a history of ginseng intake compared to 674 of the 905 controls (75%) a statistically significant difference ($p<0.01$). The odds ratio (OR) of cancer in relation to ginseng intake was 0.56 (95% confidence interval). Interestingly, ginseng extract and powder were shown to be more effective that fresh sliced ginseng, the juice, or the tea in reducing the OR ratio. A highly statistically significant preventive effect of ginseng on cancer with a dose-response relationship was observed, i.e., the higher the intake of ginseng the lower the risk of cancer. These results support the preventive effects of ginseng suggested by earlier animal studies (*Yun TK et al. A case-control study of ginseng intake and cancer. Int J Epidemiol 19(4):871-6, 1990*).

Animal Experimental Study: Korean red ginseng administered orally to newborn mice prevented the cancer causing and proliferative effects of DMBA, urethane and aflatoxin compared to control groups. Detailed histological examinations indicated that 48 weeks after DMBA treatment, the group receiving the ginseng had a 63% lower incidence of diffuse pulmonary infiltration, much lower (23%) diameter of the largest lung adenoma, and a 21% lower average lung weight. Compared to the control group receiving urethane, the group receiving urethane and ginseng had a 22% decrease in the incidence of adenoma. The group receiving ginseng and aflatoxin had a 29% lower incidence of lung cancer and a 75% lower rate of hepatoma compared to the group receiving aflatoxin alone (*Yun TK et al. Anticarcinogenic effect of long-term oral adminstration of red ginseng on newborn mice exposed to various chemical carcinogens. Cancer Det Prev 6:515-25, 1983*).

PSK and
PSP:

PSK and PSP are protein-bound polysaccharides from the cloud fungus mushroom (*Coriolus veriscolor*). Unlike lentinan (*see 'Shitake mushroom' below*), PSK and PSP are effective orally. PSK is an approved drug in Japan.

Administration may be beneficial.

Experimental Study: 11 pts. with breast cancer undergoing three cycles of chemotherapy were given PSP (1.2 g 3 times daily). There was no significant drop in their peripheral WBC and platelet counts (*Shiu WCT et al. A clinical study of PSP on peripheral blood counts during chemotherapy. Phytother Res 6:217-8, 1992*).

Experimental Controlled Study: A randomized, controlled trial of PSK in 448 curatively resected colorectal cancer pts. was studied in 35 institutions in the Kanagawa prefecture. The control group received mitomycin C intravenously on the day of and the day after surgery, followed by oral 5-fluorouracil (5-FU) administration for over six months. The PSK group received PSK orally for over three years, in addition to mitomycin C and 5-FU as in the control group. The median follow-up time for this study was four years (range, three to five years). The disease-free survival curve and the survival curve of the PSK group were better than those of the control group, and differences between the two groups were statistically significant (p = 0.013) (*Mitomi T et al. Randomized, controlled study on adjuvant immunochemotherapy with PSK in curatively resected colorectal cancer. The Cooperative Study Group of Surgical Adjuvant Immunochemotherapy for Cancer of Colon and Rectum (Kanagawa). Dis Colon Rectum 35(2):123-30, 1992*).

Experimental Controlled Study: 29 gastric and 18 colorectal cancer pts. were randomly assigned to either receive 3.0 g of PSK orally before surgery, either daily or every other day, or no PSK. The data of peripheral blood lymphocytes (PBL) were compared before and after administration of PSK, and those of the regional node lymphocytes (RNL) were compared between the control and the PSK group. The results indicate that the effects of PSK were significantly influenced by the duration of administration, but not by the frequency of administration. Oral administration of PSK leads to significant improvement in various immune parameters (*Nio Y et al. Immunomodulation by orally administered protein-bound polysaccharide PSK in patients with gastrointestinal cancer. Biotherapy 4(2):117-28, 1992*).

Experimental Double-blind Study: PSK was given to 56 pts. and a placebo to another group of 55 pts. after surgical operations on their colorectal cancers. The rate of patients in remission (or disease-free) and survival rate was significantly higher in the PSK group than in the placebo group (p<0.05). PSK-treated patients showed remarkable enhancement in white blood cells activities, such as random and/or chemotactic locomotion, and phagocytic activity, when compared with those in the control group (*Torisu M et al. Significant prolongation of disease-free period gained by oral polysaccharide K (PSK) administration after curative surgical operation of colorectal cancer. Cancer Immunol Immunother 31(5):261-8, 1990*).

Experimental Controlled Study: A controlled study using adjuvant PSK immunotherapy in pts. with nasopharyngeal carcinoma was initiated with the aim of improving survival by enhancing the host immune system against tumor cells. A total of 38 pts. were randomly selected, all of whom had previously received radiotherapy with or without chemotherapy. Eight pts. in the PSK immunotherapy group (n=21) developed local recurrence, 3 of whom later died due to distant metastasis. In the control group (n=17) 3 pts. developed local recurrence while 6 pts. developed distant metastases. All of these 6 ppts. later died due to disease progression. It seems that PSK exerts its antitumor effect systemically; the risk of distant metastases occurring is decreased, but it is apparently ineffective in improving local disease control. The estimated median survival time of the PSK-treated group compared with the control was significantly increased (35 months versus 25 months, p=0.043). The 5-year survival rate was also significantly better in the PSK immunotherapy group (28% versus 15%, p=0.043) (*Go P Chung CH. Adjuvant PSK immunotherapy in patients with carcinoma of the nasopharynx. J Int Med Res 17(2):141-9, 1989*).

See Also:

> **Experimental Controlled Study:** *Sakamoto J et al. Preoperative serum immunosuppressive acidic protein (IAP) test for the prognosis of gastric cancer: a statistical study of the threshold level and evaluation of the effect of the biological response modifier PSK. Surg Today 22(6):530-6, 1992*

> **Experimental Controlled Study:** *Kondo T et al. Alternating immunochemotherapy of advanced gastric carcinoma: a randomized comparison of carbazilquinone and PSK to carbazilquinone in patients with curative gastric resection. Biotherapy 3(4):287-95, 1991.*

Seaweed (*Undaria pinnantifida*):

Administration of an extract (Viva-Natural®) may stimulate immunological processes such as macrophage activity and enhance the antitumor effectiveness of certain chemotherapeutic agents.

> **Animal Experimental Study:** Several chemotherapeutic agents were ineffective in the treatment of Lewis lung carcinoma at lower than usual dosages. Low doses of adriamycin, cisplatin, 5-fluoruracil and vincristine, but not of BCNU, methotrexate or 6-thioguanine, became effective when combined with Viva-Natural® (*Furusawa E, Furusawa S. Antitumor potential of low-dose chemotherapy manifested in combination with immunotherapy of Viva-Natural, a dietary seaweed extract, on Lewis lung carcinoma. Cancer Lett 50:71-8, 1990*).

Shitake mushroom (*Lentinus edodes*):

The shitake mushroom is a mainstay in the Japanese diet and is regarded as a protector against cancer. Scientific research into its immune enhancing and anticancer effects have focused on shitake's polysaccharide components. One of these components, lentinan, is used in a highly purified form in cancer treatment in Japan. Lentinan must be injected because it is poorly absorbed orally and does not suppress tumor growth in animals when given orally. Another shitake polysachharide, KS-2 is absorbed orally in an active form because it is a 'peptidomannan', a polysaccharide with a small peptide component. While KS-2 was never developed into a drug, it is used by cancer patients in China and is viewed as a less expensive alternative to the expensive lentinan.

Lentinan administration may improve the prognosis in breast cancer.

> **Experimental Controlled Study:** Pts. with advanced or recurrent breast cancer who had received bilateral oophorectomy and adrenalectomy were administered lentinan. Compared to controls, they exhibited a prolongation of survival times (*Kosaka A et al. [Effect of lentinan administration on adrenalectomized rats and patients with breast cancer.] Gan To Kagaku Ryoho 9(8):1474-81, 1982) (in Japanese)*.

Lentinan administration may be effective as an adjuvant to chemotherapy in cancer therapy for gastric and colorectal cancers.

> **Experimental Controlled Study:** In a randomized study, pts. with advanced or recurrent gastric cancer were treated with the chemotherapeutic agents mitomycin C and tegafur with or without lentinan. Excellent end-point results were obtained only in lentinan-treated pts. with normal protein levels; those with protein levels below 5.9 g/dl failed to improve (*Akimoto M et al. [Modulation of anticancer effects of immunchemotherapeutic agents in various nutritional environments.] Gan To Kagaku Ryoho 15(4 Pt 2-1):827-33, 1988) (in Japanese)*.

> **Experimental Controlled Study:** In a randomized trial, 96 pts. with advanced or recurrent stomach cancer received tegafur in combination with lentinan 2 mg/wk IV while 68 pts. received only tegafur. After 4 yrs., remarkable lifespspan prolongation was found (p<0.01). Side effects of lentinan were transitional and not serious (*Taguchi T. Clinical efficacy of lentinan on patients with stomach cancer: End point results of a four-year follow-up survey. Cancer Detect Prev [Suppl]; 1:333-49, 1987)*.

> **Experimental Controlled Study:** In a randomized trial, 166 pts. with advanced gastric and colorectal cancers received mitomycin C and 5-FU with or without lentinan. Significant increases were observed in the survival rates for the lentinan gp. (p<0.05). Although the response rate in the lentinan gp. was slightly higher, the difference was not significant (*Wakui A et al. [Randomized study of lentinan on patients with advanced gastric and colorectal cancer. Tohoku lentinan study group.] Gan To Kagaku Ryoho 13(4 Pt 1):1050-59, 1986) (in Japanese)*.

KS-2 may possess similar immune enhancing effects to lentinan, but is absorbed orally.

> **Animal Experimental Study:** KS-2 inhibits the growth of Ehrlich and Sarcoma-180 tumors and prolongs the life span in mice. It was effective both orally and intraperitoneally. KS-2 itself had no direct cytotoxic effects on tumor cells. Its effects are a result of immune enhancement. In this same study, KS-2 was shown to induce circulating interferon levels in mice and cured them from influenza infection. KS-2 was also mentioned to induce interferon levels in human cancer patients as well, although no data was presented. The effective oral dose for tumor regression was between 1 and 100 mg/kg (*Fujii T et al. Isolation and characterization of a new antitumor polysaccharide, KS-2, extracted from culture mycelia of Lentinus edodes. Antibiotics 31(11):1079-90, 1978)*.

> **Animal Experimental Study:** KS-2 was labelled by flourescent isothiocyanate and given to rats. Data indicated that KS-2 was absorbed intact via the portal vein and intestinal lymphatics into the general circulation. Labeled KS-2 breakdown products

were also recovered in the urine. Histological evaluation revealed KS-2 was accumulated in the mesenteric lymph nodes, Peyer's patches, spleen, liver, and kidneys (*Yamashita A et al. Intestinal absorption and urinary excreation of antitumo peptidomannan KS-2 after oral administration in rats. Immunopharmacol 5(3):209-220, 1983*).

Solasodine glycosides:

Solasodine is the aglycone of many glycoalkaloids found in nightshade family vegetables. A cream formulation, Curaderm®, which contains 0.005% of a standardized mixture of purified glycoalkaloids known as BEC® from the apple of Sodom (*Solanum sodomeum*), is available commercially in Australia for skin cancers.

Experimental Study: In an open clinical trial, Curaderm® was shown to produce effective treatment of keratoses (56 lesions), basal cell carciomas (39 lesions), and squamous cell carcinomas (29 lesions) of the skin. Clinical and histological observations indicated that all lesions treated with Curaderm® had regressed without side effects (*Cham BE et al. Topical treatment of malignant and premalignant skin lesions by very low concentrations of a standard mixture (BEC) of solasodine glycosides. Cancer Lett 59:183-92, 1991*).

Experimental Study: Patients with various skin cancers were asked to apply a thin layer of a cetomacrogol cream containing 10% BEC® and 10% DMSO twice daily and cover it with an occlusive dressing. Histological analysis and photographic evidence taken before, during and after treatment with the cream for malignant skin cancers gave compelling evidence of the effectiveness of the formulation. The observed complete remissions were; 2/24 for basal cell carcinomas; 5/6 for squamous cell carcinomas; 23/23 for keratoes; and 9/9 for keratoacanthomas. The treated lesions did not recur for at least 3 years after cessation of therapy. The formulation produced no adverse effects during treatment and normal skin treated with the formulation was free from adverse histological or clinical effects (*Cham BE, Meares HM. Glycoalkaloids from solanum sodomaeum are effective in the treatment of skin cancers in man. Cancer Lett 36:111-8, 1987*).

See also:

> *Daunter B, Cham BE. Solasodine glycosides. In vitro preferential cytotoxicity for human cancer cells. Cancer Lett 55(3):209-20, 1990*

> *Cham BE et al. Solasodine glycosides. elective cytotoxicity for cancer cells and inhibition of cytotoxicity by rhamnose in mice with sarcoma 180. Cancer Lett 55(3):221-5, 1990*

Turmeric (*Curcuma longa*):

Turmeric and its major active component, curcumin, appear to exert powerful antioxidant effects directly as well as enhance the antioxidant system.

Animal and in Vitro Experimental Study: Curcumins were shown to inhibit cancer at initiation, promotion and progression stages of development (*Nagabhushan M, Bhide SV. Curcumin as an inhitor of cancer. J Am Coll Nutr 11(2):192-8, 1992*).

Animal Experimental Study: Anticancer activity of the rhizomes of turmeric in both *in vitro* and *in vivo* models. Initial experiments indicated that curcumin is the active compound responsible for reducing the development of animal tumors. Curcumin was shown to to cytotoxic to Dalton's lymphoma cells at a concentration of 4 mcg/ml (*Kuttan R et al. Potential anticancer activity of turmeric (Curcuma longa). Cancer Lett 29:197-202, 1985*).

See also:

> *Soudamini KK, Kuttan R. Inhibition of chemical carcinogenesis by curcumin. J Ethnopharmacol 27:227-33, 1989*

Administration may protect against environmental carcinogens, especially cigarette smoke.

Experimental Controlled Study: The level of urinary mutagens is thought to correlate with the systemic load of carcinogens and how the body deals with them. 16 chronic smokers were given two tablets containing 750 mg of turmeric daily while six nonsmokers served as a control group. At the end of the 30 day trial, the smokers had a significant reduction in the level of urinary mutagens while the control group's urinary mutagen levels remained unchanged. Due to the widespread exposure to smoke and other environmental carcinogens, these results indicate that turmeric/curcumin may be useful in cancer prevention (*Polasa K et al. Effect of turmeric on urinary mutagens in smokers. Mutagen 7(2):107-9, 1992*).

Administration may be effective in the topical treatment of oral and cutaneous cancers.

Experimental Study: Curcumin has demonstrated impressive results in experimental models of skin and epithelial cancers prompting a clinical study in 62 pts. with either ulcerating oral or cutaneous squamous cell carcinomas who had failed to respond to standard treatments like surgery, radiation, and chemotherapy. The pts. were given either an ethanol extract of turmeric (for oral cancers) or an ointment containing 9.5% curcumin in vaseline. The ointment was applied topically three times daily. At the end of the 18 month study, the treatment was found to have been very effective in reducing the smell of the lesion (90% of pts.), itching, exudate (70%), pain (50%), and size of the lesion (*Kuttan R et al. Turmeric and curcumin as topical agents in cancer therapy. Tumori 73:29-31, 1987*).

Ukrain:

Ukrain, a semi-synthetic thiophosphoric acid compound of alkaloid chelidonine isolated from *Chelidonium Majus L.*, causes a regression of tumors and metastases in many oncological patients. More than 400 documented patients with various carcinomas in different stages of development have been treated with injections of Ukrain. Ukrain can be helpful in improving the general condition and prolonging life by reduction of the tumor progression and by its immunomodulating effect (*Lohninger A Hamler F. Chelidonium majus L. (Ukrain) in the treatment of cancer patients. Drugs Exp Clin Res 18 Suppl:73-7, 1992*).

Experimental Study: Lymphocyte subsets were evaluated in 9 men with previously untreated lung cancer. Ukrain was applied as an intravenous injection every three days. One course consisted of 10 applications of 10 mg each. All immunological tests were performed before and after drug administration. The treatment was generally well tolerated. The results showed an increase in the proportion of total T-cells, and a significant decrease in the percentage of T-suppressor cells and a normalization of the helper to suppressor ratio. However, there were no signs of activation of NK, T-helper and B-cells. The restoration of cellular immunity was accompanied by an improvement in the clinical course of the disease. This effect was particularly pronounced in patients who responded to further chemotherapy. Objective tumor regression (CR+PR) was seen in 44.4% of treated patients. 4/9 pts. (44.4%) died of progressive disease during the course of this study (*Staniszewski A et al. Lymphocyte subsets in patients with lung cancer treated with thiophosphoric acid alkaloid derivatives from Chelidonium majus L. (Ukrain). Drugs Exp Clin Res 18 Suppl:63-7, 1992*).

Experimental Study: 7 pts. with various malignancies were treated with Ukrain given intravenously in a dose of 10 mg every three days. There was an increase in both total T-cells and T-helper lymphocytes, a decrease in T-suppressor cells, and normalization of the helper/suppressor ratio. A significant increase in erythrocyte-rosette-forming T-cells and NK cells was also demonstrated. Serum immunoglobulin levels, complement components (C3 and C4), and acute phase proteins were not significantly enhanced. Restoration of cellular immunity was accompanied by an improvement in the patients' performance status and in the clinical course of the disease. The treatment was generally well tolerated (*Nowicky JW et al. Evaluation of thiophosphoric acid alkaloid derivatives from Chelidonium majus L. ("Ukrain") as an immunostimulant in patients with various carcinomas. Drugs Exp Clin Res 17(2):139-43, 1991*).

See Also:

Musianowycz J et al. Clinical studies of Ukrain in terminal cancer patients (phase II). Drugs Exp Clin Res 18 Suppl:45-50, 1992

Nowicky JW et al. Ukrain both as an anti cancer and immunoregulatory agent. Drugs Exp Clin Res 18 Suppl:51-4, 1992

Danilos J et al. Preliminary studies on the effect of Ukrain (Tris(2-([5bS-(5ba,6b,12ba)]- 5b,6,7,12b,13,14-hexahydro-13-methyl[1,3] benzodioxolo[5,6-v]-1-3- dioxolo[4,5-i]phenanthridinium-6-ol]-Ethaneaminyl)Phosphinesulfide.6HCl) on the immunological response in patients with malignant tumours. Drugs Exp Clin Res 18 Suppl:55-62, 1992

Pengsaa P et al. The effects of thiophosphoric acid (Ukrain) on cervical cancer, stage IB bulky. Drugs Exp Clin Res 18 Suppl:69-72, 1992

Nowicky J et al. Biological activity of ukrain in vitro and in vivo. Chemioterapia 6(2 Suppl):683-5, 1987

CANDIDIASIS

See Also: IMMUNODEPRESSION
INFECTION

Overgrowth of *Candida albicans* in mucous membranes, or hypersensitivity to the organism, is claimed by some authors to cause a poly-symptomatic syndrome (which may include mental symptoms, irritable bowel syndrome, premenstrual syndrome, etc.) even in the absence of infection.

At the present time, however, the American Academy of Allergy and Immunology considers the concept of a 'candidiasis hypersensitivity syndrome' to be unproven. According to the Academy, "the diagnosis, the special laboratory tests, and the special aspects of treatment should be considered experimental and reserved for use with informed consent in appropriate controlled trials" (*Position statement: Candidiasis hypersensitivity syndrome. J Allergy Clin Immunol 78(2):271-3, 1986*).

GENERAL REFERENCE:

> Truss CO. *The role of candida albicans in human illness. J Orthomol Psychiatry 10:228-38, 1981*

- -

Berberine:

Berberine-containing plants like goldenseal (*Hydrastis canadensis*), barberry bark (*Berberis vulgaris*), and Oregon grape root (*Berberis aquifolium*) may be effective in the internal and topical treatment of candidiasis.

In vitro Study: Berberine sulfate in concentrations of 10-25 mcg/ml inhibited the growth of *Candida albicans* as well as 10 other fungi (*Mahajan VM, Sharma A, Rattan A. Antimycotic activity of berberine sulphate: An alkaloid from an Indian medicinal herb. Sabouraudia 20:79-81, 1982*).

Cassia alata:

Extracts of *Cassia alata* (ringworm senna) are traditionally used in West Africa to treat bacterial and fungal infections.

In vitro Study: The antibacterial and antifungal activities of water extracts of *Cassia alata* were investigated. The effectiveness of the extracts was evaluated relative to those of the standard antibacterial agent chloramphenicol and antifungal agent amphotericin B. The minimum inhibitory concentration (MIC) and minimum bactericidal concentration (MBC) for the water extract of cassia against *E. coli* were 1.6 mg/ml and 60 mg/ml respectively; corresponding data for chloramphenicol were 2 ug/ml. Similarly, the MIC and minimum fungicidal concentration (MFC) for the extract against *C. albicans* were 0.39 mg/ml and 60 mg/ml in contrast to 0.58 ug/ml and 0.98 ug/ml for amphotericin B. From the dose-response curve plots, the extract had an IC50 of 31 mg/ml for *E. coli* and 28 mg/ml for *C. albicans (Crockett CO et al. Cassia alata and the preclinical search for therapeutic agents for the treatment of opportunistic infections in AIDS patients. Cell Mol Biol 38(5):505-11, 1992).*

Echinacea:

An extract of the fresh juice (Echinacin®) of *Echinacea purpurea*, as well as preparations containing the polysaccharides, may be useful. (*See: 'IMMUNODEPRESSION'; 'INFECTION'*)

> **In vivo and In vitro Study:** Purified polysaccharides from cell cultures of the plant *Echinacea purpurea* were investigated for their ability to enhance phagocytes' activities regarding nonspecific immunity *in vitro* and *in vivo*. Macrophages from different organ origin could be activated to produce IL-1, TNF alpha and IL-6, to produce elevated amounts of reactive oxygen intermediates and to inhibit growth of *Candida albicans in vitro*. Furthermore, *in vivo* the substances could induce increased proliferation of phagocytes in spleen and bone marrow and migration of granulocytes to the peripheral blood. These effects resulted in excellent protection of mice against the consequences of lethal infections with *Listeria monocytogenes* and *C. albicans (Roesler J et al. Application of purified polysaccharides from cell cultures of the plant Echinacea purpurea to mice mediates protection against systemic infections with Listeria monocytogenes and Candida albicans. Int J Immunopharmacol 13(1):27-37, 1991).*

> **Experimental Study:** Echinacin® greatly accentuates the efficacy of a topical antimycotic agent (econazol nitrate) in preventing recurrence of vaginal candidiasis. Standardized skin tests were used to show that Echinacea's effects were due to boosting of cell-mediated immunity. Echinacin® reduced the reccurrence rate from 60.5% to between 5 and 16.7% depending on the mode of application: topical antimycotic alone (n=43) 60.5%; topical antimycotic + subcutaneous Echinacin® ampoule (n=20) 15%; topical antimycotic + intramuscular Echinacin® ampoule (n=60) 5%; topical antimycotic + intravenous Echinacin® ampoule (n=20) 15%; and topical antimycotic + oral 2 ml Echinacin® liquid (n= 60) 16.7% *(Coeugniet EG and Kuhnast R. Recurrent candidiasis: adjuvant immunotherapy with different formulations of Echinacin®. Therapiewoche 36:3352-8, 1986).*

> **Experimental Study:** Echinacin® administered intramuscularly on 4 successive days to 12 healthy males demonstrated a rapid and continous increase in granulocyte phagocytosis activity against *C. albicans (Mose J. Effect of echinacin on phagocytosis and natural killer cells. Med Welt 34:1463-7, 1983).*

See Also:

> *Steinmuller C et al. Polysaccharides isolated from plant cell cultures of Echinacea purpurea enhance the resistance of immunosuppressed mice against systemic infections with Candida albicans and Listeria monocytogenes. Int J Immunopharmacol 15(5):605-14, 1993*

Garlic (*Allium sativum*):

Administration may be beneficial.

Animal Experimental Study: Garlic treatment at 2% and 4% concentrations in feed exerted a protective effect in chickens against candidiasis. In chickens with induced candidiasis, feed containing 5% garlic was successful in eliminating candida (*Prasad G and Sharma VD. Efficacy of garlic (Allium sativum) treatment against experimental candidiasis in chicks. Br Vet J 136:448-51, 1980*).

In vitro Studies:

Adetumbi M et al. Allium sativum (garlic) inhibits lipid synthesis by Candida albicans. Antimicrob Agents Chemother 30:499-501, 1986

Sandhu DK et al. Sensitivity of yeasts isolated from cases of vaginitis to aqueous extracts of garlic. Mykosen 23:691-8, 1980

Moore GS and Atkins RD. The fungicidal and fungistatic effects of an aqueous garlic extract on medically important yeast-like fungi. Mycologia 69:341-8, 1977

Solanum nigrescens:

A cream containing the ethanol extract may be useful in the topical treatment of candida vaginitis.

Experimental Study: A cream containing a 50% ethanolic maceration of *Solanum nigrescens* was applied daily to the vagina of female guinea pigs for 15 days and observed for another 15 days. Since no inflammatory changes were observed, this preparation was used for clinical trials. Two groups of 50 non-pregnant women with confirmed *C. albicans* vaginitis were treated for 15 days, one group with intra-vaginal suppositories containing *S. nigrescens* maceration and the other with nystatin suppositories. By statistical analysis it was demonstrated that both groups behaved in a similar beneficial way suggesting that this plant may be effective for the treatment of candidal vaginitis (*Giron LM et al. Anticandidal activity of plants used for the treatment of vaginitis in Guatemala and clinical trial of a Solanum nigrescens preparation. J Ethnopharmacol 22(3):307-13, 1988*).

Tea Tree oil (*Melaleuca alternifolia*):

Local application may be effective for candida vaginitis.

Experimental Study: 28 pts. inserted a tea tree oil suppository into the vagina every evening. One wk. later, one pt. discontinued treatment due to vaginal burning. 30 days later, 21/28 pts. showed a complete recovery, while the remaining 7 pts. were clinically asymptomatic (*Belaiche P. Treatment of vaginal infections of Candida albicans with the essential oil of Melaleuca alternifolia. Phytotherapie vol.15, 1985*).

Experimental Study: A 40% solution of tea tree oil emulsified with isopropyl alcohol and water was shown to be highly effective for the treatment of vaginal candidiasis as well as cervicitis, chronic endocervicitis, and trichomonal vaginitis. Weekly in-office treatment involved thorough washing of the perineum, labia, and vagina with pHiso-Hex. Usually 4 - 6 visits were necessary. After drying, the affected areas were washed with a 1% tea tree oil solution and then a tampon (three 4X4 inch sponges) saturated with the 40% tea tree oil solution were inserted into the vagina. Patients were instructed to remove the tampon in 24 hours (*Pena EO. Melaleuca alternifolia oil. Uses for trichomonal vaginitis and other vaginal infections. Obstet Gynecol 19:793-5, 1962*).

See Also:

> *Belaiche P. Treatment of skin infection with the essential oil of Melaleuca alternifolia. Phytotherapie vol. 15, 1985*

CARDIAC ARRHYTHMIA

See Also: ATHEROSCLEROSIS

Berberine:

Berberine is an alkaloid extracted from the roots and bark of various plants such as golden-seal (*Hydrastis canadensis*), barberry root bark (*Berberis vulgaris*), and Oregon grape root (*Berberis aquifolium*).

Administration may prevent and treat ventricular arrhythmias caused by ischemia.

Animal Experimental Study: Electrical stimulation and drug-induced ventricular fibrillation, monophasic action potentials, and triggered activity were studied before and after administration of tetrahydroberberine in rabbits, dogs and guinea pigs. Results indicated that THB had a potent antifibrillatory effect, which may be attributed to its blockade of potassium, calcium and sodium currents (*Sun AY, Li DX. Antifibrillatory effect of tetrahydroberberine. Chung Kuo Yao Li Hsueh Pao 14(4):301-5, 1993*).

Animal Experimental Study: Results of studies on ischemic and reperfused myocardium in rats suggest that tetrahydroberberine could protect the myocardium from ischemic and reperfusion injury (*Zhou J, Xuan B, Li DX. Effect of tetrdroberberine on ischemic and reperfused myocardium in rats. Chung Kuo Yao Li Hsueh Pao 14(2):130-3, 1993*).

Experimental Study: 100 pts. with ventricular tachyarrhythmias received berberine. Based on 24-48 hr. ambulatory monitoring, 62% of pts. had 50% or greater, and 38% had 90% or greater, VPC suppression. The mean value of VPCs in the whole gp. was significantly decreased from 452 ± 421.8 beats/hr. to 271 ± 352.7 beats/hr. ($p<0.001$). There were no side effects except for mild gastroenterologic symptoms in some pts. (*Huang W. [Ventricular tachyarrhythmias treated with berberine.] Chung Hua Hsin Hsueh Kuan Ping Tsa Chih 18(3):155-6, 190, 1990*) (*in Chinese*).

See Also:

Animal Experimental Study: *Huang Z, Chen S, Zhang G, et al. Protective effects of berberine and phentolamine on myocardial oxygenation damage. Chin Med Sci J 7(4):221-5, 1992*

Animal Experimental Study: *Huang WM, Yan H, Jin JM, et al. Beneficial effects of berberine on hemodynamics during acute ischemic left ventricular failure in dogs. Chin Med J (Engl) 105(12):1014-9, 1992*

Animal Experimental Study: *Huang WM, Wu ZD, Gan YQ. [Effects of berberine on ischemic ventricular arrhythmia.] Chung Hua Hsin Hsueh Kuan Ping Tsa Chih 17(5):300-1,319, 1989 (in Chinese)*

Garlic (*Allium sativum*) or
Onion (*Allium cepa*):

The beneficial effects of garlic and onion are thought to be due to a variety of sulfur-containing compounds, especially allicin. Clinically, commercial garlic preparations concentrated for alliin appear to be the most useful and because alliin is relatively 'odorless' until it is converted to allicin in the body, these preparations are more socially acceptable. The compound alliin is converted to allicin by the enzyme alliinase which is activated when garlic is crushed. The dosage of the commercial product should provide a daily dose of 8 mg alliin or a total allicin potential of 4,000 mcg. (*See:* '*ATHEROSCLEROSIS*')

Administration may reduce cardiac arrythmias due to ischemia.

Animal Experimental Study: Animals fed 1% garlic powder (Kwai) in their chow demonstrated significant reduction in the incidence of ventricular tachycardia and fibrillation after ligation of the descending brand of the left ventricular artery (*Isensee H, Rietz B, Jacob R. Cardioprotective action of garlic (Allium sativum). Arzneim Forsch 43(2):94-8, 1993*).

Ginkgo biloba:

The 24% ginkgoflavonglycosides extract at a dose of 40 mg 3 times daily may be effective. Also, mixtures of ginkgolides may be of benefit. (*See:* '*CEREBROVASCULAR DISEASE*')

Administration may reduce arrhythmias due to ischemia.

Animal Experimental Study: Ginkgolide B (a major active glycoside in *Ginkgo biloba*) was comparable to metoprolol and diltiazem in preventing ischemia-induced ventricular fibrillation and against ventricular tachycardia and negative preventricular beats. It was ineffective, however, against arrhythmias caused by reperfusion after ischemia. Its antiarrhythmic effect appears related to an antagonism of an increase in slow calcium influx induced by Platelet Activating Factor in myocardial cells (*Koltai M et al. Ginkgolide B protects isolated hearts against arrhythmias induced by ischaemia but not reperfusion. Europ J Pharmacol 164:293-302, 1989*).

Animal Experimental Studies: The effects of *Ginkgo biloba* extract was studied on various models of cardiac ischemia both *in vitro* and in *vivo*. On the two *in vitro* models of ischemia-reperfusion (rat and guinea-pig hearts), the extract failed to affect cardiac function parameters, but induced a significant decrease in the intensity of ventricular fibrillation during reperfusion. On normal or hypertrophied heart *in vivo*, the extract provided effective protection against the electrocardiographic disorders induced by ischemia. On the different models of global or localized ischemia (followed or not by reperfusion), a decrease of arrhythmia without change in cardiovascular parameters was regularly noted (*Guillon JM et al. [Effects of Ginkgo biloba extract on 2 models of experimental myocardial ischemia.] Presse Med 15(31):1516-19, 1986*) (*in French*).

Hawthorn (*Crataegus oxyacantha* and *C. monogyna*):

Extracts of hawthorn berry, leaves, and flowering tops extracts are widely used by physicians in Europe for their cardiotonic effects. The beneficial effects of hawthorn extracts are due to the presence of procyanidin flavonoids. Standardized extracts, similar to those used in the clinical studies cited below are the preferred form.

The dosage for hawthorn extracts standardized to contain 1.8% vitexin-4[1]-rhamnoside or 10% procyanidins is 120-240 mg 3 times daily; for extracts standardized to contain 18% procyanidolic oligomers, the dosage is 240 to 480 mg daily. (*See: 'ATHEROSCLEROSIS'; 'CONGESTIVE HEART FAILURE'; 'HYPERTENSION'*)

Administration may be beneficial.

Review Article: Preparations of Crataegus are used in minor forms of heart disease including angina, minor forms of congestive heart failure, and cardiac arrhythmia. From experiments with animals, preparations of Crataegus exhibited the following effects: increased coronary blood flow, decreased arterial blood pressure, increased peripheral blood flow, decreased heart rate, and improved contractility of the heart muscle. Crataegus preparations are extremely well-tolerated. The acute oral toxicity (LD50) of Crataegus preparations and constituents was found to be in the range of 6 g/kg (*Ammon HPT, Handel M. [Crataegus, toxicology and pharmacology, Part I: Toxicity]. Planta Med 43(2):105-20, 1981; Part II: Pharmacodynamics. Planta Med 43(3):209-39, 1981; Part III: Pharmacodynamics and pharmacokinetics. Planta Med 43(4):313-22, 1981*) (*in German*).

Animal Experimental Study: Crude extracts of the bark and leaves of *Crataegus monogyna* prevented aconitine induced arrythmias in rabbits (*Thompson EB, Aynilian GH, Gora P, Farnsworth NR. Preliminary study of potential antiarrhythmic effects of Crataegus monogyna. J Pharm Sci 63(12):1936-7, 1974*).

CATARACT

Bilberry (*Vaccinium myrtillus*):

Bilberry, or European blueberry, is a shrubby perennial plant that grows in the woods and forest meadows of Europe.

The standard dose for bilberry extracts is based on its anthocyanoside content, as calculated by its anthocyanidin percentage. The dosage for a bilberry extract standardized for an anthocyanidin content of 25% is 80 to 160 mg three times daily.

- with Vitamin E:

Administration of bilberry extract along with vitamin E may prevent cataract progression.

Experimental Study: Bilberry extract plus vitamin E stopped progression of cataract formation in 97% of 50 pts. with senile cortical cataracts *(Bravetti G. Preventive medical treatment of senile cataract with vitamin E and anthocyanosides: clnical evaluation. Ann Ottalmol Clin Ocul 115:109, 1989).*

- -

COMBINATION TREATMENT

Hachimijiogan:

Hachimijiogan is an ancient Chinese formula used in the treatment of cataract. It contains the following 8 herbs per 22 grams: Alismatis rhizome (3.0 g), Rehmanniae root (6.0 g), Cornus fruit (3.0 g), Dioscoreae rhizome (3.0 g), Hoelen (3.0 g), Mountan bark (2.5 g), Cinnamon bark (1.0) and Aconite root (0.5 g).

The standard dose is 150-300 mg per day.

Administration may be beneficial.

Animal Experimental Study: Mice with hereditary cataracts were studied. Hachimijiogan significantly delayed cataract appearance compared to controls by 4 days, the equivalence of 13.9 yrs. in humans. It also suppressed the variation of sodium and potassium ion levels in the lens with cataractogenesis, had a slight action as a reducing agent, and dramatically reactivated the sodium-potassium ATPase activity damaged with cataract formation. Results suggest that Hachimijiogan may have a prophylactic effect in regard to cataracts caused by inhibition of sodium-potassium ATPase activity or oxidation of lens protein *(Kamei A, Hisada T, Iwata S. The evaluation of therapeutic efficacy of hachimi-jio-gan (traditional Chinese medicine) to mouse hereditary cataract. J Ocul Pharmacol 4(4):311-9, 1988).*

Animal Experimental Study: Hachimijiogan was evaluated for its effects on rat galactosemic cataracts. The formula significantly suppressed the variations of hydration rate, sodium/potassium ratios, and calcium ion level in the the lens with the advance of galactosemic cataract, especially when it was administered before or concurrently with the galactose diet. The formula was also able to delay the progressive rate of lens opacification, even though it failed to suppress the accumulation of galactitol in the lens. Results suggest the Hachimijiogan may control the balance of sodium, potassium and calcium ions which are important in the maintenance of lens transparency and thus may theoretically help to prevent diabetic cataract   (*Kamei A, Hisada T, Iwata S. The evaluation of therapeutic efficacy of hachimi-jio-gan (traditional Chinese medicine) to rat galactosemic cataract. J Ocul Pharmacol 3(3):239-48, 1987*).

Animal Experimental Study: Aged rats fed Hachimijiogan demonstrated an increase in the content of glutathione, an antioxidant, in the lens   (*Haranaka R et al. Pharmacological action of Hachimijiogan (Ba-wei-wan) on the metabolism of aged subjects. Am J Chinese Med 24:59-67, 1986*)

Experimental Study: Hachimijiogan was tested on pts. in the early stage of cataract formation. 60% improved, 20% showed no progression of their cataracts and 20% showed continued progression   (*Fujihira K. Treatment of cataract of Ba-wei-wan. J Soc Oriental Med Japan 24:465-79, 1974*).

CEREBROVASCULAR DISEASE

See Also: ATHEROSCLEROSIS
DEMENTIA
HYPERTENSION

Ginkgo biloba:

Ginkgo biloba extracts standardized to contain 24% ginkgoflavonglycosides are among the most well-studied plant-based medicines. More than 40 double-blind studies have shown it be effective in cerebral vascular insufficiency. *Ginkgo biloba* extract (GBE) is a registered drug in Germany and France for the treatment of cerebrovascular disease and is among the leading prescription medicines. Sales of GBE account for 1.0% and 1.5% of total prescription sales in Germany and France respectively. In 1989, over 100,000 physicians worldwide combined to write over 10,000,000 prescriptions.

Because of the multitude of vascular effects, *Ginkgo biloba* extract offers effective treatment for the signs, symptoms, and underlying pathophysiology of cerebrovascular insufficiency. The standard dosage for GBE is 40 mg 3 times daily *(Kleijnen J, Knipschild P. Ginkgo biloba. Lancet 340:1136-9, 1992; DeFeudis FV. Ginkgo biloba extract (EGb 761). Pharmacological Activities and Clinical Applications. Elsevier, New York, 1991; EW Funfgeld, Ed. Rokan (Ginkgo Biloba). Recent Results in Pharmacology and Clinic. Springer-Verlag, New York, 1988).*

Meta-Analysis: A meta-analysis was made on the quality of research on more than 40 clinical studies of GBE in the treatment of cerebral insufficiency. The results of the analysis indicate that the quality of the research reviewed was on par with the research methods used in investigating ergoloid mesylates an approved drug in the treatment of dementia, including Alzheimer's disease. The analysis further substantiated that GBE is effective in reducing all symptoms of cerebral insufficiency, including impaired mental function *(Kleijnen J, Knipschild P. Ginkgo biloba for cerebral insufficiency. Br J Clinical Pharmacol 34:352-8, 1992).*

Experimental Double-blind Study: GBE improved mental function in patients suffering from cerebral insufficiency. Significant improvements were noted in psychometric computer-aided examination of the short-term memory after 6 weeks and of the basic learning rate after 24 weeks in the group given GBE *(Grabel E. Cerebral insuffiency - The influence of Ginkgo biloba extract EGB 761 on basic parameters of mental performance. Placebo-controlled, randomized double-blind study with computer-aided measurement. Fortsch Med 110(5):73-6, 1992) (In German).*

Experimental Double-blind Study: 80 pts. with cerebrovascular disorders were given either GBE or dihydroergotoxine. On the basis of psychometric tests and assessment scales, it was shown that treatment with either substance improved the condition of the patients. Intergroup comparison revealed no major statistically significant differences (*Gerhardt G, Rogalla K, Jaeger J. [Drug therapy of disorders of cerebral performance. Randomized comparative study of dihydroergotoxine and Ginkgo biloba extract] Fortschr Med 108(19):384-8, 1990*) (*In German*).

Experimental Double-blind Study: 36 pts. with classical symptoms of cerebro-organic syndrome who had pathological findings on at least 2 of 4 tests (quantified EEG; saccadic eye movements; Wiener Determination Test; Number Connection Test) received either GBE (EGb 761) 40 mg 3 times daily or placebo. On both the saccadic eye movement test and the psychometric tests, a highly significant difference between gps. could be seen at 4 wks. as well as at 8 weeks. Also, a marked reduction in the theta proportion of the theta/alpha ratio was found, but only in the GBE group (*Hofferberth B. Effect of Ginkgo biloba extract on neurophysiological and psychometric measurement results in patients with cerebro-organic syndrome. A double blind study versus placebo. Arzneimittelforsch 39(II):918-20, 1989*) (*in German*).

Experimental Double-blind Study: 100 pts. aged 55-85 with CVI received either a Ginkgo preparation (30 mg ginkgo-heterosides, 112 mg Ginkgo extract) or placebo. Experimental pts. had >50% improvement in the major symptoms of cerebrovascular insufficiency such as memory loss, poor concentration, fear, tinnitus and headache (*Schmidt U. - reported in: Ginkgo biloba vermindert die Gedachtnislucken. Artezeitung 130, 17 juli, 1989*) (*in German*).

Experimental Double-blind Study: 166 pts. with moderate to severe cerebral disorders due to aging living in retirement homes randomly received either GBE or placebo. Using a specially designed geriatric clinical evaluation scale, the difference between the GBE gp. and the placebo gp. became significant by the third month and increased further over the 12 mo. of the study. Pts. on placebo had a slight initial improvement, then stagnation (*Taillandier J et al. Ginkgo biloba extract in the treatment of cerebral disorders due to aging. Longitudinal, multicenter, double blind study versus placebo, in EW Fünfgeld, Ed. Rökan (Ginkgo Biloba). Recent Results in Pharmacology and Clinic. Berlin, Springer-Verlag, 1988:291-301*).

Experimental Double-blind Study: 40 pts. aged 55-85 with mild to moderate cerebrovascular insufficiency randomly received either GBE 40 mg 3 times daily or placebo. After 12 wks., its overall efficacy was rated as 90% compared to placebo. In the GBE gp., the values for the total SCAG score (Sandoz Clinical Assessment - Geriatric) dropped by 9 points on the average, while they were unchanged in the placebo gp. (p=0.000005). Evaluation of the separate items showed a particular effect on disturbances of short-term memory and mental awareness as well as on dizziness. Superior effects were also shown in regard to headaches and tinnitus (*Halama P et al. Disturbances in cerebral performance of vascular origin. Randomized, double blind study on the efficacy of Ginkgo biloba extract. Fort Med 106:408-12, 1988*) (*in German*).

Animal Experimental Study: The gerbil is the animal model best adapted to experimental pathology studies of acute ischemia since it is devoid of any substitute vertebrobasilar vascular tissue, so that unilateral carotid artery ligature produces cerebral ischemia with quantifiable neurological signs, metabolic pertubations (especially mitochondrial) and cerebral edema development closely resembling the symptoms revealed by physiopathology in human clinical studies. Under such conditions, Gerbils given *Ginkgo biloba* extract either orally or by IV administration demonstrated clear-cut, highly significant improvements consisting of normalization of mitochondrial respiration, diminution of cerebral edema, correction of the accompanying ionic pertubations, and practically total functional restoration revealed by a normal neurological index (*Spinnewyn B et al. [Effects of Ginkgo biloba extract on a cerebral ischemia model in gerbils.] Presse Med 15 (31):1511-15, 1986*) (*in French*).

Review Article: *Ginkgo biloba* extract limits the formation of cerebral edema and suppresses its neurological consequences, whether the edema is of cytotoxic or vasogenic origin. Several membrane mechanisms could be implicated in its protective action (*Etienne A et al. [Mechanism of action of Ginkgo biloba extract in experimental cerebral edema.] Presse Med 15 (31):1506-10, 1986*) (*in French*).

Experimental Double-blind Crossover Study: 90 pts. (mean age 66.5 yrs.) with chronic cerebrovascular insufficiency randomly received GBE and placebo in either order for 45 days. Compared to placebo, GBE improved the point evaluation in the WAIS tasks sensitive to mental losses. The differences between GBE and placebo in the cube test, work recognition, Rey Figure Test and memory performance test are significant. Based on the psychological test battery, GBE effects a distinct improvement in memory efficiency, logical thinking and vigilance. Based on the patients' subjective assessment of changes on GBE, the extract is particularly active against those symptoms with a presumed rheological or vascular-oriented pathogenesis. GBE improved the anxiety-relieving effects of placebo, and significantly reduced anxious behavior. In the GBE gp., there was also a significant reduction in the number of cases with symptoms of dizziness, headache and asthenia. The multifactorial action of GBE clearly inhibits the progressive reduction in intellectual and cognitive ability, with significant improvement in ability to concentrate, recollection capacity and ability to make logical allocations (*Arrigo A. Treatment of chronic cerebrovascular insufficiency with Ginkgo biloba extract. Therapiewoche 36:5208-18, 1986*) (*in German*).

Experimental Study: 112 ambulant pts. (mean age 71 yrs.) with signs of chronic cerebral insufficiency (such as vertigo, headache, tinnitus, short-term memory disturbances, restricted vigilance and depressed mood) received GBE 120 mg daily. After 1 yr., there was a statistically significant ($p<0.001$) regression of all symptoms. Initial improvement continued for the duration of the study, making a placebo response unlikely, and there were no adverse side-effects (*Vorberg G. Ginkgo biloba extract: a long-term study of chronic cerebral insufficiency in geriatric patients. Clin Trials J 22(2):149-57, 1985*).

Experimental Double-blind Study: 33 pts. (mean age 59) with vertigo and ataxia randomly received either GBE 120 mg/d or placebo. After 6 wks., cranio-corpography showed a statistically significant decrease in the lateral sway amplitude in the Underberger 'stepping on the spot' test for the treatment gp., while the placebo gp. showed only a slight decrease. After 12 wks., the mean amplitude of the treatment gp. approached normal values for healthy persons, while the placebo gp. showed no further improvement. (GBE vs. placebo after 6 wks.: $p<0.020$; after 12 wks.: $p<0.005$). 50% of pts. in the treatment gp. vs. 20% of pts. in the placebo gp. reported a subjective decrease in vertigo.   There were no adverse side effects (*Claussen C-F, Kirtane MV. Randomized double blind study on the effect of Ginkgo biloba extract in dizziness and unstable gait in the elderly, in C-F Claussen, Ed. Presbyvertigo, Presbyataxie, Presbytinnitus, Gleichgewichts-störungen im Alter. Berlin, Springer-Verlag, 1985:103-115*) (*in German*).

Experimental Double-blind Study: 189 hospitalized female pts. aged 49-95, with half being older than 76, with various atherosclerotic conditions were studied. All were inpatients for several mo. or yrs. due to disabling conditions, frequently of vascular origin, plus inability to live alone due to age or social conditions. After 6 mo., clinical and psychometric measures showed significant differences in favor of GBE. Pts. receiving the extract showed increased intellectual and operational performance in the context of improved mood; these changes were found to be statistically significant as compared to pts. receiving placebo. There were no significant side effects (*Augustin P. Ginkgo biloba extract in geriatrics. Clinical and psychometric study of 189 patients. Psychologie Médicale 8:123-30, 1976*) (*in French*).

Administration may improve blood viscosity in patients with completed strokes.

Experimental Controlled Study: Compared to 90 pt. controls, administration of GBE to 60 pts. with completed strokes improved hematocrit and blood and plasma viscosity (*Anadere et al. Hemorheological findings in patients with completed stroke and the influence of Ginkgo biloba extract. Clin Hemorheo 5:411-20, 1985*).

CONGESTIVE HEART FAILURE

See Also: ATHEROSCLEROSIS
HYPERTENSION

Coleus forskohlii:

The root of _Coleus forskohlii_, an herb used in Ayurvedic medicine, contains a diterpene molecule known as forskolin which is a powerful activator of adenylate cyclase in various tissue leading to elevation of cAMP. In the heart, this causes an increased force of contraction (positive inotropic effect) which may be effective in congestive heart failure.

The forskolin content of Coleus root is typically 0.2-0.3%; thus the forskolin content of Coleus products may not be sufficient to produce a pharmacological effect. Therefore, it is best to use standardized extracts which have concentrated the forskolin content. The dosage of the extract should provide a daily intake of 5-10 mg of forskolin, although oral administration of 50 mg/kg of an ethanol extract of Coleus was as effective as 10 mg/kg of pure forskolin in reducing blood pressure in rats, suggesting that the activity of the extract is higher than would be expected from its forskolin content alone.

> **Experimental Study:** In 7 pts. with dilated cardiomyopathy (DCM) with normal (gp. A) and 8 DCM pts. with pathological dP/dtmax-values (gp. B), the pressure/volume (P/V) effects of the administration of dobutamine, 10 mcg/kg/min IV, and forskolin, 3 mcg/kg/min IV, were analyzed. For the total gp. (A + B) there was no change of contractility with forskolin (p=0.05); with dobutamine; however, contractility rose by an average of +25%. The preload decline was more pronounced with forskolin (LVEDP by -27%) as compared to dobutamine (-19%), while left ventricular (LV)-function improved only moderately with forskolin (+9%) and significantly (+34%) with dobutamine. Thus, forskolin improved LV-function primarily via reduction of preload in DCM-hearts and without rising metabolic costs. Beneficial hemodynamic effects with forskolin are quantitatively less as compared to those with dobutamine (accompanied by higher MVO_2-costs). It is concluded that residual myocardial reserves in DCM are mobilized by dobutamine rather than forskolin. Serial P/V-loop and on-line MVO_2 registration aided in the demonstration of forskolin efficacy as compared to dobutamine. Higher doses of forskolin may be required to produce a positive inotropic effect (_Kramer W, et al. Effects of forskolin on left ventricular function in dilated cardiomyopathy. Arzneim Forsch 37(3):364-7, 1987_).

> **Animal Experimental Study:** The main pharmacological action of coleonol (forskolin) in animals is a blood pressure-lowering effect due to relaxation of the vascular smooth muscle. In small doses it has a positive inotropic effect on isolated rabbit heart as well as on cat heart _in vivo_ (_Dubey MP et al. Pharmacological studies on coleonol, a hypotensive diterpene from Coleus forskohlii. J Ethnopharmacol 3:1-13, 1981_).

Animal Experimental Study: Forskolin exerts positive inotropic effects which are not blocked by beta-blockers. Forskolin also lowers blood pressure in dogs, cats, spontaneously hypertensive rats, and renal hypertensive rats (*Lindner E, Dohadwalla AN, Bhattacharya BK. Positive inotropic and blood pressure lowering activity of a diterpene derivative from Coleus forskohli: Forskolin. Arznneim Forsch 28(2):284-9, 1978*).

Digitalis and other Cardioactive Glycosides:

Digitalis and other plants containing cardioactive glycosides have a long history of use in congestive heart failure. Despite centuries of use, the verdict is still not in regarding the role of cardiac glycosides in the long-term management of mild to moderate cases of congestive heart failure.

Due to the risk of toxicity, only well-defined preparations should be used according to established guidelines. Digitalis is best reserved for severe cases of congestive heart failure.

Plants with cardioactive glycosides:

> *Adonis vernalis* (yellow pheasant's eye)
> *Convallaria majalis* (lily of the valley)
> *Digitalis* spp. (foxglove)
> *Scilla maritima* or *Urginea maritima* (squill)
> *Strophanthus* spp.

Review Article: In the United States, the number of admissions for congestive heart failure increased from 51,000 in 1955 to 274,000 by 1988. Even accounting for population growth and an increase in the number of elderly, this represents a 2-fold increase. Additionally, CHF was responsible for about 643,000 hospitalizations in 1988. In 1990, digoxin was one of the most commonly prescribed drugs in the US, accounting for greater than 21 million prescriptions. There has been little decline in the drug's use over the last 5 years, indicating that newer treatments for CHF have not replaced the widespread use of digitalis. Despite these findings, considerable controversy surrounds the appropriateness of its role and value in treating CHF patients who are in sinus rhythm. A number of recent, uncontrolled and controlled studies have arrived at apparently contradictory conclusions concerning the effects of digitalis on mortality in post-myocardial infarction and heart failure patients. A large, double-blind, randomized, controlled clinical trial to evaluate the effects of digitalis on mortality, morbidity and quality of life is currently underway (*Yusuf S et al. Need for a large randomized trial to evaluate the effects of digitalis on morbidity and mortality in congestive heart failure. Am J Cardiol 69(18):64G-70G, 1992*).

Review Article: Limitations and contraindications for the use of digitalis substances are reported, especially in the treatment of ischemic heart disease. Preliminary data regarding the effects of digitalis on the diastolic phase are unfavorable, although the relationship between digitalis and diastolic function ought to be studied in greater depth in various clinical conditions. In spite of many recent trials, the old question of the usefulness of digitalis in the chronic treatment of patients in sinus rhythm and heart failure is still debated. An important clinical benefit in the chronic use of digitalis appears restricted to a relatively small proportion of patients with severe congestive heart failure, while in the majority of chronically treated subjects the effects of the drug are scanty or insignificant. The beneficial effect of digitalis used chronically is essentially believed to be due to its positive inotropic action. Since the vagomimetic and the antiadrenergic effects of digitalis have been demonstrated to be independent from its inotropic action, they could be considered determinants of the clinical benefits of digitalis. These indirect effects may be useful in the control of the negative neuroendocrine response developing during congestive heart failure. Thus the statement that digitalis is essentially an inotropic agent seems restrictive; its definition should reflect the favorable effects obtained in some cases of congestive heart failure rather than its various and contrasting underlying mechanisms of action (*Bolognesi R, Tsialtas D, Manca C. Digitalis and heart failure: does digitalis really produce beneficial effects through a positive inotropic action? Cardiovasc Drugs Ther 6(5):459-64, 1992*).

Review Article: Although the cardiac glycosides are universally acknowledged to be important agents in the drug therapy of advanced congestive heart failure (CHF), their role in the treatment of more moderate CHF, particularly in patients in sinus rhythm, remains controversial. Over the past decade, several randomized clinical trials have been undertaken to help clarify the appropriate use of the cardiac glycosides in these patients. Although the data are not conclusive, the available evidence indicates that digoxin is efficacious and relatively safe in patients with CHF whether given alone or in combination with vasodilators. Ongoing myocardial ischemia, hypokalemia and reduced drug clearance due to renal disease or drug interactions remain the clinical parameters most closely associated with digitalis toxicity. The introduction of Fab fragments of antidigoxin antibodies has increased the margin of safety in the use of the cardiac glycosides (*Kelly RA. Cardiac glycosides and congestive heart failure. Am J Cardiol 65(10):10E-16E,22E-23E, 1990*).

Experimental Double-blind Study: 433 pts. aged 29-80 with mild to moderate CHF were given digoxin 0.125 mg, xamoterol 200 mg, or placebo twice daily. Patients were assessed at baseline and after 3 months. Compared with placebo, xamoterol significantly increased exercise tolerance and improved breathlessness and feelings of tiredness. Digoxin showed no statistically significant over placebo on exercise tolerance, but did improve symptom scores on the Likert scale (*The German and Austrian Xameterol Study Group. Double-blind placebo-controlled comparison of digoxin and xamoterol in chronic heart failure. Lancet i:488-93, 1988*).

Review Article: A search of the medical literature from 1960 to 1982 identified 736 articles, of which 16 specifically addressed the clinical evaluation of digitalis therapy for patients with congestive heart failure and sinus rhythm. Only two double-blind, placebo-controlled trials provided clinically useful information. One study showed that digoxin therapy could be withdrawn successfully in elderly patients with stable congestive heart failure. The other showed that patients with chronic heart failure and an S3 gallop benefited from digoxin therapy (*Mulrow CD, Feussner JR, Velez R. Reevaluation of digitalis efficacy. New light on an old leaf. Ann Intern Med 101(1):113-7, 1984*).

Hawthorn (*Crataegus oxyacantha*; *C. monogyna*):

Extracts of hawthorn berry, leaves, and flowering tops extracts are widely used by physicians in Europe for their cardiotonic effects. The beneficial effects of hawthorn extracts are due to the presence of proyanidin flavonoids. Standardized extracts, similar to those used in the clinical studies cited below are the preferred form. The dosage for hawthorn extracts standardized to contain 1.8% vitexin-4[1]-rhamnoside or 10% procyanidins is 120-240 mg three times daily; for extracts standardized to contain 18% procyanidolic oligomers, the dosage is 240 to 480 mg daily. *(See: 'ATHEROSCLEROSIS'; 'CARDIAC ARRHYTHMIA'; 'HYPERTENSION')*

Administration may be effective in mild to moderate CHF.

Experimental Double-blind Study: In 30 pts. with cardiac insufficiency, a randomized double-blind study was carried out to determine the efficacy of the Crataegus special extract WS 1442 (Crataegutt® forte), an extract standardized to contain 15 mg procyanidin oligomers per 80 mg capsule. Treatment duration was 8 weeks, and the substance was administered at a dose of 1 capsule taken twice a day. The main target parameters were alteration in the pressure-x-rate product (PRP) under standardised loading on a bicycle ergometer, and a score of subjective improvement of complaints elicited by a questionnaire. Secondary parameters were exercise tolerance and the change in heart rate and arterial blood pressure. The active substance gp. showed a statistically significant advantage over placebo in terms of changes in PRP (at a load of 50 W) and the score, but also in the secondary parameter heart rate. In both groups, systolic and diastolic blood pressure was mildly reduced. No adverse reactions occurred *(Leuchtgens H. [Crataegus Special Extract WS 1442 in NYHA II heart failure. A placebo controlled randomized double-blind study]. Fortschr Med 111(20-21):352-4, 1993) (in German).*

Review Article: The effectiveness of Crataegus preparations have been demonstrated in numerous pharmacological studies. These effects, produced mainly by the flavonoids, indicate a simultaneous cardiotropic and vasodilatory action, as confirmed clinically in double-blind studies. This means that Crataegus can be employed for cardiological indications for which digitalis is not yet indicated. Prior to use, however, a Crataegus preparation must meet certain preconditions with respect to dosage, pharmaceutical quality of the preparation, and an accurate definition of the latter *(Blesken R. [Crataegus in cardiology]. Fortschr Med 110(15):290-2, 1992) (in German).*

Experimental Double-blind Study: 36 pts. suffering from decreasing cardiac performance given Crataegutt® (an extract standardized to contain 3 mg procyanidin oligomers per 60 mg capsule) demonstrated significant improvement in cardiac function as determined by exercise tolerance, pressure heart rate product, and physician's rating. Patients also noted an increased sense of wellbeing *(O'Conolly VM et al. [Treatment of cardiac performance (NYHA stages I to II) in advanced age with standardized crataegus extract]. Fortschr Med 104:805-8, 1986) (in German).*

Review Article: Preparations of Crataegus are used in minor forms of heart disease including angina, minor forms of congestive heart failure, and cardiac arrythmia. From experiments with animals, preparations of Crataegus exhibited the following effects: increased coronary blood flow, decreased arterial blood pressure, increased peripheral blood flow, decreased heart rate, and improved contractility of the heart muscle. Crataegus preparations are extremely well-tolerated. The acute oral toxicity (LD50) of Crataegus preparations and constituents was found to be in the range of 6 g/kg *(Ammon HPT, Handel M. [Crataegus, toxicology and pharmacology, Part I: Toxicity]. Planta Med 43(2):105-20, 1981; Part II: Pharmacodynamics. Planta Med 43(3):209-39, 1981; Part III: Pharmacodynamics and pharmacokinetics. Planta Med 43(4):313-22, 1981) (in German).*

See Also:

> **Animal Experimental Study:** *Nasa Y et al. Protective effect of Crataegus extract on the cardiac mechanical dysfunction in isolated perfused working rat heart. Arzniem Forsch 43(3):945-9, 1993.*

- with digitalis or other cardiac glycoside:

> **Experimental Study:** Of 170 pts. with various forms of cardiac insufficiency treated with Crataelanat® (32 mg of Crataegus extract with 1/8th mg strophantin), 126 with severe decompensations experienced improved cardiac function. Good results were also achieved in pts. with decompensated cor pulmonale *(Wolkerstorfer H. [Treatment of heart disease with a digoxin-crataegus combination] Munch Med Wochenschr 108(8):438-41, 1966) (in German).*

CONSTIPATION

See Also: IRRITABLE BOWEL SYNDROME

Anthraquinone-containing stimulant laxatives:

Stimulant laxatives act on the large intestine by increasing peristalsis. Preparations containing senna have emerged as the most popular as senna is better tolerated (less griping) and is perhaps the most physiologic compared to other sources of anthraquinones and non-fiber laxatives (*Godding EW. Laxatives and the special role of senna. Pharmacology 36(Suppl 1):230-6, 1988*).

Other sources of anthraquinones include *Aloe spp.*, Cascara sagrada (*Rhamnus purshiana*), rhubarb (*Rheum officinale*), and frangula (*Rhamnus frangula*).

It is generally recommended that commercial over-the-counter sources be used rather than crude plant material, because the former contain standardized concentrates of anthraquinones and allow for more accurate dosages.

Anthraquinone-containing stimulant laxatives usually produce a soft to semifluid stool in 6-12 hrs. after ingestion.

> WARNINGS: Although extremely effective in promoting bowel movements, the use of stimulant laxatives should be minimized. They should never be used as an initial treatment of constipation, and they should be discontinued as soon as normal bowel function is restored. Anthraquinone laxatives can produce severe cramping, electrolyte and fluid deficiencies, and malabsorption of nutrients. Since anthraquinones are absorbed into breast milk, they may cause diarrhea in breast-fed infants. Stimulant laxatives should not be used if symptoms of appendicitis are present (abdominal pain, nausea, and vomiting). In general, long-term use of stimulant laxatives can lead to a poorly functioning colon and dependence on the laxative for relief. Anthaquinone-containing stimulant laxatives may impart a yellowish-brown color to acid urine and a reddish color to alkaline urine. Prolonged use may produce benign pigmentation of the colonic mucosa (melanosis coli) that may regress after discontinuation.

See Also:

> **Review Article:** *K Ewe et al, Eds. Proceedings of the Second International Symposium on Senna. Pharmacology 47(Suppl 1), 1993.*

> **Review Article:** *E Leng-Peschlow, Ed. Senna and its rational use. Pharmacology 44(Suppl 1), 1992.*

Castor oil:

A stimulant laxative.

Produces one or more copious, watery evacuations 2-6 hrs. after ingestion.

WARNINGS: Because of its strong cathartic effect, castor oil should not be used to treat common constipation. It may produce colic, dehydration and electrolyte imbalance.

Citrus seed extract:

Administration may be beneficial.

Experimental Study: 25 pts. with severe atopic eczema were treated. 14/25 complained of intermittent diarrhea, constipation, flatulence, intestinal rushes, bloating and abdominal discomfort (particularly after carbohydrate-rich meals). 10/25 received 2 drops of a 0.5% oral solution (2 drops in 200 ml water) of citrus seed extract (Para Mycrocidin) twice daily, while the other 15 pts. received capsules containing 50 mg extract each at a dosage of 3 caps 3 times daily. After 1 mo., 2/10 pts. on the liquid improved, while all 15 of the pts. on the capsules (which contained a higher dosage of the extract) noted definite improvement of constipation, flatulence, abdominal discomfort and night rest. There were no side effects, although the dosage of the liquid extract that pts. would ingest was limited due to the bitter taste. The extract was mostly effective against Candida, Geotrichum sp. and hemolytic E. coli (*Ionescu G et al. Oral citrus seed extact in atopic eczema: In vitro and in vivo studies on intestinal microflora. J Orthomol Med 5(3):155-8, 1990*).

Psyllium (Ispaglula; *Plantago ovata*):

A bulk-forming laxative which stimulates intestinal motility and water retention.

Available as whole or powdered seeds (which are rich in mucilage, a hemicellulose) and as a refined hydrophilic colloid obtained from the seeds.

Most effective when taken with 2 glasses of water.

May take 2 to 3 days to be effective.

Experimental Double-blind Study: In a study of 80 pts. with irritable bowel syndrome, 82% improved following active treatment compared to 53% following placebo (p<0.02). Constipation significantly improved in the ispaglula gp. (p=0.026) while it was unchanged in the controls (*Prior A, Whorwell PJ. Double blind study of ispaglula in irritable bowel syndrome. Gut 28(11):1510-13, 1987*).

COMBINATION TREATMENT

<u>Psyllium</u> and
<u>Senna</u>:

Combined administration may be more effective.

Experimental Blinded Study: 42 pts. who had ≤ 3 bowel movements during 1 wk. of single-blind placebo treatment randomly received either psyllium alone (7.2 g/d) or psyllium and senna (6.5 + 1.5 g/d). Both laxatives increased defacation frequency and wet and dry stool weights, although the added effect of senna was clearly evident. 7/19 pts. in the combination gp. formed a sub-population of high-responders to senna and were responsible for most of the increase in stool frequency and dry weight in this gp., while laxation in the remaining 12/19 pts. in the gp. was similar to those receiving psyllium alone. Both laxatives provided a similarly high degree of subjective relief and improvement in stool consistency. As assessed by stool frequency and weight, laxation was attained by 63% of the psyllium and senna gp. compared to 48% of the psyllium gp. (*Marlett JA et al. Comparative laxation of psyllium with and without senna in an ambulatory constipated population. <u>Am J Gastroenterol</u> 82(4):333-7, 1987*).

DEMENTIA

See Also: CEREBROVASCULAR DISEASE

Ginkgo biloba:

Ginkgo biloba extracts standardized to contain 24% ginkgoflavonglycosides are among the most well-studied plant-based medicines. _Ginkgo biloba_ extract (GBE) is a registered drug in Germany for the treatment of cerebral dysfunction. Although preliminary studies in established Alzheimer's patients are promising, at this time it appears that GBE only helps delay mental deterioration in the early stages of Alzheimer's disease. In cases of severe dementia due to Alzheimer's disease, GBE is of little value. However, if the mental deficit is due to vascular insufficiency or depression and not Alzheimer's disease, GBE will usually be effective in improving mental function. The standard dosage for GBE is 40 mg 3 times daily _(Kleijnen J Knipschild P. Ginkgo biloba. Lancet 340:1136-9, 1992; DeFeudis FV. Ginkgo biloba extract (EGb 761). Pharmacological Activities and Clinical Applications. New York, Elsevier, 1991; EW Funfgeld, Ed. Rokan (Ginkgo Biloba) Recent Results in Pharmacology and Clinic. New York, Springer-Verlag, 1988)._

Experimental Placebo-controlled Crossover Study: 18 pts. (mean age, 69.3 years) with slight age-related memory impairment received GBE (320 mg or 600 mg) or placebo 1 hour before performing a dual-coding test that measures the speed of information processing. The test consisted of several coding series of drawings and words presented at decreasing times of 1920, 960, 480, 240, and 120 ms. The dual-coding phenomenon (a break point between coding verbal material and images) was demonstrated in all the tests. After placebo, the break point was observed at 960 ms and dual coding beginning at 1920 ms. After each dose of the Ginkgo extract, the break point (at 480 ms) and dual coding (at 960 ms) were significantly shifted toward a shorter presentation time, indicating an improvement in the speed of information processing _(Allain H, Raoul P, Lieury A, et al. Effect of two doses of ginkgo biloba extract (EGb 761) on the dual-coding test in elderly subjects. Clin Ther 15(3):549-58, 1993)._

Experimental Double-blind Study: Two experiments were conducted to assess the EEG effects of (1) three different dosages of GBE and (2) three different extractions of _G. biloba_ (GBE and two fractions from it). Medication or placebo were administered for 3 days preceding the recording sessions. 25 parameters were computed from the EEG spectra. Medication-related effects were obtained for most of the power measures, whereas dominant frequencies of the respective frequency band remained largely unchanged _(Kunkel H. EEG profile of three different extractions of Ginkgo biloba. Neuropsychobiology 27(1):40-5, 1993)._

Meta-Analysis: A meta-analysis was made on the quality of research on more than 40 clinical studies of GBE in the treatment of cerebral insufficiency. The results of the analysis indicate that the quality of the research reviewed was on par with the research methods used in investigating ergoloid mesylates an approved drug in the treatment of dementia, including Alzheimer's disease. The analysis further substantiated that GBE is effective in reducing all symptoms of cerebral insufficiency, including impaired mental function (*Kleijnen J, Knipschild P. Ginkgo biloba for cerebral insufficiency. Br J Clinical Pharmacol 34:352-8, 1992*).

Experimental Double-blind Study: GBE improved mental function in patients suffering from cerebral insufficiency. Significant improvements were noted in psychometric computer-aided examination of the short-term memory after 6 weeks and of the basic learning rate after 24 weeks in the group given GBE (*Grabel E. Cerebral insuffiency - The inflence of Ginkgo biloba extract EGB 761 on basic parameters of mental performance. Placebo-controlled, randomized double-blind study with computer-aided measurement. Fortsch Med 110(5):73-6, 1992*).

Animal Experimental Study: The effect of tacrine and *Ginkgo biloba* extract on choline uptake into hippocampal synaptosomes was studied. While ginkgo increased an uptake of choline, tacrine actually decreased choline uptake (*Kristofikova Z et al. Changes of high-affinity choline uptake in the hippocampus of old rats after long-term administration of two nootropinc drugs (tacrine and Ginkgo biloba extract). Dementia 3:304-7, 1992*).

Experimental Double-blind Study: 31 pts. over the age of 50 years and showing a mild to moderate degree of memory impairment oral doses of 40 mg GBE or identical placebo 3-times daily. Assessments were made at baseline and after 12 and 24 weeks of treatment using a range of psychometric tests. Statistical analysis of the data as compared to baseline suggests that GBE had a beneficial effect on cognitive function in this group of patients (*Rai GS, Shovlin C, Wesnes KA. A double-blind, placebo controlled study of Ginkgo biloba extract ("Tanakan") in elderly outpatients with mild to moderate memory impairment. Curr Med Res Opin 12(6):350-5, 1991*).

Experimental Double-blind Study: 36 pts. with cerebro-organic syndrome were administered either GBE (EGb 761) 40 mg 3 times daily or placebo. After 4 and 8 wks., a highly significant difference was seen in both saccadic eye movements and psychometric tests in the GB gp. compared to controls; also a marked reduction in the theta proportion of the alpha/theta ratio was found in the experimental subjects. Side effects were minimal (*Hofferberth B. [Effect of Ginkgo biloba extract on neurophysiological and psychometric measurement results in patients with cerebro-organic syndrome: A double-blind study versus placebo.] Arzneimittelforschung 39:918-22, 1989*) (*in German*).

Animal Experimental Study: *Ginkgo biloba* extract was shown to normalize the muscarinic acetylcholine receptor in the hippocampus of aged animals, to increase cholinergic transmission, and to address many of the other major elements of Alzheimer's disease (*Allard M. Treatment of old age disorders with Ginkgo biloba extract - From pharmacology to clinic, in EW Funfgeld, Ed. Rokan (Ginkgo Biloba) - Recent Results in Pharmacology and Clinic. New York, Springer-Verlag, 1988:201-11*).

Experimental Double-blind Study: 54 elderly pts. with mild signs of impairment in everyday function on the Crichton Geriatric Rating Scale randomly received either GBE or placebo. Cognitive efficiency was measured monthly using a battery of tests of mental ability, while the quality of life was assessed using a behavioral questionnaire administered before and after the study. Not only did general accuracy on the tests improve with GBE, but the speed of performance also increased, indicating a general improvement in mental efficiency. In addition, the pts. in the treatment gp. reported an increase in their degree of interest in everyday activities. Results suggest that GBE could prove effective in the treatment of the early stages of primary degenerative dementia (*Wesnes K et al. A double blind placebo-controlled trial of Ginkgo biloba extract in the treatment of idiopathic cognitive impairment in the elderly. Hum Psychopharmacol 2:159-69, 1987*).

Experimental Double-blind Study: 60 pts. with mild to moderate primary degenerative dementia randomly received either GBE or placebo. In comparison with placebo, GBE administered over a period of 4-12 wks. significantly improved the clinical condition and the results of psychometric tests. By 4 wks., there were significant improvements in psychometric tests, subjective assessments of both physician and patients, and in the global scores of the clinical-geriatric scales which showed a drop of about 30%, demonstrating that pts. were better able to handle every-day problems. On the Number-Symbol Test and Number-Repeat Test, initial test values did not differentiate between the gps.; however the test values of the GBE gp. increased significantly compared to the placebo gp., showing that short-term memory and vigilance are considerably improved (*Weitbrecht WU, Jansen W. Primary degenerative dementia: therapy with Ginkgo biloba extract. Fortschr Med 104:199-202, 1986*) (*in German*).

Experimental Study: In a study of both young, healthy volunteers and elderly pts. with dementia, signal analysis of EEGs as related to psychometric tests confirmed clinical trials suggesting that GBE adds to alertness (*Pidoux B. [Effects of ginkgo biloba extract on functional activity of the brain.] Presse Med 15 (31):1588-91, 1986*) (*in French*).

Experimental Double-blind Study: 166 elderly pts. with cerebral disorders causing mild mental deterioration received either GBE or placebo. After about 3 mo., the experimental gp. began to demonstrate significant positive differences from the control group. After 1 yr., pts. receiving the extract demonstrated significantly improved mental function when tested for memory, alertness, attention, mood and sociability. Improvement among treated pts. was twice that of the placebo gp. (*Taillandier J. Gingko biloba extract in the treatment of cerebral disorders due to aging, in EW Funfgeld, Ed. Rokan. New York, Springer-Verlag, 1988, pp. 291-301; Taillandier J et al. [Ginkgo biloba extract in the treatment of cerebral disorders due to aging. A longitudinal multicenter double-blind drug vs. placebo study.] Presse Med 15 (31):1583-7, 1986*)

Experimental Study: GBE was found to specifically reactivate the noradrenergic system in the cerebral cortex and to affect the beta-receptors. It had no effect on alpha-2 receptors or on serotonin uptake (*Racagni G et al. [Neuromediator changes during cerebral aging. The effect of Ginkgo biloba extract. Presse Med 15 (31):1488-90, 1986*) (*in French*).

Review Article: Several studies have shown that GBE has a pharmacodynamic dose-related effect on vigilance (as demonstrated by EEG analysis), that GBE significantly increases the speed of memory scanning without effect on performance, that GB extract increases cerebral blood flow and enhances glucose consumption, and that it has a markedly beneficial effect upon sociability, vigilance, mood, memory and intellectual efficiency (*Michel PF. Chronic cerebral insufficiency and Gingko biloba extract, in A*

Agnoli et al, Eds. Effects of Ginkgo Biloba Extracts on Organic Cerebral Impairment. John Libbey Eurotext Ltd., 1985:71-6).

Experimental Double-blind Study: 40 pts. aged 60-80 with slight to moderate primary degenerative dementia randomly receiving either GBE 120 mg/day or placebo. Starting the eighth wk. there was an improvement in the experimental gp. which appeared to be clinically relevant, with statistically significant improvement in both psychometric tests and clinical scales *(Weitbrecht WV, Jansen W. Doubleblind and comparative (Ginkgo biloba versus placebo) therapeutic study in geriatric patients with primary degenerative dementia - a preliminary evaluation, in A Agnoli et al, Eds. Effects of Ginkgo Biloba Extracts on Organic Cerebral Impairment John Libbey Eurotext Ltd., 1985:91-9).*

Experimental Study: Elderly pts. who demonstrated deteriorated mental performance and vigilance and who were given GBE showed restoration of vigilance towards normal levels and improved performance on psychometric procedures along with improvements in EEG tracings. Pts. with a more unfavorable initial clinical condition (based on resting EEG activity) displayed the most improvement *(Gebner B et al. Study of the long-term action of a ginkgo biloba extract on vigilance and mental performance as determined by means of quantitative pharmaco-EEG and psychometric measurements. Arzneim Forsch 35:1459-65, 1985).*

See Also:

Experimental Double-blind Study: *Grassel E. [Effect of Ginkgo-biloba extract on mental performance. Double-blind study using computerized measurement conditions in patients with cerebral insufficiency]. Fortschr Med 110(5):73-6, 1992 (in German)*

Experimental Double-blind Study: *Herrschaft H. [The clinical application of Ginkgo biloba in dementia syndromes (restoration of brain performance in vascular or degenerative CNS disease)]. Pharm Unserer Zeit 21(6):266-75, 1992 (in German)*

Experimental Double-blind Study: *Arrigo A, Cattaneo S. Clinical and psychometric evaluation of Ginkgo biloba extract in chronic cerebro-vascular diseases, in A Agnoli et al, Eds. Effects of Ginkgo Biloba Extracts on Organic Cerebral Impairment. John Libbey Eurotext Ltd., 1985:71-6*

Experimental Double-blind Study: *Eckmann VF, Schlag H. Knotrollierte doppelblind-studie zum wirksamkeitsnachweis von Tebonin forte bei patienten mit zerebrovakularer insuffizienz. Fortschr Med 31:1474-8, 1982*

DEPRESSION

See Also: ANXIETY
                CEREBROVASCULAR DISEASE
                INSOMNIA

Ginkgo biloba:

Ginkgo biloba extracts (GBE) standardized to contain 24% ginkgoflavonglycosides may be effective for depression, especially in cases of cerebrovascular insufficiency (_DeFeudis FV. Ginkgo biloba extract (EGb 761). Pharmacological Activities and Clinical Applications. Paris, Elsevier, 1991; EW Funfgeld, Ed. Rokan (Ginkgo Biloba) Recent Results in Pharmacology and Clinic. New York, Springer-Verlag, 1988_).

> **Animal Experimental Study:** GBE exerts anxiolytic and antidepressant activity in various animal models (_Porsolt RD et al. Effects of an extract of Ginkgo biloba (EGB 761) on "learned helplessness" and other models of stress in rodents. Pharmacol Biochem Behav 36:963-71, 1990_).

> **Animal Experimental Study:** Chemical changes in rat cerebral cortex after administration of GBE indicate a possible antidepressant effect (_Brunello N et al. Effects of an extract of Ginkgo biloba on noradrenergic system of rat cerebral cortex. Pharmacol Res Commun 17:1063-72, 1985_).

St. John's Wort (_Hypericum perforatum_):

A St. John's wort extract standardized to contain 0.125% hypericin content has been administered in clinical studies at a dosage of 300 mg three times daily.

> > WARNING: _The use of St. John's wort extract at prescribed levels is not associated with any significant side effects; however, there is considerable evidence that it can cause severe photosensitivity in animals grazing extensively on the plant and there is some evidence that, at high levels, it can produce photosensitivity in humans. Individuals taking larger amounts of St. John's wort extracts (or hypericin) should therefore avoid exposure to strong sunlight._

> **Experimental Double-blind Study:** Out-pts. with mild to moderately severe depression randomly received either an extract of St. John's wort (LI 160) or placebo. 66.6% improved on the extract compared to 26.7% on placebo. 2 pts. had transient minor side effects, and no impairment of cognitive performance was observed (_Schmidt U, Sommer H. [St. John's wort extract in the ambulatory therapy of depression. Attention and reaction ability are preserved.] Fortschr Med 111(19):339-42, 1993_) (in German).

Experimental Double-Blind Crossover Study: 12 healthy subjects given St. John's wort extract demonstrated improved cortical function. Cortical evoked potential and EEG were used as parameters *(Johnson D. Effects of St. John's wort extract Jarsin. 4th International Congress on Phytotherapy. Munich, Germany. September 10-13, 1992, abstract SL53).*

Experimental Double-Blind Study: Results of classic psychometric scales in depressive patients indicated that St. John's wort extract produced a 55% improvement in the Clinical-Global-Impression-Scale within four weeks *(Woelk H. Multicentric practice-study analyzing the functional capacity in depressive patients. 4th International Congress on Phytotherapy. Munich, Germany. September 10-13, 1992, abstract SL54).*

Experimental Double-Blind Study: An impressive improvement was found in depression and the psychovegetative complaints of disturbed sleep, headache, and fatigue in patients given given St. John's wort extract. The responder rate as determined by the raw sum value of the Hamilton Depression Scale was 66.6% for St. John's wort and only 27.6% for the placebo. There were no side effects *(Sommer H. Improvement of psychovegetative complaints by hypericum. 4th International Congress on Phytotherapy. Munich, Germany. September 10-13, 1992, abstract SL55).*

Experimental Study: 15 female pts. took a standardized hypericin extract and demonstrated improvement in subjective ratings of anxiety, dysphoric mood, loss of interest, hypersomnia, anorexia, depression (worse in the morning), insomnia, obstipation, psychomotor retardation, and feelings of worthlessness. There were no adverse side-effects *(Muldner H, Zoller M. Antidepressive effect of a hypericum extract standardized to the active hypericine complex]. Arzneim Forsch 34:918-20, 1984) (in German).*

Hypericin may enhance the function of norepinephrine neurons in the brain.

Experimental Study: 6 female pts. aged 55-65 took a standarized (hypericin) extract of *Hypericum perforatum*. Urinary 3-methoxy-4-hydroxyphenylglycol (MHPG) rose indicating an antidepressive action *(Muldner H, Zoller M. Antidepressive effect of a hypericum extract standardized to the active hypericine complex]. Arzneim Forsch 34:918-20, 1984) (in German).*

Hypericin may inhibit monamine oxidase.

Experimental Study: Hypericin from *H. perforatum* was found to irreversibly inhibit types A and B MAO *in vivo (Suzuki O et al. Inhibition of monoamine oxidase by hypericin. Planta Medica 50:272-4, 1984).*

See Also:

Animal Experimental Studies: *Okpanyi SN, Weischer ML. Experimental animal studies of the psychotropic activity of a Hypericum extract. Arzneim Forsch 37:10-13, 1987*

Siberian Ginseng (*Eleutherococcus senticosus*):

Siberian ginseng has consistently demonstrated an ability to increase the sense of well-being in a variety of psychological disturbances including depression, insomnia, hypochondriasis, and various neuroses. A possible explanation is improved balance of monoamines as Siberian ginseng has been shown to increase monoamine content in the brain, adrenals, and urine of rats *(Farnsworth NR et al. Siberian ginseng (Eleutherococcus senticosus): Current status as an adaptogen. Econ Med Plant Res 1:156-215, 1985).*

DIABETES MELLITUS

See Also: ATHEROSCLEROSIS
RETINOPATHY

Aloe vera:

Administration may combat hyperglycemia.

Animal Experimental Study: The hypoglycemic effect of aloe and its bitter principle may be mediated through a direct effect as well as by stimulating the synthesis and/or release of insulin (*Beppu H, Nagamura Y, Fujita K. Hypoglycaemic and antidiabetic effects in mice of Aloe arborescens Miller var. natalensis Berger. Phytother Res 7:S37-S42, 1993*).

Experimental Study: 5 pts. with type II diabetes given the dried sap of aloe (1/2 tsp. daily) experienced a reduction from a mean glucose level of 273 to 151 mg/dl (*Ghannam N: The antidiabetic activity of aloes: Preliminary clinical and experimental observations. Hormone Res 24:288-94, 1986*).

Animal Experimental Study: Diabetic mice given aloe (500 mg/kg) for 7 days had blood glucose levels of 394 mg/dl compared to 646 mg/dl in the control gp. and 726 in a gp. receiving glibenclamide (*Ghannam N: The antidiabetic activity of aloes: Preliminary clinical and experimental observations. Hormone Res 24:288-94, 1986*).

See Also:

Animal Experimental Study: *Ajabnoor MA. Effect of aloes on blood glucose levels in normal and alloxan diabetic mice. J Ethnopharm 28:215-20, 1990*

Topical application of the gel may foster local wound healing. (*See: 'WOUND HEALING'*)

Experimental Study: Topically applied *Aloe vera* gel may help wound healing in diabetics and is especially useful in the treatment of diabetic foot problems (*Davis RH et al. Aloe vera, a natural approach for treating wounds, edema, and pain in diabetes. J Am Pod Med Assoc 78:60-8, 1988*).

Bilberry (*Vaccinium myrtillus*):

Bilberry or European blueberry contains flavonoid compounds known as anthocyanosides. Bilberry anthocyanosides are potent antioxidants that improve the microcirculation and protect the vascular endothelium in diabetes. (*See: 'PERIPHERAL VASCULAR DISEASE'; 'RETINOPATHY'; 'VASCULAR FRAGILITY'*)

The standard dose for *Vaccinium myrtillus* extract (VME) is based on its anthocyanoside content, as calculated by its anthocyanidin percentage. Most studies have used a bilberry extract standardized for an anthocyanidin content of 25% at a dosage of 160 mg to 480 mg daily.

Administration of VME may reduce microangiopathy.

> **Experimental Study:** VME given to 54 diabetic pts. at a dose of 500-600 mg/d for 8 to 33 months produced almost total normalization of polymeric collagen and a 30% decrease in structural glycoprotein (*Lagrue G et al. Pathology of the microcirculation in diabetes and alterations of the biosynthesis of intracellular matrix molecules. Front Matrix Biol S Karger 7:324-35, 1979*).
>
> > *Note: Diabetics suffer thickening of capillaries due to increased polymeric collagen and structural glycoprotein synthesis.*

See Also:

> **Experimental Study:** *Boniface R et al. Pharmacological properties of myrtillus anthocyanosides: Correlation with results of treatment of diabetic microangiopathy. Stud Org Chem 23:293-301, 1986.*

Administration of VME may reduce diabetic retinopathy.

> **Experimental Study:** 31 pts. with various types of retinopathy (diabetic retinopathy n=20; retinitis pigmentosa n=5; macular degeneration n=4; hemorrhagic retinopathy due to anti-coagulant therapy) were treated with VME. A tendency towards reduced vascular permeability and tendency to hemorrhage was observed in all pts., expecially those with diabetic retinopathy (*Scharrer A, Ober M. [Anthocyanosides in the treatment of retinopathies]. Klin Monatsbl Augenheilkd 178:386-9, 1981*) (*in German*).

Bitter melon:

Bitter melon (*Momordica charantia*), also known as balsam pear, is a tropical fruit widely cultivated in Asia, Africa and South America. The unripe fruit is edible and has been used extensively in folk medicine as a remedy for diabetes. The fresh juice of the unripe fruit, as well as the dried fruit or seeds, has demonstrated oral hypoglycemic activity. Several compounds with hypoglycemic activity have been identified, including an insulin-like polypeptide known as p-insulin [the 'p' is for plant] (*Cunnick J, Takemoto D. Bitter melon (Momordica charantia). J Naturopath Med 4(1):16-21, 1993*).

Unripe bitter melon is available primarily at Asian grocery stores. While commercial bitter melon extracts are available, prescribing 100 ml of a decoction (*see below*) or 2 oz. of fresh juice may be the best form to use. The dosage of other forms should approximate this dose.

Administration may improve glucose tolerance.

> *Note: The effects are gradual and cumulative.*

> **Experimental Study:** Type II diabetic pts. were given either 5 g of dried bitter melon powder 3 times daily or 100 ml of an aqueous extract of bitter melon as a single dose

in the morning. The aqueous extract was produced by chopping 100 g of the fruit and boiling it in 200 ml of water until the volume was reduced to 100 ml. After 3 weeks, pts. receiving the dried powder (n=5) experienced a drop of 25% in blood sugar levels. The gp. (n=7) receiving the aqueous extract experienced a statistically significant drop of 54% after 3 weeks and a drop in glycosylated hemoglobin from 8.37 to 6.95 after 7 weeks (*Srivastava Y et al. Antidiabetic and adaptogenic properties of Momordica charantia extract: An experimental and clinical evaluation. Phytother Res 7:285-9, 1993*).

Animal Experimental Study: Oral administration of the juice of bitter melon (10 ml/kg for 30 days) did not show a significant effect, either acute or cumulative, on the ability of rats with streptozotin-induced diabetes to tolerate an external glucose load. The glycosylated hemoglobin concentrations were significantly elevated in both juice-treated and untreated diabetic rats and there was no significant difference between the two groups. Viable beta-cells capable of secreting insulin upon stimulation appear to be required for *M. charantia* to exert its oral hypoglycemic activity (*Karunanayake EH et al. Effect of Momordica charantia fruit juice on streptozotocin-induced diabetes in rats. J Ethnopharmacol 30(2):199-204, 1990*).

Animal Experimental Study: In normal mice, an aqueous extract (A) of bitter melon lowered the glycemic response to both oral and intraperitoneal glucose without altering the insulin response. This aqueous extract (A) and the residue after alkaline chloroform extraction (B) reduced the hyperglycemia in diabetic mice at 1 hour. Material recovered by acid water wash of the chloroform extract remaining after an alkaline water wash (D) produced a more slowly generated hypoglycaemic effect. The results suggest that orally administered karela extracts lower glucose concentrations independently of intestinal glucose absorption and involve an extrapancreatic effect. Two types of hypoglycemic substances with different time-dependent effects are indicated (*Day C et al. Hypoglycaemic effect of Momordica charantia extracts. Planta Med 56(5):426-9, 1990*).

Animal Experimental Study: An acetone extract of bitter melon given orally daily lowered the blood glucose and serum cholesterol levels to the normal range after 15 to 30 days in alloxan diabetic rats. Once the blood sugar level was lowered after 30 days of treatment it did not increase even after 15 days of discontinuation of the treatment (*Singh N et al. Effects of long term feeding of acetone extract of Momordica charantia (whole fruit powder) on alloxan diabetic albino rats. Ind J Physiol Pharmac 33(2):97-100, 1989*).

Animal Experimental Study: In the test gp., bitter melon powder was given at a dose of 4 g/kg/Day/rat for a period of 2 months. While the control gp. of rats developed cataract in 90 to 100 days, the bitter melon treated rats showed cataract in 140 to 180 days. Cataract formation was found to be dependant on blood sugar levels since the control gp. with blood sugar 307 +/- 81 (mg%) was blind 2 months earlier than bitter melon treated gp. which showed blood sugar 149 +/- 66.37 (mg%) (*Srivastava Y, Venkatakrishna-Bhatt H, Verma Y. Effect of Momordica charantia Linn. pomous aqueous extract on cataractogenesis in murrin alloxan diabetics. Pharmacol Res Commun 20(3):201-9, 1988*).

Experimental Study: Administration of 100 ml of the fresh juice of unripe bitter melon to 18 newly diagnosed type II diabetics led to significant improvements in glucose tolerance in 73% of pts. (*Welihinda J et al. Effect of Momardica charantia on the glucose tolerance in maturity onset diabetes. J Ethnopharmacol 17:277-82, 1986*).

Animal Experimental Study: Molecules with insulin-like bioactivity are present in *Momordica charantia* seeds (*Ng TB et al. Insulin-like molecules in Momordica charantia seeds. J Ethnopharmacol 15(1):107-17, 1986*).

Experimental Study: 7 pts. with type II diabetes given 50 mg/kg body weight of dried bitter melon powder demonstrated improved glucose tolerance (*Akhtar MS. Trial of Momordica charantia Linn (Karela) powder in patients with maturity-onset diabetes. J Pak Med Assoc 32(4):106-7, 1982*).

Experimental Study: Bitter melon juice at a dose of 50 ml/d significantly reduced blood glucose concentrations during a 50 g oral glucose tolerance test in type II diabetics. Fried bitter melon consumed as a daily supplement to the diet produced a small but significant improvement in glucose tolerance. Improvement in glucose tolerance was not associated with an increase in serum insulin responses (*Leatherdale BA et al. Improvement in glucose tolerance due to Momordica charantia (karela). Br Med J 282(6279):1823-4, 1981*).

See Also:

>   **Experimental Study:** *Qijun L et al. Influence of balsam pear (the fruit of Momordica charantia L.) on blood sugar level. J Tradit Chin Med 5(2):99-106, 1985*

>   **Animal Experimental Study:** *Welihinda J et al. The insulin-releasing activity of the tropical plant Momordica charantia. Acta Biol Med Germ 41:1229-40, 1982*

Administration may delay the formation of diabetic cataracts and other complications of diabetes. (*See: 'CATARACT'*)

Animal Experimental Study: Bitter melon was shown to delay the development of cataracts and other secondary complications of diabetes in rats (*Srivastava Y et al. Antidiabetic and adaptogenic properties of Momordica charantia extract: An experimental and clinical evaluation. Phytother Res 7:285-9, 1993*).

Capsaicin:

Capsaicin is the active component of cayenne pepper (*Capsicum frutescens*). When topically applied, capsaicin is known to stimulate and then block small-diameter pain fibers by depleting them of the neurotransmitter substance P. Substance P is thought to be the principle chemomediator of pain impulses from the periphery (*Cordell GA, Araujo OE. Capsaicin: Identification, nomenclature, and pharmacotherapy. Ann Pharmacother 27:330-6, 1993*).

Commercial ointments containing 0.025% or 0.075% are available over-the-counter.

Topical application may relieve the pain of diabetic neuropathy.

Experimental Controlled Study: 75 diabetic pts. with chronic (12 mo.) painful distal symmetrical polyneuropathy participated in the study. 22 pts. were untreated and 53 pts. were treated with imipramine ± mexiletine for deep pain, capsaicin for superficial pain, and stretching exercises and metaxalone ± piroxican for muscular pain. Each type of pain was scored separately on a scale of 0 (none) to 19 (worst), and the total of all three types was used as an index of overall pain. Ability to sleep through the night was scored by a scale of 1 (never) to 5 (always). No significant differences were observed in initial pain scores, sleep scores, demographics, biochemistries, or physical findings between the two groups. After 3 mo., significant improvements in scores were noted in the treated but not the untreated patients. In addition, a significant difference was found in the change of scores between the treated and untreated pts.: total pain (-18 vs. 0) deep pain (-7 vs. -1), superficial pain (-5 vs. 0), muscular pain (-6 vs. 0), and sleep (1.2 vs. 0.2). In treated pts. 21% became pain-free (total pain), 66% had improvement (decrease in total pain: 5, but not total elimination of painful symptoms), and 13% were considered treatment failures. This compares with 0% (p), 10% (p), and 90% (p), respectively, in the untreated pts. (*Pfeifer MA et al. A highly successful and novel model for treatment of chronic painful diabetic peripheral neuropathy. Diabetes Care 16(8):1103-15, 1993*).

Experimental Double-blind Study: Investigators at 12 sites enrolled 277 men and women with painful diabetic peripheral polyneuropathy and/or radiculopathy in an 8-wk double-blind vehicle-controlled study with parallel randomized treatment assignments. Participants were unresponsive or intolerant to conventional therapy and were experiencing pain that interfered with functional activities and/or sleep. Either 0.075% capsaicin cream or vehicle cream was applied to the painful areas 4 times/day. A visual analogue scale of pain intensity and baseline measurements of the pain's interference with the ability to walk, work, participate in recreational activities, use shoes and socks, sleep, and eat were recorded at onset and at 2-wk intervals. A physician's global evaluation scale assessed changes in pain status from baseline. Statistically significant differences in favor of capsaicin versus vehicle were observed: 69.5 vs 53.4% of pts. with clinical improvement in pain status (p=0.012), 26.1 vs. 14.6% with improvement in walking (p=0.029), 18.3 vs. 9.2% with improvement in working (p=0.019), 29.5 vs. 20.3% with improvement in sleeping (p=0.036), and 22.8 vs. 12.1% with improvement in participating in recreational activities (p=0.037) (*The Capsaicin Study Group. Effect of treatment with capsaicin on daily activities of patients with painful diabetic neuropathy. Diabetes Care 15(2):159-65, 1992*).

Experimental Double-blind Study: 22 pts. applied either capsaicin (0.075%) or vehicle cream was to painful areas 4 times/day. Pain measurements were recorded at baseline and at 2-wk intervals for 8 wk. Capsaicin treatment was more beneficial than vehicle treatment in the overall clinical improvement of pain status, as measured by physician's global evaluation (p=0.038) and by a categorical pain severity scale (p=0.057). Decrease in mean pain intensity by a visual analogue scale was 16% in capsaicin-treated and 4.1% in vehicle-treated subjects. Mean pain relief on visual analogue scale was 44.6 and 23.2%, respectively. In a follow-up open-label study, approximately 50% of subjects reported improved pain control or were cured, and 25% each were unchanged or worse. A burning sensation at the application site was noted by some subjects but both its magnitude and duration decreased with time (*Tandan R et al. Topical capsaicin in painful diabetic neuropathy. Controlled study with long-term follow-up. Diabetes Care 15(1):8-14, 1992*).

Experimental Study: 22 pts. with painful diabetic neuropathy were given either capsaicin (0.075%) or vehicle-only cream. After 8 wk of use, there was no significant change in warm and vibration thresholds, but the cold threshold was significantly reduced by capsaicin and vehicle creams to an equal degree. In fewer subjects who used capsaicin cream in an open-label study, there was no significant effect on sensory thresholds after up to 32 wk of use. No adverse effects of topical 0.075% capsaicin were noted on human sensory function, even in subjects with preexisting neuropathic sensory impairment (*Tandan R et al. Topical capsaicin in painful diabetic neuropathy. Effect on sensory function. Diabetes Care 15(1):15-8, 1992*).

Experimental Double-blind Study: 15 pts. with painful diabetic neuropathy applied either capsaicin 0.075% or vehicle-only cream. 12 pts. completed the eight-week study. 9/12 pts. reported symptomatic relief; 5 of them used the drug and 4 used the vehicle. The 3 pts. who reported no relief of symptoms applied the vehicle (*Basha KM, Whitehouse FW. Capsaicin: a therapeutic option for painful diabetic neuropathy. Henry Ford Hosp Med J 39(2):138-40, 1991*).

Experimental Double-blind Study: A multicenter study was conducted to establish the efficacy of topical 0.075% capsaicin cream in relieving the pain associated with diabetic neuropathy. Capsaicin or vehicle cream was applied to painful areas four times per day for 8 weeks in pts. randomly assigned to one of two groups. Pain intensity and relief were recorded at 2-week intervals using physician's global evaluation and visual analog scales. Analysis at final visit for 252 pts. showed statistical significance favoring capsaicin compared with vehicle for the following: 69.5% vs 53.4% pain improvement by the physician's global evaluation scale, 38.1% vs 27.4% decrease in pain intensity, and 58.4% vs 45.3% improvement in pain relief. With the exception of transient burning, sneezing, and coughing, capsaicin was well tolerated. Study results suggest that topical capsaicin cream is safe and effective in treating painful diabetic neuropathy (*The Capsaicin Study Group. Treatment of painful diabetic neuropathy with topical capsaicin. A multicenter, double-blind, vehicle-controlled study. Arch Intern Med 151(11):2225-9, 1991*).

Experimental Double-blind Study: 40 pts. applied either 0.075% capsaicin cream (Zostrix®, GenGerm) or placebo to their affected extremities daily. After 4 wks., 76% of treated pts. had some pain relief, compared to 50% of placebo patients. In addition, those responding to capsaicin said their pain was cut in half, while those on placebo averaged between 15% and 20% relief (*David Chad, associate professor of neurology and pathology, U. of Massachusetts at Worcester - reported in Med World News, February 27, 1989*).

Case Reports: 2 diabetic pts. with severe neuropathy responded dramatically within 2 wks. to topical applications of capsaicin cream (Zostrix®, GenDerm) 3-4 times daily (*Ross DR, Varipapa RJ. Treatment of painful diabetic neuropathy with topical capsaicin. Letter. N Engl J Med 321(7):474-5, 1989*).

See Also:

   Experimental Study: *Scheffler NM et al. Treatment of painful diabetic neuropathy with capsaicin 0.075%. J Am Podiatr Med Assoc 81(6):288-93, 1991.*

Coccinia indica:

The leaves of *Coccinia indica* have been used since ancient times as an antidiabetic drug by Ayurvedic physicians. The active component appears to be pectin.

Experimental Double-blind Study: Out of the 16 pts. who received a preparation from the leaves of Coccinia for 6 weeks, 10 showed marked improvement in their glucose tolerance while none out of the 16 pts. in the placebo gp. showed such a marked improvement (*Khan AK, Akhtar S, Mahtab H. Treatment of diabetes mellitus with Coccinia indica. Br Med J 280(6220):1044, 1980; Khan AK, Akhtar S, Mahtab H. Coccinia indica in the treatment of patients with diabetes mellitus. Bangladesh Med Res Counc Bull 5(2):60-6, 1979*).

Animal Experimental Study: An ethanol extract of *Coccinia indica* leaves was administered orally at a dose of 200 mg/kg body wt. after 18 h of fasting to normal fed and streptozotocin-induced male diabetic rats (180-250 g). Blood sugar was depressed by 23% (p) and 27% (p) in the normal fed and streptozotocin-diabetic rats respectively compared with controls which were given distilled water. Hepatic glucose-6-phosphatase and fructose-1,6-bisphosphatase activities were depressed by 32% (p) 30% (p 0.05) respectively in the streptozotocin-diabetic rats, compared with 19% (p 0.02) and 20% (p) depression in the normal fed controls, whereas both the red-cell and hepatic G6PDH activities were found to be elevated by feeding the extract in the streptozotocin-diabetic and in the normal fed controls. Taken together, these results indicate that *Coccinia indica* extract lowered blood glucose by depressing its synthesis through depression of the key gluconeogenic enzymes and by enhancing glucose oxidation by the shunt pathway through activation of its principal enzyme G6PDH (*Shibib BA et al. Hypoglycaemic activity of Coccinia indica and Momordica charantia in diabetic rats: depression of the hepatic gluconeogenic enzymes glucose-6-phosphatase and fructose-1,6-bisphosphatase and elevation of both liver and red-cell shunt enzyme glucose-6-phosphate dehydrogenase. Biochem J 292:267-70, 1993*).

Fenugreek:

Fenugreek (*Trigonella foenum graecum*) seeds or debitterized fenugreek seed powder may be effective in improving glucose tolerance.

Experimental Double-blind Study: Isocaloric diets with and without fenugreek were each given randomly for 10 days to type I diabetics. Defatted fenugreek seed powder (100 g), divided into two equal doses, was incorporated into the diet and served during lunch and dinner. The fenugreek diet significantly reduced fasting blood sugar and improved the glucose tolerance test. There was also a 54% reduction in 24-h urinary glucose excretion (*Sharma RD et al. Effect of fenugreek seeds on blood glucose and serum lipids in type I diabetes. Eur J Clin Nutr 44(4):301-6, 1990*).

Experimental Double-blind Study: The addition of powdered fenugreek seed (15 g) soaked in water significantly reduced the subsequent postprandial glucose levels in pts. with type II diabetes. The plasma insulin also tended to be lower in the fenugreek gp. but without a statistical difference (*Madar Z et al. Glucose-lowering effect of fenugreek in non-insulin dependent diabetics. Eur J Clin Nutr 42(1):51-4, 1988*).

Experimental Study: Fenugreek seeds given at a dose of 25 g/d for 3 weeks to type II diabetics led to significant improvements in blood sugar control and insulin responses. The 24 hr urinary glucose output and serum cholesterol levels were also reduced (*Sharma RD. Effect of fenugreek seeds and leaves on blood glucose and serum insulin responses in human subjects. Nutr Res 6:1353-64, 1986*).

Animal Experimental Study: Administration of the defatted fenugreek seed (in daily doses of 1.5-2 g/kg) to both normal and diabetic dogs reduced fasting and after-meal blood levels of glucose, glucagon, somatostatin and insulin (*Ribes G et al. Antidiabetic effects of subfractions from fenugreek seeds in diabetic dogs. Proc Soc Exp Biol Med 182(2):159-66, 1986*)

See Also:

> **Animal Experimental Study:** *Riyad MA et al. Effect of fenugreek and lupine seeds on the development of experimental diabetes in rats. Planta Med 54(4):286-90, 1988.*

Fenugreek seeds may normalize serum lipids in diabetics. (*See 'ATHEROSCLEROSIS'*)

Garlic (*Allium sativum*) or
Onion (*Allium cepa*):

> Garlic and onion have significant blood sugar-lowering action. The active principles are believed to be sulfur-containing compounds, allicin and allyl propyl disulphide (APDS), although other constituents such as flavonoids may play a role as well.

> Experimental and clinical evidence suggests that allicin and APDS lower glucose levels by competing with insulin (also a disulphide) for insulin-inactivating sites in the liver. This results in an increase of free insulin (*Bever BO, Zahnd GR. Plants with oral hypoglycemic action. Quart J Crude Drug Res 17:139-96, 1979*).

> The beneficial cardiovascular effects of garlic and onion in diabetics on blood lipids and blood pressure also argue for the liberal intake of garlic and onions by the diabetic patient. (*See: 'ATHEROSCLEROSIS'*)

Consumption may lower blood sugar levels.

> **Animal Experimental Study:** S-allyl cysteine sulphoxide (SACS), a sulfur-containing amino acid of garlic which is the precursor of allicin and garlic oil, was found to show significant antidiabetic effects in alloxan diabetic rats. Administration at a dose of 200 mg/kg body weight decreased significantly the concentration of blood glucose and the activities of serum enzymes such as alkaline phosphatase, acid phosphatase and lactate dehydrogenase and liver glucose-6-phosphatase. It increased significantly liver and in-testinal HMG CoA reductase activity and liver hexokinase activity (*Sheela CG, Augusti KT. Antidiabetic effects of S-allyl cysteine sulphoxide isolated from garlic Allium sativum Linn. Indian J Exp Biol 30(6):523-6, 1992*).

> **Experimental Study:** Graded doses of onion extracts (1 ml of extract = 1 g of whole onion) at levels sometimes found in the diet, i.e., 1 to 7 ounces of onion, reduced blood sugar levels during oral and intravenous glucose tolerance in a dose-dependent manner, i.e., the higher the dose the greater the effect. The effects were similar in both raw and boiled onion extracts (*Sharma KK et al. Antihyperglycemic effect of onion: Effect on fasting blood sugar and induced hyperglycemia in man. Ind J Med Res 65:422-9, 1977*).

Experimental Study: An onion extract administered to 3 diabetic pts. inhibited post-prandial hyperglycemia *(Mathew PT, Augusti KT. Hypoglycaemic effects of onion, Allium cepa Linn. on diabetes mellitus - a preliminary report. Indian J Physiol Pharmacol 19(4):213-7, 1975).*

Experimental Study: In a 4-h test of 6 fasting normal subjects, APDS administered orally at a dose of 125 mg/kg caused a marked fall in blood glucose levels and an increase in serum insulin *(Augusti KT. Studies on the effects of a hypoglycemic principle from Allium Cepa Linn. Indian J Med Res 61(7):1066-71, 1973).*

See Also:

> **Experimental Study:** *Augusti KT. Gas chromatographic analyses of onion principles and a study on their hypoglycemic action. Indian J Exp Biol 14(2):110-2, 1976.*

Ginkgo biloba:

Administration may be helpful in treating diabetic peripheral vascular disease. *(See: 'PERIPHERAL VASCULAR DISEASE')*

Administration may protect against diabetic retinopathy.

In vitro Animal Experimental Study: Rats were made diabetic by the injection of alloxan. After 1 mo., the electroretinogram amplitude in response to a light stimulus (as measured in the isolated rat retina maintained by perfusion) significantly decreased in the diabetic rats compared to controls; it was even more pronounced after 2 months. Compared to untreated diabetic rats, the electroretinograms of rats treated with *Ginkgo biloba* extract had a significantly greater amplitude after 2 months of diabetes. These results are attributed to the free radical scavenger property of the extract *(Doly M et al. [Effect of Ginkgo biloba extract on the electrophysiology of the isolated retina from a diabetic rat.] Presse Med 15 (31):1480-3, 1986) (in French).*

Gymnema sylvestre:

The leaves of this woody climber, which grows in the tropical forests of central and southern India, have been employed as an adjunct in the treatment of diabetes mellitus for many centuries.

GS4, a water-soluble extract of the leaves, may enhance endogenous insulin production in both type I and type II diabetics.

> *Note: 'Mangala Gymnema', the GS4 extract used in these studies, in contrast to the crude extract, has concentrated its 'antidiabetic principle', and two contaminants' have been removed which inhibit nutrient absorption and inactivate the taste buds that identify sweetness (Shanmugasundaram ERB - reported in Brown DJ. Phytotherapy review and commmentary. Townsend Letter for Doctors, Aug/Sept 1991:714).*

Experimental Study: GS4 400 mg daily was administered for 18-20 mo. to 22 type II diabetic pts. on oral hypoglycemic agents. There was a significant reduction in blood glucose, glycosylated hemoglobin and glycosylated plasma proteins, and insulin levels were increased. The dosage of medication could be decreased, and 5/22 pts. were able to discontinue the oral hypoglycemic agent. As compared to oral hypoglycemic drugs, GS4 was superior in regard to subjective reports of well-being, lon-term glycemic control, and the lowering of plasma lipids (*Baskaran K et al. Antidiabetic effect of a leaf extract from Gymnema sylvestre in non-insulin-dependent diabetes mellitus patients. J Ethnopharmacol 30:295-305, 1990*).

Experimental Controlled Study: GS4 400 mg daily was administered to 27 pts. with insulin-dependent DM. Insulin requirements came down by almost 50% together with fasting blood glucose and glycosylated hemoglobin and glycosylated plasma protein levels. Serum lipids returned to near normal levels, while glycosylated hemoglobin and glycosylated plasma protein levels of treated pts. remained higher than in normal controls. C-peptide levels were increased, suggesting greater availability of endogenous insulin. Subjective measures of well-being (alertness, work and school performance, etc.) were improved. There were no side effects. Serum lipids, glycosylated hemoglobin and glycosylated plasma protein levels in diabetic controls were unchanged (*Shanmugasundaram ERB et al. Use of Gymnema sylvestre leaf extract in the control of blood glucose in insulin-dependent diabetes mellitus. J Ethnopharmacol 30:281-94, 1990*).

GS4 may increase the number of islets of Langerhans and the number of beta cells.

Animal Experimental Study: Rats made diabetic with steptozotocin were administered GS4 orally. After 20 days, fasting blood glucose levels returned to normal. During glucose tolerance testing, there was a rise in serum insulin to levels closer to normal fasting levels. In the pancreas, the number of islets and the number of beta cells both doubled and pancreatic weight increased by about 30% (*Shanmugasundaram ERB et al. Possible regeneration of the islets of Langerhans in streptozotocin-diabetic rats given Gymnema sylvestre leaf extracts. J Ethnopharmacol 30:265-79, 1990*)

Inulin:

Burdock root (*Arctium lappa*), dandelion root (*Taraxacum officinalis*), and Jerusalem artichokes (*Helianthus tuberosa*) contain inulin, a polyfructosan or fructose oligosaccharide that exerts beneficial effects on blood sugar control. Consumption of these roots, as vegetables or as teas, may be effective in reducing postprandial hyperglycemia.

Experimental Study: A 20 g oral dose of fructose oligosaccharides produced only a mild blood glucose and insulin rise which was lower than that of fructose. When 10 g were combined with a 50 g wheat-starch meal, areas under blood glucose curves tended to be much smaller compared to meals without the fructose oligosaccharide (*Rumessen JJ et al. Fructans of Jerusalem artichokes: Intestinal transport, absorption, fermentation, and influence on blood glucose, insulin, and C-peptide responses in healthy subjects. Am J Clin Nutr 52:675-81, 1990*).

Experimental Study: Powdered burdock root fed to diabetics in the form of palatable crackers inhibited postprandial hyperglycemia after a starch meal (*Silver AA, Krantz JC. The effect of the ingestion of burdock root on normal and diabetic individuals. A preliminary report. Ann Intern Med 5:274-84, 1931*).

Prickle-pear Cactus (*Opuntia ficus indica*):

The stems of the prickle-pear cactus or nopal has a long folk-use in Mexico in the treatment of diabetes.

Experimental Double-blind Study: Three experiments were performed comparing the effects of 30 capsules a day of a commercial Opuntia product (Nopal) to a placebo in diabetic and healthy individuals. Results indicated the intake of 30 Opuntia capsules daily in pts. with diabetes mellitus had a discrete beneficial effect on glucose and cholesterol. However this dosage is unpractical and is not currently recommended in the management of diabetes (*Frati Munari AC et al. [Evaluation of nopal capsules in diabetes mellitus]. Gac Med Mex 128(4):431-6, 1992*) (*in Spanish*).

Experimental Double-blind Study: The gp. of type II diabetic pts. (n=16) taking 500 g of broiled nopal stems experienced a mean reduction of glucose (17%) and insulin (50%) levels after 180 minutes compared to placebo (*Frati-Munari AC et al. Hypoglycemic effect of Opuntia streptacantha Lemaire in NIDDM. Diabetes Care 11:63-6, 1988*).

Procyanidolic Oligomers:

Procyanidolic oligomers (PCOs), also known as leukocyanidins or pycnogenols, are complexes of flavonoids (polyphenols). Most commercial preparations use PCOs extracted from grape seed skin (*Vitis vinifera*), although PCOs can also be extracted from the bark of Landes pine, the bracts of the lime tree, and the leaves of the hazel-nut tree. (*See: 'PERIPHERAL VASCULAR DISEASE'; 'RETINOPATHY'; 'VASCULAR FRAGILITY'*)

The standard therapeutic dosage of PCOs is 150 to 300 mg per day.

Similar to the action of bilberry anthocyanosides (*see above*), administration may be effective in diabetic microangiopathy and retinopathy as they may improve the microcirculatory disturbances and vascular fragility noted in diabetes.

Experimental Double-blind Study: In a double-blind trial of 150 mg daily of procyanidol oligomers versus placebo in 25 in diabetic and hypertensive pts., capillary resistance rose from 14.6 cm Hg to 18 cm Hg in the treated gp., while no significant variation was observed in the placebo gp. (*Lagrue G, Olivier-Martin F, Grillot A. [A study of the effects of procyanidol oligomers on capillary resistance in hypertension and in certain nephropathies. Sem Hop Paris 57(33-36):1399-401, 1981*) (*in French*).

Experimental Study: The effects of 150 mg/d of procyanidol oligomers on capillary resistance disorders in hypertensive and diabetic pts. were studied in an open trial. In a gp. of 28 pts., capillary resistance rose from 15.4 cm Hg to 18.1 cm Hg (*Lagrue G, Olivier-Martin F, Grillot A. [A study of the effects of procyanidol oligomers on capillary resistance in hypertension and in certain nephropathies. Sem Hop Paris 57(33-36):1399-401, 1981*) (*in French*).

See Also:

Experimental Study: *Soyeux A et al. [Endotelon. Diabetic retinopathy and hemorheology (preliminary study)]. Bull Soc Ophtalmol Fr 87(12):1441-4, 1987 (in French)*

DIARRHEA

See Also: IRRITABLE BOWEL SYNDROME

Diarrhea can be sub-divided into osmotic and secretory forms:

Osmotic diarrhea: The result of the accumulation of non-absorbale solutes in the gut lumen.

    1. Ingestion of poorly absorbable solutes

        Examples: Magnesium sulfate, sodium sulfate, citrate-containing laxatives, some laxatives (such as $Mg(OH)_2$), mannitol, sorbitol

    2. Maldigestion

    3. Mucosal transport defects

Secretory diarrhea: The result of the effect of a secretory stimulus on the intestinal mucosa.

    1. Inhibition of absorption

    2. Secretion of water and electrolytes resulting in a net luminal gain.

Generally, osmotic diarrhea stops upon fasting or upon discontinuation of ingestion of the poorly absorbable solute, while secretory diarrhea persists despite fasting and the stools are larger in volume and more watery. For acute diarrhea, traveler's diarrhea, and some cases of chronic diarrhea, the most imporant aspect of therapy is prevention or correction of salt and water depletion (*Krejs GJ. Diarrhea, in JB Wyngaarden & LH Smith Jr., Eds. Cecil, Textbook of Medicine. 18th edition. Philadelphia, W. B. Saunders, 1988*).

– –

Berberine:

    An isoquinoline alkaloid found in goldenseal (*Hydrastis canadensis*), barberry bark (*Berberis vulgaris*) and Oregon grape root (*Berberis aquifolium*).

    Berberine is an effective antimicrobial against a wide range of pathogenic organisms (*Amin AH et al. Berberine sulfate: antimicrobial activity, bioassay, and mode of action. Can J Microbiol 15:1067-76, 1969; Hahn FE, Ciak J. Berberine. Antibiotics 3:577-88, 1976; Kaneda Y et al. In vitro effects of berberine sulfate on the growth of Entamoeba histolytica, Giardia lamblia and Tricomonas vaginalis. Annals Trop Med Parasitol 85:417-25, 1991*).

Administration may be beneficial for treating infectious secretory diarrheas (*Desai AB et al. Berberine in treatment of diarrhea. Indian Pediatr 8:462-65, 1971; Sharma R et al. Berbrine tannate in acute diarrhea. Indian Pediatr 7:496-501, 1970*).

> *Note: Dosage of crude herb or extract should approximate the dosage of berberine. Standardized extracts will provide more accurate levels of berberine.*

Cholera

Experimental Controlled Study: Pts. with acute diarrhea due to *Vibrio cholerae* randomly received berberine sulfate (BS) 400 mg in a single dose or served as controls. In treated pts., the mean 8-hr. stool volume during the second 8-hr. period after treatment declined to 2.22 L, which was significantly less than the 2.79 L found in the controls ($p<0.05$). However, pts. who specifically received BS plus tetracycline did not have a significant reduction in stool output compared to pts. who received tetracycline alone. No side effects of BS were noted. Results suggest that the activity of BS against cholera is slight and not additive with tetracycline (*Rabbani GH et al. Randomized controlled trial of berberine sulfate therapy for diarrhea due to enterotoxigenic Escherichia coli and Vibrio cholerae. J Infect Dis 155:979-84, 1987*).

Experimental Double-blind Study: 185 pts. with acute watery diarrhea due to cholera received either berberine, tetracycline, tetracycline and berberine, or placebo. Those given tetracycline or tetracycline and berberine had considerably reduced volume and frequency of diarrheal stools, duration of diarrhea, and volumes of required intravenous and oral rehydration fluid. Berberine did not produce an antisecretory effect; however, analysis by factorial design equations showed a reduction in diarrheal stools by one liter and a reduction in cyclic adenosine monophosphate concentrations in stools by 77% in the groups given berberine. Considerably fewer pts. given tetracycline or tetracycline and berberine excreted vibrios in stools after 24 hours than those given berberine alone (*Khin-Maung U et al. Clinical trial of berberine in acute watery diarrhoea. Br Med J 291:1601-5, 1985*).

Giardiasis

Experimental Placebo-controlled Study: 40 children ages 1-10 infected with Giardia lamblia received either berberine 5 mg/kg/d, metronidazole 10 mg/kg/d or a placebo of vitamin B syrup in 3 divided doses. After 6 days, 48% of pts. treated with berberine were asymptomatic and, on stool analysis, 68% were Giardia-free. 33% of pts. treated with metronidazole were asymptomatic and, on stool analysis, all were Giardia-free. 15% of pts. on placebo were asymptomatic and, on stool analysis, 25% were Giardia-free (*Choudhry VP, Sabir M, Bhide VN. Berberine in giardiasis. Indian Pediatr 9:143-6, 1972*).

See Also:

> **Experimental Study:** *Gupte S. Use of berberine in treatment of giardiasis. Am J Dis Child 129:866, 1975*

Non-specific gastroenteritis

Experimental Controlled Study: Pts. with acute diarrhea due to enterotoxigenic *E. coli* randomly received berberine sulfate 400 mg in a single dose or served as controls. In treated pts., the mean stool volumes were significantly less than those of controls during 3 consecutive 8-hr. periods after treatment ($p<0.05$). At 24 hrs. after treatment, significantly more treated pts. stopped having diarrhea as compared to controls (42% vs. 20%; $p<0.05$). No side effects of BS were noted. Results suggest that BS is effective for *E. coli* diarrhea (*Rabbani GH et al. Randomized controlled trial of berberine sulfate therapy for diarrhea due to enterotoxigenic Escherichia coli and Vibrio cholerae. J Infect Dis 155:979-84, 1987*).

Negative Experimental Double-blind Study: 215 pts. with acute watery diarrhea not due to cholera received either berberine, tetracycline, tetracycline and berberine, or placebo. Neither tetracycline nor berberine had any benefit over placebo (*Khin-Maung U et al. Clinical trial of berberine in acute watery diarrhoea. Br Med J 291:1601-5, 1985*).

Experimental Controlled Study: 65 children below 5 years of age with acute diarrhea responded better to berberine tannate (25 mg/every 6 hrs.) than to standard antibiotic therapy. Berberine was found to be effective for diarrhea caused by *E. coli, Shigella, Salmonella, Klebsiella* and *Faecalis aerogenes* (*Sack RB, Froehlich JL. Berberine inhibits intestinal secretory response of Vibrio cholerae toxins and Escherichia coli enterotoxins. Infect Immun 35:471-5, 1982*).

Experimental Controlled Study: 200 adult pts. with acute diarrhea were given standard antibiotic treatment with or without berberine hydrochloride at a dose of 150 mg/d. Pts. receiving berberine recovered quicker. An additional 30 cases of acute diarrhea were treated with berberine alone. Berberine arrested diarrhea in all of these cases with no mortality or toxicity (*Kamat SA. Clinical trial with berberine hydrochloride for the control of diarrhoea in acute gastroenteritis. J Assoc Physicians India 15:525-9, 1967*).

See Also:

Experimental Study: *Bhakat MP et al. Therapeutic trial of Berberine sulphate in nonspecific gastroenteritis. Ind Med J 68:19-23, 1974*

Carob Pod Powder (*Ceratonia siliqua*):

Since the early 1950s, there have been several reports in the medical literature that decoctions (brewed teas) of roasted carob powder are effective and without side effects in the treatment of acute-onset diarrhea. Carob is rich in dietary fiber (26%) and polyphenols (21%). These components are thought to be responsible for the beneficial effects.

Experimental Double-blind Study: 41 infants aged 3-21 months with acute diarrhea of bacterial and viral origin were treated in a hospital setting with oral rehydration fluid and randomly received for up to 6 days either carob pod powder (1.5 g/kg body weight/day) or an equivalent placebo. The powders were either diluted in the oral rehydration solution or in milk. The duration of diarrhea in the carob group was 2 days and 3.75 days in the placebo group. Normalizations in defecation, body temperature, and weight and cessation of vomiting were also reached much more quickly in the carob group. No side effects to carob were reported (*Loeb H et al. Tannin-rich carob pod for the treatment of acute-onset diarrhea. J Ped Gastroenterol Nutr 8:480-5, 1989*).

Citrus Seed Extract:

Administration may be beneficial.

Experimental Study: 25 pts. with severe atopic eczema were treated. 14/25 complained of intermittent diarrhea, constipation, flatulence, intestinal rushes, bloating and abdominal discomfort (particularly after carbohydrate-rich meals). 10/25 received 2 drops of a 0.5% oral solution (2 drops in 200 ml water) of citrus seed extract (Para Mycrocidin) twice daily, while the other 15 pts. received capsules containing 50 mg extract each at a dosage of 3 caps 3 times daily. After 1 mo., 2/10 pts. on the liquid improved, while all 15 of the pts. on the capsules (which contained a higher dosage of the extract) noted definite improvement of constipation, flatulence, abdominal discomfort and night rest. There were no side effects, although the dosage of the liquid extract that pts. would ingest was limited due to the bitter taste. The extract was mostly effective against Candida, Geotrichum sp. and hemolytic E. coli (*Ionescu G et al. Oral citrus seed extact in atopic eczema: In vitro and in vivo studies on intestinal microflora. J Orthomol Med 5(3):155-8, 1990*).

DYSMENORRHEA

Bilberry (*Vaccinium myrtillus*):

Extracts of anthocyanosides, flavonoid components of bilberry, have demonstrated significant vascular smooth muscle relaxing effects in experimental models (*Bettini V et al. Mechanical responses of isolated coronary arteries to barium in the presence of Vaccinium myrtillus anthocyanosides. Fitoterapia 56:3-10, 1985; Bettini V et al. Inhibition by Vaccinium myrtillus anthocyanosides of barium-induced contractions in segments of internal thoracic vein. Fitoterapia 55:323-7, 1984; Bettini V et al. Effects of Vaccinium myrtillus anthocyanosides on vascular smooth muscle. Fitoterapia 55:265-72, 1984*).

Administration may be beneficial (*Colombo D, Vescovini R. Controlled trial of anthocyanosides from Vaccinium myrtillus in primary dysmenorrhea. G Ital Obstet Ginecol 7:1033-8, 1985*).

Bromelain:

Bromelain refers to the mixture of sulfur containing proteolytic enzymes or proteases obtained from the stem pineapple plant (*Ananas comosus*).

The standard dosage of bromelain (1,800-2,000 m.c.u.) is 125-450 mg 3 times daily on an empty stomach.

A smooth muscle relaxant believed to decrease prostaglandins of the 2 series while increasing levels of PGE_1-like compounds (*Felton G. Does kinin released by pineapple stem bromelain stimulate production of prostaglandin E_1-like compounds? Hawaii Med J 36:39-47, 1977; Taussig SJ, Batkin S. Bromelain, the enzyme complex of pineapple (Ananas comosus) and its clinical application. An update. J Ethnopharmacol 22:191-203, 1988*).

Vaginal instillation may be beneficial.

> **Experimental Study:** 27 pts. with primary dysmenorrhea and 8 normal women received local bromelain applications (using a phosphate buffer solution of pH 5.6), and 8 pts. were examined by isthmography immediately before and after the application of the enzyme solution. Bromelain brings about definite dilatation of isthmus and relaxation of its sphincters when the uterus is under estrogen but not when it is under progestin effect. In primary dysmenorrhea, local bromelain treatment given just before or just after the onset of menstruation always results in dramatic relief of pain and associated symptoms due to its effect on the isthmus, not to its effect on the cervix (*Youssef AH. The uterine isthmus and its sphincter mechanism: a clinical and radiographic study. III. The effect of bromelain on the uterine isthmus. Am J Obstet Gynecol 79(6):1161-8, 1960*).

Experimental Study: 30 pts. with spasmodic dysmenorrhea received local applications of a bromelain solution when in pain. 42/48 treatments had good results. Probable reasons for failure were found in 5/6 unsuccessful treatments. The local application of bromelain usually caused dilatation of the cervical canal as observed by radiography and confirmed by palpation. Within a few minutes, softening and increased vascularity of the cervix was noted. The optimum time for application was just at the onset of or shortly before the period (*Simmons CA. The relief of pain in spasmodic dysmenorrhoea by bromelain. Lancet ii:827-30, 1958*).

Experimental Study: 64 pts. with dysmenorrhea so disabling as to require narcotics for relief were treated when in pain with vaginal instillation of a bromelain solution which had been mixed earlier and freeze dried until needed (each 50 cc of phosphate buffer containing 0.075 g bromelain). All 40 pts. with primary dysmenorrhea obtained immediate relief, while the 24 pts. with secondary dysmenorrhea had poor to fair results. The best results were in teen-agers, young nulliparas, and a few older pts. without concurrent gynecologic disease (*Hunter RG et al. The action of papain and bromelain on the uterus. Am J Obstet Gynecol 73:867-80, 1957*).

Dong Quai (*Angelica sinensis*):

Dong quai is the root of *Angelica sinensis*. Japanese Angelica (*Angelica acutiloba*) has similar properties.

Dong quai has demonstrated good uterine tonic activity, causing an initial increase in uterine contraction followed by relaxation.

The standard dosage is 1 gram 3 times daily.

Administration may be beneficial.

Animal Experimental Study: Intraduodenal administration of 70% MeOH extract of Japanese Angelica root (3 g/kg) increased uterine contractile activities in anesthetized rabbits.The activity of the extract shifted to the aqueous layer (positive at a dose of 1 g/kg) with successive fractionation of the extracts with hexane and BuOH, indicating contribution of a hydrophilic principle(s) to the effect. In some animal preparations, inhibiting effect of the extract on uterine contraction was noted after the uterotonic effect terminated (*Harada M, Suzuki M, Ozaki Y. Effect of Japanese Angelica root and peony root on uterine contraction in the rabbit in situ. J Pharmacobiodyn 7(5):304-11, 1984*).

Feverfew (*Tanacetum parthenium*):

Extracts have been shown to inhibit the synthesis of prostaglandins, leukotrienes, and thromboxanes at the initial stage of synthesis (*Makheja AM, Bailey JM. A platelet phospholipase inhibitor from the medicinal herb feverfew (Tanacetum parthenium). Prostagland Leukotri Med 8:653-60, 1982; Makheja AM, Bailey JM. The active principle in feverfew. Lancet ii:1054, 1981*).

Note: The efficacy of feverfew is dependent upon adequate levels of parthenolide, the active ingredient. (The preparations used in clinical trials has a parthenolide content of 0.4-0.66%.)

Animal Ex vivo Study: Extracts of fresh feverfew caused a dose- and time-dependent, irreversible inhibition of the contractile response of rabbit aortic rings to all receptor-acting agonists tested. The presence of potentially SH reacting parthenolide and other sesquiterpene alpha-methylenebutyrolactones in these extracts, and the close parellelism of pure parthenolide, suggest that the inhibitory effects are due to these compounds. Extracts of the dry leaves were not inhibitory and actually caused potent and sustained contractions of aortic smooth muscle; these extracts were found to be devoid or parthenolide or butyrolactones (*Barsby RWJ, Salan U, Knight BW, Hoult JRS. Feverfew and vascular smooth muscle: Extracts from fresh and dried plants show opposing pharmacological profiles, dependent upon sesquiterpene lactone content. Planta Medica 59:20-5, 1993*).

Chemical Analysis: The parthenolide content of over 35 different commercial preparations of feverfew was determined by bioassay, 2 HPLC methods, and NMR. The results indicate a wide variation in the amts. of parthenolide in commercial preparations. The majority of products contained no parthenolide or only traces (*Heptinstall S et al. Parthenolide content and bioactivity of feverfew (Tanacetum parthenium (L.) Schultz-Bip.). Estimation of commercial and authenticated feverfew products. J Pharm Pharmacol 44:391-5, 1992*).

WARNING: No long-term toxicity studies have been conducted. While feverfew is extremely well-tolerated and no serious side effects have ever been reported, chewing the leaves can result in small ulcerations in the mouth and swelling of the lips and tongue in about 10% of users (*Awang DVC. Feverfew. Can Pharm J 122:266-70, 1989*).

Administered traditionally for the treatment of dysmenorrhea (*Duke JA. Handbook of Medicinal Herbs. Boca Raton, FL, CRC Press, 1985:118*).

Papain:

An extract of proteolytic enzymes derived from papaya may offer similar benefits to bromelain (*see above*).

Administration may be effective (*Hunter RG et al. The action of papain and bromelain on the uterus. Am J Obstet Gynecol 73:867-80, 1957*).

ECZEMA
(ATOPIC DERMATITIS)

<u>Chamomile</u> (*Matricaria chamomilla*):

Chamomile preparations are widely used in Europe for the treatment of a variety of common skin complaints including eczema, psoriasis, and dry, flaky, irritated skin. The flavonoid and essential oil components of chamomile possess significant anti-inflammatory and anti-allergy activity (*Mann C, Staba EJ. The chemistry, pharmacology, and commercial formulations of chamomile. <u>Herbs, Spices, and Medicinal Plants</u> 1:235-80, 1984*).

Topical application may be beneficial.

> **Animal Experimental Study:** Chamomile extracts exerted anti-inflammatory effects when applied topically in animal models of inflammation (*Della Loggia R et al. Evaluation of the anti-inflammatory activity of chamomile preparations. <u>Planta Med</u> 56:657-8, 1990*).

See Also:

> **Animal Experimental Study:** *Tubaro A et al. Evaluation of antiinflammatory activity of a chamomile extract after topical application. <u>Planta Med</u> 51:359, 1984*

<u>*Euphorbia acaulis*</u>:

The root of *Euphorbia acaulis* has been used in Ayurvedic medicine for eczema.

Administration may be beneficial.

> **Experimental Double-blind Study:** Of the 23 pts. given 50 mg of powdered Euphorbia acaulis root 3 times daily for 2-6 weeks, 18 experienced complete relief and 3 experienced 75% relief (*Agrawal DK, Chandra J, Raju TV. Clinical studies of Euphorbia acaulis, Rox b. in cases of eczema—a preliminary report. <u>Indian J Dermatol</u> 16(3):57-9, 1971*).

<u>*Ginkgo biloba*</u>:

Ginkgo biloba contains several unique terpene molecules known collectively as ginkgolides that antagonize platelet activating factor (PAF), a key chemical mediator in atopic dermatitis. PAF plays a central role in many inflammatory and allergic processes including neutrophil activation, increasing vascular permeability, smooth muscle contraction including bronchoconstriction, and reduction in coronary blood flow. Ginkgolides compete with PAF for binding sites and inhibit the various events induced by PAF (*Koltai M et al. Platelet activating factor (PAF). A review of its effects, antagonists and possible future clinical implica-*

tions (Part I). Drugs 42(1):9-29, 1991; Koltai M et al. PAF. A review of its effects, antagonists and possible future clinical implications (Part II). Drugs 42(2):174-204, 1991).

Administration of mixtures of ginkgolides (BN 52063), as well as *Ginkgo biloba* extract standardized to contain 24% ginkgoflavonglycosides, may be beneficial.

Experimental Study: Clinical and histopathologic responses to intradermal PAF were evaluated in 12 atopic subjects, without evidence of atopic dermatitis, before and after administration of 120 mg BN 52063. Without BN 52063 pretreatment, PAF produced an immediate acute wheal and flare reaction. The reaction was characterized by a predominantly neutrophilic response, which was seen at 30 minutes and was maximal at 4 hours. Eosinophils were observed in the infiltrate as early as 30 minutes after injection, and were maximal by 12 hours. BN 52063 antagonized the acute flare response to intradermal PAF but had little effect on cellular recruitment at the site of injection (*Markey AC et al. Platelet activating factor-induced clinical and histopathologic responses in atopic skin and their modification by the platelet activating factor antagonist BN52063. J Am Acad Dermatol 23(2):263-8, 1990*).

Licorice root (*Glycyrrhiza glabra*):

Glycyrrhetinic acid isolated from licorice exerts an effect similar to that of topical hydrocortisone in the treatment of eczema, contact and allergic dermatitis, and psoriasis.

Experimental Clinical and In vitro Study: Glycyrrhetinic acid potentiated the activity of hydrocortisone by inhibiting the 11-beta-hydroxysteroid dehydrogenase which catalyses the conversion of hydrocortisone to an inactive form (*Teelucksingh S et al. Potentiation of hydrocortisone activity in skin by glycyrrhetinic acid. Lancet 335:1060-3, 1990*).

Topical administration may be beneficial.

Experimental Studies: 9 of 12 pts. with intractable eczema noted marked improvement and 2 pts. noted mild improvements when an ointment containing glycyrrhetinic acid was applied topically. In a separate study, 93% of pts. applying glycyrrhetinic acid demonstrated improvement compared to 83% using cortisone (*Evans FQ. The rational use of glycyrrhetinic acid in dermatology. Br J Clin Pract 12:269-79, 1958*).

See Also:

In Vitro Study: *Okimasa E et al. Inhibition of phospholipase A2 by glycyrrhizin, an anti-inflammatory drug. Acta Med Okayama 37:385-91, 1983.*

Lupine Seed extract (*Lupinus termis*):

Topical application of the ethanol extract of lupine seeds may be beneficial.

Experimental Double-blind Study: The study compared a 10% ointment prepared from a 95% ethanol extract of lupine seeds with a 0.02% flumethasone pivalate ointment and a placebo showed that the lupine seed extract was effective in the treatment of chronic eczema. The results obtained with the extract were statistically comparable to those obtained with corticoid therapy (*Antoun MD, Taha OM. Studies on Sudanese* *medicinal plants. II. Evaluation of an extract of Lupinus termis seeds in chronic eczema. J Nat Prod 44(2):179-83, 1981)*

Witch Hazel (*Hamamelis virginiana*):

Topical application may be beneficial.

Experimental Double-blind Study: Two groups of patients with atopic dermatitis (n=36) and contact dermatitis (n=80) were treated with a witch hazel preparation (Hametum Salbe®) and a control preparation. Hametum Salbe® was superior in effectiveness in treatment of atopic dermatitis compared to the control preparation. There was no difference in therapeutic efficacy in the treatment of primary irritant contact dermatitis. For treatment and interval therapy as well as for long-term treatment of chronic dermatoses Hametum Salbe® is a valuable dermatological preparation which can be used without any risk in long-term therapy *(Pfister R. [Problems in the treatment and after care of chronic dermatoses. A clinical study on hametum ointment]. Fortschr Med 99(31-32):1264-8, 1981) (in German).*

- -

COMBINATION TREATMENT

Licorice-containing Chinese Herbal Formula:

A Chinese herbal formula containing licorice (*Glycyrrhiza glabra*) along with *Ledebouriealla seseloides, Potentilla chinensis, Clematis chenisis, Clematis armandi, Rehmania glutinosa, Paeonia lactiflora, Lophatherum gracile, Dictamnus dasycarpus, Tribulus terrestris,* and *Schizonepeta tenuiflora* has been the subject of several studies by a group of researchers after one of their patients with atopic dermatitis experienced remarkable improvement after taking a decoction prescribed by a Chinese doctor.

Administration may be beneficial.

Experimental Double-blind Study: 40 adult pts. with longstanding, refractary, widespread, atopic dermatitis were randomized to receive 2 month's treatment of either the active formula or placebo, followed by a crossover to the other treatment after a 4-week washout period. Of the 31 pts. completing the study, 20 preferred the active formula while only 4 pts. preferred the placebo. There was also a subjective improvement in itching (p) and sleep (p) during the active treatment phase. No side effects were reported although many complained about the unpalatability of the decoction *(Sheehan MP et al. Efficacy of traditional Chinese herbal therapy in adult atopic dermatitis. Lancet 340:13-7, 1992).*

Experimental Double-blind Study: 47 children were given active treatment and placebo in random order, each for 8 weeks, with an intervening 4-week wash-out period. 37 children tolerated the treatment and completed the study. Response to active treatment was superior to response to placebo, and was clinically valuable. There was no evidence of haematological, renal or hepatic toxicity. These findings anticipate a wider therapeutic potential for traditional Chinese medicinal plants in this disease, and other skin diseases *(Sheehan MP, Atherton DJ. A controlled trial of traditional Chinese medicinal plants in widespread non-exudative atopic eczema. Br J Dermatol 126(2):179-84, 1992).*

See Also:

Review Article: *Atherton DJ et al. Treatment of atopic eczema with traditional Chinese medicinal plants. Pediatr Dermatol 9(4):373-5. 1992*

Atherton DJ et al. Traditional Chinese plants for eczema. Letter. Lancet 338(8765):510, 1991

Atherton DJ et al. Chinese herbs for eczema. Letter. Lancet 336(8725):1254, 1990

FATIGUE

<u>Caffeine-containing Herbs</u>:

Caffeine-containing beverages and herbs (coffee, tea, guarana, cola nut, and cocoa) are used worldwide to reduce fatigue.

> WARNING: Caffeine ingestion can result in significant side effects, including 'caffeinism' (*Chou T. Wake up and smell the coffee. Caffeine, coffee, and the medical consequences. <u>West J Med</u> 157:544-53, 1992*).

Caffeine consumption may delay physical fatigue and improve performance.

Review Article: Three principal cellular mechanisms have been proposed to explain the ergogenic potential of caffeine during exercise: (a) increased myofilament affinity for calcium and/or increased release of calcium from the sarcoplasmic reticulum in skeletal muscle; (b) cellular actions caused by accumulation of cyclic-$3^1,5^1$-adenosine monophosphate (cAMP) in various tissues including skeletal muscle and adipocytes; and (c) cellular actions mediated by competitive inhibition of adenosine receptors in the central nervous system and somatic cells. The relative importance of each of the above mechanisms in explaining *in vivo* physiological effects of caffeine during exercise continues to be debated. However, growing evidence suggests that inhibition of adenosine receptors is one of the most important, if not the most important, mechanism to explain the physiological effects of caffeine at nontoxic plasma concentrations. Numerous animal studies using high caffeine doses have reported increased force development in isolated skeletal muscle in both *in vitro* and *in situ* preparations. In contrast, *in vivo* human studies have not consistently shown caffeine to enhance muscular performance during high intensity, short term exercise. Further, recent evidence supports previous work that shows caffeine does not improve performance during short term incremental exercise. Although controversy exists, the major part of published evidence evaluating performance supports the notion that caffeine is ergogenic during prolonged (30 min), moderate intensity (approximately 75 to 80% VO2max) exercise. The mechanism to explain these findings may be linked to a caffeine-mediated glycogen sparing effect secondary to an increased rate of lipolysis (*Dodd SL, Herb RA, Powers SK. Caffeine and exercise performance. An update. <u>Sports Med</u> 15(1):14-23, 1993*).

Experimental Double-blind Study: The effects of breakfast and caffeine on performance, mood and cardiovascular functioning in the late morning and after lunch were studied. 48 subjects were tested at 07:45 and then assigned to one of the four conditions formed by combining caffeine and breakfast conditions. Subjects in the caffeine condition were given a dose of 4 mg/kg, the caffeine manipulation being double blind. At 11:15 subjects were given another coffee (subjects remained in the same caffeine condition) and had lunch at 12:30. Performance was examined prior to lunch (11:30) and after lunch (14:00). Effects of breakfast on recognition memory (lower false alarm rate) and logical reasoning (reduced accuracy) were found in the late morning but not after lunch. However, a semantic processing task was performed more slowly by the breakfast group after lunch. Caffeine improved performance on a sustained attention task, the logical reasoning task and semantic memory task. Subjects given caffeine also reported greater alertness and feelings of well-being, whereas the effects of breakfast on mood changed from the late morning to early afternoon. Few interactions between breakfast and caffeine conditions were obtained *(Smith AP, Kendrick AM, Maben AL. Effects of breakfast and caffeine on performance and mood in the late morning and after lunch. Neuropsychobiology 26(4):198-204, 1992).*

See Also:

> **Review Article:** *Clarkson PM. Nutritional ergogenic aids: caffeine. Int J Sport Nutr 3(1):103-11, 1993*

> **Review Article:** *Jacobson BH, Kulling FA. Health and ergogenic effects of caffeine. Br J Sports Med 23(1):34-40, 1989*

Panax ginseng:

Administration of *Panax ginseng* (Chinese or Korean ginseng) root may improve performance, reduce mental fatigue from mental stress and delay physical fatigue from prolonged exercise.

Experimental Double-blind Crossover Study: Ginseng extract (Ginsana) at a dose of 100 mg twice a day for 12 weeks was compared with placebo in various tests of psychomotor performance in university students. A favorable effect of ginseng relative to baseline performance was observed in attention (cancellation test), mental arithmetic, logical deduction, integrated sensory-motor function (choice reaction time), and auditory reaction time. However, statistically significant superiority over the placebo group was noted only for mental arithmetic. It is interesting to note that in the course of the trial the students taking ginseng reported a greater sensation of well-being *(D'Angelo L et al. A double-blind, placebo controlled clinical study on the effect of a standardized ginseng extract on psychomotor performance in healthy volunteers. J Ethnopharmacol 16:15-22, 1986).*

Experimental Double-blind Study: Nurses who had switched from day to night duty rated themselves for competence, mood, and general well-being, and were given an objective test of psychophysical performance, blood counts, and blood chemistry. The group administered ginseng demonstrated higher scores in competence, mood parameters, and objective psychophysical performance when compared with those receiving a placebo *(Hallstrom C, Fulder S, Carruthers M. Effect of ginseng on the performance of nurses on night duty. Comp Med East & West 6:277-82, 1982).*

Animal Experimental Study: Ginseng spares glycogen utilization in exercising muscle by enhancing the utilization of oxygen in fatty acid oxidation. During prolonged exercise, the development of fatigue is closely related to the depletion of glycogen stores and the build-up of lactic acid, both in skeletal muscle and the liver. When an adequate supply of oxygen is available to the working muscle, nonesterified fatty acids are the preferred energy substrate, thus sparing utilization of muscle glycogen, blood glucose, and, consequently, liver glycogen. The greater the ability to conserve body carbohydrate stores by mobilizing and oxidizing fatty acids, the greater the amount of time to exhaustion (*Avakia EV, Evonuk E. Effects of Panax ginseng extract on tissue glycogen and adrenal cholesterol depletion during prolonged exercise. Planta Med 36:43-8, 1979*).

Animal Experimental Study: Ginseng possessed significant antifatigue activity in exercising mice, as a clear dose-dependent increase in time to exhaustion was noted in mice receiving ginseng. The time to exhaustion was increased up to 183% in the mice given ginseng 30 minutes prior to exercising, compared with controls (*Brekhman II, Dardymov IV. Pharmacological investigation of glycosides from ginseng and Eleutherococcus. Lloydia 32:46-51, 1969*).

See Also:

> **Review Article:** *Hikino H: Traditional remedies and modern assessment: The case of ginseng, in ROB Wijeskera, Ed. The Medicinal Plant Industry. Boca Raton, FL, CRC Press, 1991:149-66*

> **Review Article:** *Chong SK, Oberholzer VG. Ginseng—is there a use in clinical medicine? Postgrad Med J 64(757):841-6, 1988*

> **Animal Experimental Study:** *Petkov VD, Mosharrof AH. Effects of standardized ginseng extract on learning, memory and physical capabilities. Am J Chin Med 15:19-29, 1987*

> **Review Article:** *Shibata S et al. Chemistry and pharmacology of Panax. Econ Medicinal Plant Res 1:217-84, 1985*

> **Animal Experimental Study:** *Kaku T et al. Chemicopharmacological studies on saponins of Panax ginseng C.A. Meyer. Arzniem Forsch 25:539-47, 1975*

> **Animal Experimental Study:** *Saito H, Yoshida Y, Takagi K. Effect of Panax ginseng root on exhaustive exercise in mice. Jap J Pharmacol 24:119-27, 1974*

> **Animal Experimental Study:** *Sterner W, Kirchdorfer AM. [Comparative work load tests on mice with standardized ginseng extract and a ginseng containing pharmaceutical preparation.] Z Gerontol 3:307-12, 1970 (in German)*

Siberian Ginseng (*Eleutherococcus senticosus*):

Administration may improve work capacity, athletic performance and mental alertness.

> **Review Article:** The results of clinical trials designed to evaluate the 'adaptogenic' effects of Eleutherococcus were reviewed. In these studies the fluid extract of *Eleutherococcus senticosus* root was administered to more than 2,100 healthy human subjects. The data indicated that Eleutherococcus: (1) increased the ability of humans to withstand many adverse physical conditions (i.e., heat, noise, motion, work load increase, exercise, and decompression); (2) increased mental alertness and work output; and (3) improved the quality of work under stressful conditions and athletic performance. The male and female subjects ranged in age from 19 to 72 years. Dosages of the fluid extract (33% ethanol) ranged from 2.0-16.0 ml, one to three times a day, for periods of up to 60 consecutive days (*Farnsworth NR et al. Siberian ginseng*

(Eleutherococcus senticosus): Current status as an adaptogen. Econ Med Plant Res 1:156-215, 1985).

Experimental Placebo-controlled Crossover Study: 6 adolescent males displayed significant increases in maximal work test, maximal working capacity, VO$_2$max, and oxygen pulse compared to the placebo when given 2 ml of Eleutherococcus fluid extract twice daily for 8 days *(Asano K et al. Effect of Eleutherococcus senticosus extract on human physical working capacity. Planta Med 53:175-7, 1986).*

GALLBLADDER DISEASE
(CHOLECYSTITIS AND CHOLELITHIASIS)

<u>Curcumin</u>:

The yellow pigment and active component of turmeric (*Curcuma longa*).

Administration may increase the solubility of the bile.

> **Animal Experimental Study:** Curcumin increases bile acid output by over 100% and greatly increases the solubility of the bile, suggesting a possible benefit in the prevention and treatment of gallstones (*Ramprasad C and Sirsi M. Curcuma longa and bile secretion - Quantitative changes in the bile constituents induced by sodium curcuminate.* <u>J Sci Indust Res</u> *16C:108-10, 1957*).

<u>Silymarin</u>:

Silymarin, the flavonoid complex from milk thistle (*Silybum marianum*), may be beneficial by increasing the solubility of the bile.

> **Experimental Double-blind Study:** Biliary lipid composition was assayed in 4 gallstone and 15 cholecystectomy pts. before and after silymarin (420 mg/d for 30 days) or placebo. Silymarin treatment led to significant reduction in the biliary cholesterol concentration and bile saturation index (*Nassauto G, Lemmolo RM, et al. Effect of silibinin on biliary lipid composition. Experimental and clinical study.* <u>J Hepatol</u> *12:290-5, 1991*).

Silybin, the main active component of silymarin, bound to phosphatidylcholine may be more effective. (*See: 'HEPATITIS'*)

> **Experimental Study:** The biliary excretion of silybin was evaulated in 9 cholecystectomy pts. with T-tube drainage following a single oral dose of silybin-phosphatidylcholine complex (IdB 1016) and silymarin. The amount of silybin recovered in the bile in free and conjugated form within 48h was 11% for the silybin-phosphatidylcholine and 3% for silymarin (*Schandalik R, Gatti G, Perucca E. Pharmacokinetics of silybin in bile following administration of silipide and silymarin in cholecystectomy patients.* <u>Arzneim Forsch</u> *42(7):964-8, 1992*).

> **Experimental Study:** In order to assess the pharmacokinetic profile in man, plasma silybin levels were determined after administration of single oral doses of a silibin-phosphatidylcholine complex (IdB 1016) and silymarin (equivalent to 360 mg silybin) to 9 healthy volunteers. Although absorption was rapid with both preparations, the bioavailability of the silibin-phosphatidylcholine complex was much greater than that of silymarin, as indicated by higher plasma silybin levels at all sampling times after

intake of the complex. Regardless of the preparation used, the terminal half-life was relatively short (generally less than 4 h). In a subsequent study, 9 healthy volunteers received IdB 1016 (120 mg twice daily expressed as silybin equivalents) for 8 consecutive days. The plasma silybin level profiles and kinetic parameters on day 1 were similar to those determined on day 8. Most of the silybin present in the systemic circulation was in conjugated form. Less than 3% of the administered dose was accounted for by urinary recovery of free plus conjugated silybin, a significant proportion of the dose probably being excreted in the bile. It is concluded that complexation with phosphatidylcholine in IdB 1016 greatly increases the oral bioavailability of silybin, probably by facilitating its passage across the gastrointestinal mucosa (*Barzaghi N et al. Pharmacokinetic studies on IdB 1016, a silybin-phosphatidylcholine complex, in healthy human subjects. Eur J Drug Metab Pharmacokinet 15(4):333-8, 1990*).

- -

COMBINATION TREATMENT

Plant Terpenes:

A mixture of plant terpenes (Rowachol®) has been shown to help dissolve gallstones in several studies. Although effective alone, better results appear to be achieved when plant terpene complexes are combined with bile acid therapy.

Each 100 mg capsule of Rowachol® contains:

> Menthol 32 mg
> Menthone 6 mg
> Pinene 17 mg
> Borneol 5 mg
> Camphene 5 mg
> Cineol 2 mg
> Olive oil 33 mg

> Dosage: 2 to 3 capsules with meals (3 times daily) if used alone or 1 capsule 3 times daily if used in combination with chenodeoxycholic acid (750 mg/per day).

Experimental Study: 31 pts. with radiolucent common bile duct stones received medical treatment for 3 to 48 months. Of 19 pts. given Rowachol alone, 8 (42%) had complete stone disappearance. Of 15 pts. given Rowachol and chenodeoxycholic acid or ursodeoxycholic acid, 11 (73%) had complete dissolution within 18 months (*Somerville KW et al. Stones in the common bile duct: experience with medical dissolution therapy. Postgrad Med J 61:313-6, 1985*).

Experimental Study: The effect of Rowachol (200 mg 3 times daily) on biliary lipid secretion and serum lipids was measured in 6 healthy male volunteers before and after 4 weeks of treatment. Biliary cholesterol and phospholipid secretion increased significantly from 113 mumol/h to 155 mumol/h (p) and from 409 mumol/h to 587 ± 185 mumol/h (p), respectively. Bile acid secretion increased from 1519 mumol/h to 2287 mumol/h ($p < 0.05$ and $p < 0.10$). This marked increase in biliary lipid secretion was not followed by a change in molar composition of biliary lipids and lithogenicity of bile. Serum cholesterol and triglycerides declined from 4.9 mmol/l to 4.1 mmol/l (p) and from 1.2 mmol/l to 0.9 mmol/l (p) respectively. The ratio of HDL cholesterol to total cholesterol increased from 0.22 to 0.31 (p) (*Leiss O, von Bergmann K. Effect of Rowachol on biliary lipid secretion and serum lipids in normal volunteers. Gut 26(1):32-7, 1985*).

Experimental Study: 30 pts. with gallstones were given Rowachol (1 capsule twice daily) and chenodeoxycholic acid (750 mg/d) for up to 2 years. Stone disappeared completely in 11 pts. within 1 year and in 15 within 2 years (*Ellis WR et al. Pilot study of combination treatment for gall stones with medium dose chenodeoxycholic acid and a terpene preparation. Br Med J 289:153-6, 1984*).

Experimental Study: 6 of 23 pts. with gallstones had complete dissolution after taking 3 capsules of Rowachol and 750-1,000 mg of chenodeoxycholic acid daily for 6 months (*Bell GD et al. How does Rowachol, a mixture of plant monterpenes, enhance the cholelithic potential of low and medium dose chenodeoxycholic acid? Br J Pharmacol 13:278-9, 1982*).

Negative Animal Experimental Study: 80 hamsters were allocated to 8 groups. One group received only standard rodent chow. The other 7 groups received the lithogenic regime (standard chow containing ethinyl estradiol and increased cholesterol), either alone or with 20 mg/kg/day of UDCA, or 5, 10, or 20 mg/kg/day of mixed terpenes in olive oil, 10 mg/ kg/day of Rowachol or 0.2 cc/day of olive oil. The animals were sacrificed after 12 weeks. Two additional groups of 6 hamsters each received the lithogenic regime for 12 weeks, and then were switched to the standard diet, alone or with 10 mg/kg/day of Rowachol for 8 weeks at which time they were sacrificed. Rowachol decreased HMGCoA reductase activity 18%, but did not dissolve gallstones. Neither the terpenes nor Rowachol altered the biliary cholesterol saturation index, bile acid pool size or the activity of cholesterol 7-alpha hydroxylase or prevented formation of gallstones. UDCA unsaturated bile, increased the total bile acid pool size 38%, depressed the activity of HMGCoA reductase 29%, and prevented formation of gallstones (*Handelsman B et al. Rowachol and ursodeoxycholic acid in hamsters with cholesterol gallstones. Am J Med Sci 84(3):16-22, 1982*).

Experimental Study: 46 pts. with gallstones were given either Rowachol, chenodexoycholic acid, or both. At 6 months, the response rate was 2/13, 0/6, and 11/21 respectively (*Ellis WR et al. Adjunct to bile-acid treatment for gall-stone dissolution: low dose chenodeoxycholic acid combined with a terpene preparation. Br Med J 282:611-2, 1981*).

Experimental Study: Rowachol's effect on the lipid composition of (1) samples of fasting gall bladder bile obtained at the time of cholecystectomy, and (2) T-tube bile on the tenth post-operative day were studied. In a dose of 2 capsules 3 times daily. for only 48 hours, Rowachol significantly enhanced the cholesterol solubility of both gallbladder and T-tube bile. Rowachol in a dose of one capsule 3 times a day for 48 hours did not alter bile composition, while 4 capsules 4 times daily for a similar period caused a significant reduction in biliary cholesterol saturation index (*Doran J, Keighley MR, Bell GD. Rowachol—a possible treatment for cholesterol gallstones. Gut 20(4):312-7, 1979*).

Experimental Study: 23 pts. were treated with Rowachol (1 capsule/10 kg body weight/d). After 6-12 mo., 3 had complete and 4 had partial dissolution of their gallstones (*Bell GD, Doran J. Gallstone dissolution in man using an essential oil prepara-tion. Br Med J 278:24, 1979*).

Experimental Study: Of 4/151 pts. with x-ray confirmed gallstones treated with Rowachol for 6 months experienced complete gallstone dissolution; the other pts. showed no change in the size of their gallstones. There was no change in liver, blood or urine tests in any pt. (*Hordinsky BZ. Terpenes in the treatment of gallstones. Minn Med 54:649-51, 1971*).

Enteric-coated peppermint oil may produce similar results to Rowachol® and is more readily available in the United States and Canada. The components of peppermint oil are as follows:

Menthol 42%
Menthone 27%
Neo-menthone 7%
Cineole 6%
Menthyl acetate 6%

Dosage: 1 to 2 capsules (0.2 ml peppermint oil per capsule) with meals (3 times daily) if used alone, or 1 capsule 3 times a day if used in combination with che-nodeoxycholic acid (750 mg/per day).

Animal Experimental Study: In guinea pigs, peppermint oil produced the greatest spasmolytic effect on Oddi's sphincter compared to other essential oils. It also pro-moted the release of cholecystokinin which led to unblockage of Oddi's sphincter pro-duced by morphine (*Giachetti D, Taddei E, Taddei I. Pharmacological activity of es-sential oils on Oddi's sphincter. Planta Med 54:389-92, 1988*).

GLAUCOMA

Coleus forskohlii:

The root of _Coleus forskohlii_, an herb used in Ayurvedic medicine, contains a diterpene molecule known as forskolin, a powerful activator of adenylate cyclase in various tissue that leads to elevation of cAMP. In the the eye, elevation of cAMP may reduce intraocular pressure.

Topically applied forskolin may be effective.

Experimental Double-blind Study: Two studies were performed to investigate the effects of forskolin on intraocular pressure (IOP). In the first study two 1.0% formulations of forskolin eye drops were compared with placebo in 10 healthy volunteers. Oxybuprocaine eye drops were used for local anaesthesia before measurement of IOP by applanation tonometry. This was followed by instillation of either medication or placebo on a randomized crossover basis and hourly measurement of IOP. For 6 hours after drug application a definite decrease in IOP relative to baseline values was observed after each of the forskolin treatments as well as after placebo. In a subsequent study only one formulation of 1% forskolin was compared with placebo. Proxymetacaine eye drops were used for local anaesthesia. Forskolin resulted in a significant reduction in IOP relative to placebo. It is concluded that forskolin reduces IOP in healthy volunteers, and that oxybuprocaine reduces IOP in its own right (_Meyer BH et al. The effects of forskolin eye drops on intraocular pressure. S Afr Med J 71(9):570-1, 1987_).

Negative Experimental Double-blind Study: A 1% forskolin suspension produced no statistically significant effects on the rate of aqueous flow in human volunteers (_Brubaker RF et al. Topical forskolin (Colforsin) and aqueous flow in humans. Arch Ophthalmol 105:637-41, 1987_).

Experimental Controlled Study: A single instillation of a 1% forskolin suspension produced no statistically significant effects on the rate of aqueous flow or intraocular in human volunteers. A second instillation, however, resulted in significant reduction in maximum IOP (a drop of 2.4 mm Hg in 1 hour) and aqueous flow rate (87% of the control rate) (_Seto C et al. Acute effects of topical forskolin on aqueous humor dynamics in man. Jap J Ophthalmol 30:238-44, 1986_).

Experimental Human and Animal Study: A 1% forskolin suspension lowered intraocular pressure in humans, rabbits, and monkeys. The outflow pressure fell by an average of 70% (_Caprioli J, Sears M. Forskolin lowers intraocular pressure in rabbits, monkeys, and man. Lancet i:958-60, 1983_).

169

Ginkgo biloba:

Ginkgo biloba extract (GBE) standardized to contain 24% ginkgoflavonglycosides may be effective. The standard dose of GBE is 40 mg 3 times daily. (*See: 'CEREBROVASCULAR DISEASE'; 'PERIPHERAL VASCULAR DISEASE'; 'RETINOPATHY'*).

Experimental Study: 46 pts. with, in most cases, severe vascular degenerative retinochoroidal circulatory disturbances or with glaucomatous visual field defects were treated with *Ginkgo biloba* extract 160 mg/day for 4 weeks, then 120 mg/day. Treatment success was assessed monthly by measuring visual acuity, visual field, funduscopy, pulse rate and blood pressure, sometimes including intraocular pressure, fluorescence angiography and ODG. Mild improvements were noted, but were deemed relevant due to the largely bad prognosis of these serious disorders (*Merte HJ, Merkle W. [Long-term treatment with Ginkgo biloba extract of circulatory disturbances of the retina and optic nerve.] Klin Monatsbl Augenheilkd 177(5):577-83, 1980*) (*in German*).

Salvia miltiorrhiza:

A traditional Chinese herbal medicine.

Administration may be beneficial.

Experimental Study: 121 pts. (153 eyes) with middle or late stage glaucoma for whom intraocular pressure was controlled to within the normal range by surgery or miotics received daily intramuscular injections of *Salvia miltiorrhiza* root alone (2 g in 1 ml solution) or in combination with other Chinese herbs for a 30 day course of treatment. Visual acuity improved in 43.8% of the eyes treated, and 30.9% of eyes improved to a point where pts. could see more than 2 more lines on the visual acuity test than prior to treatment. Visual acuity was unchanged in 43.1% of eyes, and decreased by 1 line in 13%. Based on the Ben Esterman Grid, visual fields improved in 49.7% of eyes, and increased more than 11% in 33.3%. Visual fields were unchanged in 37.9% of eyes and reduced in 12.4%. There were no statistically significant differences among the 4 preparations. Compared to 23 eyes not treated with herbs, the traditional Chinese herbal therapy was more effective in regard to changes in visual field ($p < 0.01$). On follow-up 7-30 months later, for 14/19 eyes examined, the visual fields were unchanged or improved, suggesting that the benefits of herbal treatment can be maintained for a long period of time (*Zhen-zhong W, You-qin J, Su-mo Y, MIng-ti X. Radix Salviae Miltiorrhizae in middle and late stage glaucoma. Chin Med J (Engl) 96(6):445-7, 1983*).

HEADACHE

Capsaicin:

Capsaicin is the active component of cayenne pepper (*Capsicum frutescens*). When topically applied, capsaicin is known to stimulate and then block small-diameter pain fibers by depleting them of the neurotransmitter substance P. Substance P is thought to be the principle chemomediator of pain impulses from the periphery.

Commercial ointments containing 0.025% or 0.075% capsaicin are available over-the-counter.

Intranasal application of capsaicin ointment may relieve cluster headaches.

Experimental Double-blind Study: Pts. in acute cluster were randomized to receive either capsaicin or placebo in the ipsilateral nostril for 7 days. Pts. recorded the severity of each headache for 15 days. Headaches on days 8-15 of the study were significantly less severe in the capsaicin group vs the placebo group. There was also a significant decrease in headache severity in the capsaicin group on days 8-15 compared to days 1-7, but not in the placebo group. Episodic CH pts. appeared to benefit more than chronic CH patients. These results indicate that intranasal capsaicin may provide a new therapeutic option for the treatment of this disease (*Marks DR et al. A double-blind placebo-controlled trial of intranasal capsaicin for cluster headache. Cephalalgia 13(2):114-6, 1993*).

Feverfew (*Tanacetum parthenium*):

Feverfew appears to work in the treatment and prevention of migraine headaches by inhibiting the release of blood vessel dilating substances from platelets (serotonin and histamine), inhibiting the production of inflammatory substances (leukotrienes, serine proteases, etc.), and re-establishing proper blood vessel tone. Commercial sources providing assurance of botanical identity and minimum required level of parthenolides are needed (*Awang DVC. Feverfew. Can Pharm J 122:266-70, 1989*).

In vitro Study: Feverfew was found to contain a factor that inhibits prostaglandin synthesis, but differs from salicylates by not inhibiting cyclo-oxygenase by prostaglandin (PG) synthase. "The ability of feverfew to inhibit PG production may account for its effectiveness as a herbal remedy in conditions responding to acetylsalicylate and like-acting drugs" (*Collier HOJ, Butt NM, McDonald-Gibson WJ, Saeed SA. Extract of feverfew inhibits prostaglandin biosynthesis. Letter. Lancet October 25, 1980*).

The dosage of feverfew used in one double-blind study was one capsule containing 25 mg of the freeze-dried pulverized leaves twice daily; in another double-blind study it was one capsule containing 82 mg of dried powdered leaves once daily. While these low dosages may be effective in preventing an attack, a higher dose (1 to 2 grams) may be necessary during an acute attack.

> *Note: The efficacy of feverfew is dependent upon adequate levels of parthenolide, the active ingredient. (The preparations used in successful clinical trials have a parthenolide content of 0.4-0.66%.)*

Animal Ex vivo Study: Extracts of fresh feverfew caused a dose- and time-dependent, irreversible inhibition of the contractile response of rabbit aortic rings to all receptor-acting agonists tested. The presence of potentially SH reacting parthenolide and other sesquiterpene alpha-methylenebutyrolactones in these extracts, and the close parellelism of pure parthenolide, suggest that the inhibitory effects are due to these compounds. Extracts of the dry leaves were not inhibitory and actually caused potent and sustained contractions of aortic smooth muscle; these extracts were found to be devoid or parthenolide or butyrolactones (*Barsby RWJ, Salan U, Knight BW, Hoult JRS. Feverfew and vascular smooth muscle: Extracts from fresh and dried plants show opposing pharmacological profiles, dependent upon sesquiterpene lactone content. Planta Medica 59:20-5, 1993*).

Chemical Analysis: The parthenolide content of over 35 different commercial preparations of feverfew was determined by bioassay, 2 HPLC methods, and NMR. The results indicate a wide variation in the amts. of parthenolide in commercial preparations. The majority of products contained no parthenolide or only traces (*Heptinstall S et al. Parthenolide content and bioactivity of feverfew (Tanacetum parthenium (L.) Schultz-Bip.). Estimation of commercial and authenticated feverfew products. J Pharm Pharmacol 44:391-5, 1992*).

WARNING: No long-term toxicity studies have been conducted. While feverfew is extremely well-tolerated and no serious side effects have ever been reported, chewing the leaves can result in small ulcerations in the mouth and swelling of the lips and tongue in about 10% of users (*Awang DVC. Feverfew. Can Pharm J 122:266-70, 1989*).

An inhibitor of serotonin release from platelets (which contain over 90% of blood serotonin stores) (*Heptinstall S et al. Extracts of feverfew inhibit granule secretion in blood platelets and polymorphonuclear leucocytes. Lancet i:1071-4, 1985*).

Said to have similar analgesic properties as the non-steroidal anti-inflammatory drugs.

Administration may reduce migraine headaches.

Experimental Double-blind Crossover Study: 72 pts. were randomly allocated to receive either 1 capsule dried feverfew leaves daily or placebo. After 4 mo., pts. were transferred to the other treatment for another 4 months. Treatment with feverfew was associated with a reduction in the mean number and severity of attacks and in the degree of vomiting; duration of single attacks was unaltered. There were no serious side-effects (*Murphy JJ et al. Randomised double-blind placebo-controlled trial of feverfew in migraine prevention. Lancet ii:189-92, 1988*).

Experimental Double-blind Study: 17 pts. who ate fresh leaves of feverfew daily as prophylaxis (ave. of 2.44 leaves or 60 mg) received either feverfew 50 mg in capsules or placebo. The pts. in the 2 gps. did not differ in the amt. of feverfew usually consumed or in the duration of consumption. The mean frequency of attacks in pts. receiving placebo increased from 1.22 monthly prior to the study to 3.43 attacks during the final 3 mo. of the 6 mo. study, while pts. taking feverfew showed no change. In addition, those taking feverfew reported a far lower incidence of nausea and vomiting during episodes than those taking placebo. There was one report each of transient palpitations, colicky abdominal pain and heavier menstruation. Pts. in the placebo gp. reported symptoms of nervousness, tension and insomnia which are believed to be due to withdrawal effects   (*Johnson ES et al. Efficacy of feverfew as prophylactic treatment of migraine. B. Med J 291:569-73, 1985*).

Observational Study: A survey of 270 pts. who had taken feverfew for prolonged periods suggested that the herb decreased the frequency and severity of migraine attacks with only minor side-effects   (*Mahaja AN, Bailey JM. A platelet phospholipase inhibitor from the medicinal herb feverfew (Tanacetum parthenium). Prostaglandins Leukotrienes Med 8:653-60, 1982*).

Ginger (*Zingiber officinale*):

Administration may reduce and relieve migraine headaches.

> *Note: Ginger may be particularly effective for the nausea and vomiting associated with migraine headaches as it has been reported to be effective for both the nausea of motion sickness (Mowrey D, Clayson D. Motion sickness, ginger and psychophysics. Lancet i:655-58, 1982) and for the nausea of early pregnancy (Roach B. Townsend Letter for Doctors July, 1983, September, 1984 & June, 1986).*

Case Report: A 42 year-old woman with a long history of classical migraines discontinued all medications for 2-3 mo. prior to a trial of ginger. For the trial, 500-600 mg of dried ginger was taken mixed with water at the onset of the visual aura and repeated every 4 hrs. for 4 days. Improvement was evident within 30 min. and there were no side effects. She subsequently began to use uncooked fresh ginger in her daily diet. Migraines became less frequent and, when they did occur, they were at a "much lower intensity" than previously   (*Mustafa T, Srivastava KC. Ginger (Zingiber officinale) in migraine headache. J Ethnopharmacol 29(3):267-73, 1990*).

HEARTBURN
(REFLUX ESOPHAGITIS)

See Also: PEPTIC ULCER (DUODENAL AND GASTRIC)

Avoid carminatives (such as peppermint and spearmint).

These volatile oils have been shown to decrease pressure in the lower esophageal sphincter (*Sigmund CJ, McNally EF. The action of a carminative on the lower esophageal sphincter. Gastroenterology 56:13-18, 1969*).

Licorice root (*Glycyrrhiza glabra*):

Licorice root contains about 6-14% glycyrrhizin, which in the body is cleaved to form glycyrrhetinic acid. Glycyrrhetinic acid (carbenoxolone) preparations have been shown to be useful in esophagitis and peptic ulcer. Licorice root may offer similar benefit.

> WARNING: If ingested regularly, licorice root (>3 g/d for more than 6 weeks) or glycyrrhizin (>100 mg/d) may cause sodium and water retention, hypertension, hypokalemia, and suppression of the renin-aldosterone system through a pseudo-aldosterone action of glycyrrhetinic acid. Monitoring of BP and electrolytes and increasing potassium intake is suggested (*Farese RV et al Licorice-induced hypermineralocorticoidism. N Engl J Med 325(17):1223-7, 1991; MacKenzie MA et al. The influence of glycyrrhetinic acid on plasma cortisol and cortisone in healthy young volunteers. J Clin Endocrinol Metab 70:1637-43, 1990*).

DGL may offer the benefits of licorice and glycyrrhetinic acid without the risk of side effects. (*See: 'PEPTIC ULCER'*)

> *Note: Side effects of glycyrrhizin (pseudo-aldosteronism) from crude licorice root or glycyrrhetinic acid (carbenoxolone) preparations may be prevented by following a high-potassium, low-sodium diet. Although no formal trial of either of these guidelines has been performed, patients who normally consume high-potassium foods and restrict sodium intake, even those with hypertension and angina, have been reported to be free from the aldosterone-like side effects of glycyrrhizin (Baron J et al. Metabolic studies, aldosterone secretion rate and plasma renin after carbonoxolone sodium as biogastrone. Br Med J 2:793-5, 1969*).

The dosage of licorice root is based on the content of glycyrrhetinic acid. Positive clinical studies with glycyrrhetinic acid or carbenoxolone typically used a dosage of 150-300 mg/d. This amount would correspond to about 3 to 6 grams of crude licorice root daily.

The following study utilized Pyrogastrone[®], a commercial product containin carbenoxolone sodium 20 mg, alginic acid 600 mg, aluminum hydroxide 240 mg, magnesium trisilicate 60 mg, and sodium bicarbonate 210 mg per capsule:

Experimental Study: 80 pts. with reflux esophagitis were randomized to receive either Pyrogastrone® 5 tabs daily or cimetidine 400 mg twice daily for 6 weeks, extended to 12 if necessary. At 6 weeks, 49% of the Pyrogastrone®-treated pts. and 37% of the cimetidine-treated pts. were healed. After 12 weeks the cumulative healing rates were 64% for Pyrogastrone® and 66% for cimetidine. Compared with baseline both drugs achieved similarly significant improvements in symptom score, endoscopic and histological grading, even in those who did not heal completely. Response was not related to length of symptoms or initial severity of esophagitis. At six weeks, 5 cimetidine-treated pts. had relapsed compared to none in the Pyrogastrone® group (p=0.05). 11/25 (44%) pts. healed with Pyrogastrone® relapsed within one year compared with 15 of 27 (56%) healed with cimetidine. Although this trend in favor of Pyrogastrone® was not significant at one year, the early relapse rate was significantly greater in cimetidine-treated patients (*Maxton DG et al. Controlled trial of pyrogastrone and cimetidine in the treatment of reflux oesophagitis. Gut 31(3):351-4, 1990*)

The following two studies demonstrate that the glycyrrhetinic acid portion of the formula is the major active component of Pyrogastrone:

Experimental Double-blind Study: 37 pts. with esophagitis, confirmed endoscopically and histologically, were given either Pyrogastrone® or the alginate-antacid compound used alone. The total daily dosage of glycyrrhetinic acid was 100 mg. During the 8-week period of the trial pts. were seen every 2 weeks and endoscoped at 4 and 8 weeks. Response to treatment was assessed symptomatically and endoscopically using 6-point grading scales, and multiple esophageal biopsies were taken at each endoscopy. The addition of glycyrrhetinic acid to the alginate antacid compound was shown to enhance symptomatic relief and to increase healing of esophagitis and esophageal ulceration significantly. No serious side-effects were reported in either group (*Reed PI, Davies WA. Controlled trial of a carbenoxolone/alginate antacid combination in reflux oesophagitis. Curr Med Res Opin 5(8):637-44, 1978*).

Experimental Double-blind Study: 29 pts. were treated with Pyrogastrone® and 30 with antacid/alginate alone four times each day for 8 weeks to ascertain the value of carbenoxolone in the treatment of patients with endoscopically confirmed reflux oesophagitis. Symptom review every 2 weeks and endoscopic findings every 4 weeks were converted to a 6-point grading system to facilitate statistical comparison, using a stochastic model for predicting the rate of change in grades during treatment. Glycyrrhetinic acid-treated patients showed an 82% improvement in symptom grades over 8 weeks and improved 50% faster (p) than did control patients, who showed a 63% improvement. Endoscopic improvement was not significantly different in the first 4 weeks, although healing was better maintained in carbenoxolone-treated patients during the second 4 weeks (p). At the low doses used (5 X 20 mg daily) no significant side effects of glycyrrhetinic acid were encountered (*Young GP et al. Treatment of reflux oesophagitis with a carbenoxolone/antacid/alginate preparation. A double-blind controlled trial. Scand J Gastroenterol 21(9):1098-104, 1986*).

HEPATITIS

See Also: ALCOHOLISM

Catechin:

Catechin is a flavonoid that is found in high concentrations in *Acacia catechu* (black cate-chu, black cutch) and *Uncaria gambier* (pale catechu, gambier).

Administration of catechin or plant extracts concentrated for catechin may be beneficial.

WARNING: Administration can induce autoimmune hemolysis. Use with caution.

Case Reports: 5 pts. who received catechin for 4-36 months are presented. Three developed both hemolytic anemia and thrombocytopenia, while 2 had only thrombocytopenia. After suspending the drug the hematological values returned to normal in all of the pts. Catechin-dependent platelet antibodies were detected in 4 of the 5 pts. and catechin-dependent red blood cell anti-bodies were present in 3 (*Gandolfo GM et al Hemolytic anemia and throm-bocytopenia induced by cyanidanol.* Acta Haematol *88(2-3):96-9, 1992*).

Case Reports: 6 pts. who developed hemolysis while receiving catechin were studied. The disorder was episodic in all pts. and resolved after discon-tinuing the drug. The causative antibodies could be demonstrated in all 6 cases, even when the hemolytic episode had preceded analysis by more than 1 year. It seems that the stable association of catechin with RBC generates antigenic sites against which a heterogeneous immune response is elicited giving rise to long-lasting drug-dependent antibodies as well as autoantibod-ies (*Salama A, Mueller-Eckhardt C. Cianidanol and its metabolites bind tightly to red cells and are responsible for the production of auto- and/or drug-dependent antibodies against these cells.* Br J Haematol *66(2):263-6, 1987*).

Experimental Double-blind Study: 338 pts. with HBeAg-positive chronic hepatitis received either catechin in a daily dose of 1.5 g for 2 weeks, followed by 2.25 g for a further 14 weeks, or a placebo. The HBeAg titer decreased by at least 50% in 44 of 144 cases treated with catechin compared to 21 of 140 cases treated with placebo (p). The HBeAg disappeared in 16 of the catechin cases and four of the placebo (p) and a seroconversion was observed in 6 catechin pts. and 3 placebo patients. The mean HBeAg titer in the catechin gp. was significantly lower than that in the placebo gp. at the end of the 16 weeks of therapy (p<0.05). The pts. whose HBeAg titer was lowered were largely those with chronic active hepatitis and had higher initial values of SGPT, SGOT and gamma-globulin than the pts. whose HBeAg titers remained unchanged. The mean values for these liver function tests also fell significantly in the former sub-group. Catechin was well tolerated, the only notable side effect being a transient febrile reaction in 13 pts. (*Suzuki H et al. Cianidanol therapy for HBe-antigen-positive chronic hepatitis: a multicentre, double-blind study. Liver 6(1):35-44, 1986*).

Negative Experimental Double-blind Study: 40 pts. with biopsy proven chronic active hepatitis were studied, 22 received catechin in a dose of 3 g daily and 18 received placebo. Side effects related to cyanidanol were fever (4 pts.), haemolysis (1 pt.) and urticaria (1 pt.). All side effects subsided on discontinuation of the medication. Catechin had an effect no better than placebo on symptoms, laboratory tests, and histological findings on liver biopsy (*Bar-Meir S et al. Effect of (+)-cyanidanol-3 on chronic active hepatitis: a double blind controlled trial. Gut 26(9):975-9, 1985*).

Experimental Double-blind Study: 160 pts with acute viral hepatitis type B were given either catechin 3 g/d or placebo for 8 weeks. The mean time for serum bilirubin to decrease to 1.3 mg/dl was 30.8 days in the treated gp. and 52.2 days in the control gp. (p). The time for SGOT to decrease to 100 IU/L was 17.98 in the treated gp. and 26.53 in the control gp. (p). The elimination rate of HBsAg was identical in both groups. Treatment did not alter the incidence of chronicity (*Schomerus H et al. Catechin in the treatment of acute viral hepatitis: a randomized controlled trial. Hepatology 4(2):331-5, 1984*).

Negative Experimental Double-blind Study: The effects of catechin 1.5-2.0 g/d versus placebo, each combined with continuous prednisolone therapy (10-15 mg/d), was studied over the course of 1 yr. in pts. with chronic active hepatitis (CAH). The results showed a more favorable, but not significantly better, response in pts. receiving catechin versus placebo (*Abonyi M, Kisfaludy S, Szalay F. Therapeutic effect of (+)-cyanidanol-3 in toxic alcoholic liver disease and in chronic active hepatitis. Acta Physiol Hung 64(3-4):455-60, 1984*).

Experimental Double-blind Study: 124 pts. with actue viral hepatitis were treated with catechin or placebo. In 35 pts. with hepatitis A, there were no significant differences. In 58 pts. with hepatitis B and 31 pts. with non-A, non-B viral hepatitis, pts. receiving catechin (3 g/d) demonstrated reduced SGPT and SGOT activity after 45 days compared to those pts. receiving placebo (*Piazza M et al. Effect of (+)-cyanidanol-3 in acute HAV, HBV, and non-A, non-B viral hepatitis. Hepatology 3(1):45-9, 1983*).

Experimental Double-blind Study: 100 pts. with acute viral hepatitis received either catechin (2 g/day) or placebo. Catechin accelerated the disappearance of HBsAg from the blood, lowered serum bilirubin, and relieved symptoms such as anorexia, nausea, and pruritus. Catechin was well tolerated. None of the pts. had a relapse of acute hepatitis. Chronic active hepatitis developed in one of the placebo-treated pts (*Blum AL et al. Treatment of acute viral hepatitis with (+)-cyanidanol-3. Lancet ii:1153-5, 1977*).

Licorice Root (*Glycyrrhiza glabra*):

Licorice root contains glycyrrhizin, which in the body is cleaved to form glycyrrhetinic acid. Glycyrrhetinic acid exhibits profound pharmacological activity including anti-viral and anti - inflammatory properties.

The dosage of licorice root is based on the content of glycyrrhetinic acid. Positive clinical studies with glycyrrhizin typically used a dosage of 800-2,000 mg/d. This amount would correspond to about 5 to 12 grams of crude licorice root daily.

> WARNING: If ingested regularly, licorice root (>3 g/d for more than 6 weeks) or glycyrrhizin (>100 mg/d) may cause sodium and water retention, hypertension, hypokalemia, and suppression of the renin-aldosterone system through a pseudo-aldosterone action of glycyrrhetinic acid. Monitoring of BP and electrolytes and increasing potassium intake is suggested (*Farese RV et al. Licorice-induced hypermineralocorticoidism. N Engl J Med 325(17):1223-7, 1991; MacKenzie MA et al. The influence of glycyrrhetinic acid on plasma cortisol and cortisone in healthy young volunteers. J Clin Endocrinol Metab 70:1637-43, 1990).*

> *Note: Side effects of glycyrrhizin (pseudo-aldosteronism) from crude licorice root or glycyrrhetinic acid (carbenoxolone) preparations may possibly be prevented by following a high-potassium, low-sodium diet. Although no formal trial of either of these guidelines has been performed, patients who normally consume high-potassium foods and restrict sodium intake, even those with hypertension and angina, have been reported to be free from the aldosterone-like side effects of glycyrrhizin (Baron J et al. Metabolic studies, aldosterone secretion rate and plasma renin after carbenoxolone sodium as biogastrone. Br Med J 2:793-5, 1969).*

Administration may be beneficial.

> *Note: Intravenous administration may not be necessary as glycyrrhizin is easily absorbed and well-tolerated.*

> **Experimental Study:** Glycyrrhetinic acid (GA) was administered as a single oral dose (100-500 mg) to 10 healthy female volunteers who had previous diagnoses of breast cancer. Plasma GA levels were measured 1, 2, 4 and 6 hr after oral doses using solid-phase extraction and HPLC. At doses less than 500 mg/m^2 (n=7), levels of GA in plasma were less than 900 ng/ml for all sampling times. In 3 subjects given 500 mg/m^2, plasma levels peaked at 4.6 mcg/ml at 4 hr. GA has mineralocorticoid properties, but no changes (compared to baseline) were observed in systolic or diastolic BP, serum sodium, or plasma renin concentrations. A decrease in serum potassium of 0.3 mEq/L (p=0.03) was seen at 4 hr, but the fall was not related to dose or plasma level of GA. No subject reported side effects. GA was well tolerated at doses up to 500 mg, and the drug was detectable at peak concentrations in plasma 4 hr after a single oral dose (*Vogel VG. Phase I pharmacology and toxicity study of glycyrrhetinic acid as a chemopreventive drug. Proc Annu Meet Am Assoc Cancer Res 33:A1245, 1992).*

- with <u>Cysteine</u> and <u>Glycine</u>:

A glycyrrhizin-containing product, Stronger Neominophagen C (SNMC), consisting of 0.2% glycyrrhizin, 0.1% cysteine and 2.0% glycine in physiological saline solution, is widely used intravenously in Japan for the treatment of hepatitis. The other components, glycine and cysteine, appear to modulate glycyrrhizin's actions. Glycine has been shown to prevent the aldosterone effects of glycyrrhizin, while cysteine aids in detoxification via increased glutathione synthesis and cystine conjugation.

Experimental Controlled Study: The biochemical, virus-serological and histomorphological data (blind liver aspiration, laparoscopy) during and following 12 mo. of IV administration of glycyrrhizin to 7 pts. with chronic hepatitis B, and a comparison with the course of the disease over the 12 mo. prior to treatment, was evaluated in a prospective study. During or after treatment, 4 pts. experienced a regression of biochemical disease activity. In 2/4 pts., during treatment, an HBe-Ag seroconversion occurred for the first time and has persisted (to date 10 months); in another pt. with no detectable HBe-Ag prior to treatment, HBe antibodies were formed under treatment, and have persisted to the present time. In 2 of these responders, histology also revealed an unequivocal reduction in disease activity. On the basis of the results obtained so far (30-40% success rate), IV glycyrrhizin compares quite favorably with interferon (*Eisenburg J. [Treatment of chronic hepatitis B. Part 2: Effect of glycyrrhizinic acid on the course of illness]. Fortschr Med 110(21):395-8, 1992*) (*in German*).

Experimental Double-blind Study: Daily intravenous injections of 40 ml of SNMC over a month was examined in a randomized double-blind study of 133 pts. with chronic active hepatitis. SNMC improved liver function (p) and lowered levels of serum transaminases (p) (*Suzuki H et al. Effects of glycyrrhizin on biochemical tests in patients with chronic hepatitis - Double blind trial. Asian Med J 26:423-38, 1984*).

SNMC administration may be effective for subacute hepatic failure, an often fatal consequence of viral hepatitis.

Experimental Study: 18 pts. with subacute hepatic failure due to viral hepatitis were given IV SNMC at a dose of 40 or 100 ml daily for 30 days followed by thrice weekly thereafter. The survival rate was 72.2% as compared to the reported rate of 31.1% (*Acharya SK et al. A preliminary open trial on interferon stimulator (SNMC) derived from Glycyrrhiza glabra in the treatment of subacute hepatic failure. Ind J Med Res 98:75-8, 1993*).

Phyllanthus amarus:

Administration may reverse the carrier state in hepatitis B.

Negative Experimental Double-blind Study: 59 and 57 carriers of hepatitis B virus were received either 400 mg 3 times daily of *P. amarus* or placebo, respectively, for 30 days and were evaluated on days 15, 30, 60, and 180. HBsAg was detected during treatment and follow-up in every case but 1 in each gp. at day 180 (*Leelarasamee A et al. Failure of Phyllanthus amarus to eradicate hepatitis B surface antigen from symptomless carriers. Lancet 335:1600-1, 1990*).

Experimental Placebo-controlled Study: Hepatitis B carriers were treated with a preparation of *Phyllanthus amarus* (the dried, powdered, sterilized plant in a 200 mg cap 3 times daily) or placebo for 30 days. 22/37 (59%) pts. had lost the hepatitis B surface antigen when tested 15-20 days after treatment compared to only 1/23 (4%) of placebo-treated controls. Some pts. were followed for up to 9 mo. and the surface antigen has not returned. There were few or no toxic effects (*Thyagarajan SP et al. Effect of Phyllanthus amarus on chronic carriers of hepatitis B virus. Lancet ii:764-6, 1988*).

See Also:

> **Negative Experimental Study:** *Berk L et al. Beneficial effects of Phyllanthus amarus for chronic hepatitis B, not confirmed. J Hepatol 12(3):405-6, 1991*

> **Experimental Study:** *Blumberg BS et al. Hepatitis B virus and primary hepatocellular carcinoma: treatment of HBV carriers with Phyllanthus amarus. Vaccine 8:S86-92, 1990*

> **Experimental Study:** *Blumberg BS et al. Hepatitis B virus and hepatocellular carcinoma—treatment of HBV carriers with Phyllanthus amarus. Cancer Detect Prev 14(2):195-201, 1989*

Silymarin:

Silymarin, the flavonolignan complex of milk thistle (*Silybum marianum*), is a potent antioxidant that is concentrated within liver tissue to exert significant hepatoprotection.

Administration may be beneficial, especially in chemical and alcohol-induced liver disease. (*See: 'ALCOHOLISM'*)

Experimental Controlled Study: Abnormal results of liver function tests (elevated levels of AST, ALT activity) and/or abnormal hematological values (low platelet counts, leucocytosis, relative lymphocytosis) were observed in 49 of 200 workers exposed to toluene and/or xylene vapors for 5-20 years. 30 of the affected workers were treated with silymarin (Legalon) at a dose of 70 mg 3 times daily for 30 days. The remaining 19 were left without treatment. Under the influence of silymarin the liver function tests and the platelet counts significantly improved. The leukocytosis and relative lymphocytosis showed a nonsignificant tendency towards improvement (*Szilard S, Szentgyorgyi D, Demeter I. Protective effect of Legalon in workers exposed to organic solvents. Acta Med Hung 45(2):249-56, 1988*).

Experimental Double-blind Study: 106 consecutive pts. with liver disease were selected on the basis of elevated transaminase levels. In general, pts. had relatively slight acute and subacute liver disease, mostly induced by alcohol abuse. They randomly received either silymarin or placebo. There was a statistically highly significant greater decrease of serum SGPT (ALAT) and SGOT (ASAT) in the treated gp. than in controls. Serum total and conjugated bilirubin decreased more in the treated gp. than in controls, but the differences were not significant. BSP retention returned to normal significantly more often in the treated gp., and the mean percentage decrease of BSP was markedly higher. Finally, normalization of histological changes occurred significantly more often in the treated gp. than in controls (*Salmi HA, Sarna S. Effect of silymarin on chemical, functional, and morphological alterations of the liver. A double-blind controlled study. Scand J Gastroenterol 17:517-21, 1982*).

Experimental Double-blind Study: 29 pts. with acute viral hepatitis treated with sily-marin at a dosage of 140 mg 3 times daily showed a definite therapeutic influence on the characteristic increased serum levels of bilirubin, GOT and GPT associated with acute viral hepatitis compared with a placebo group. The laboratory parameters in the silymarin gp. regressed more than in the placebo gp. after the 5th day of treatment. The number of pts. having attained normal values after 3 weeks' treatment was significantly higher in the silymarin gp. than in the placebo gp. *(Magliulo E, Gagliardi B, Fiori GP. [Results of a double blind study on the effect of silymarin in the treatment of acute viral hepatitis, carried out at two medical centres.] Med Klin 73(28-29):1060-5, 1978) (in German).*

Administration of silybin, the main active component of silymarin, bound to phosphatidyl-choline may be beneficial. *(See: 'ALCOHOLISM').*

Experimental Study: 8 pts. with chronic viral hepatitis (3 anti-HBV positive, 3 anti-HBV and anti-HCV positive, and 2 anti-HCV positive) were given one capsule (equivalent to 120 mg silybin) between meals for 2 months. After treatment, serum malondialdehyde levels (an indicator of lipid peroxidation) decreased by 36%, and the quantitiative liver function evaluation, as expressed by galactose elimination capacity, increased by 15%. A statistically significant (p) of transaminases was also seen: AST decreased 17% and ALT decreased 16% *(Mascarella S et al. Therapeutic and an-tilipoperoxidant effects of silybin-phosphatidylcholine complex in chronic liver disease: Preliminary results. Curr Ther Res 53(1):98-102, 1993).*

The silybin-phosphatidylcholine complex may be more effective than silymarin.

Experimental Pharmacokinetic Study: The biliary excretion of silybin was evaulated in 9 cholecystectomy pts. with T-tube drainage following a single oral dose of silybin-phosphatidylcholine complex (IdB 1016) and silymarin. The amount of silybin recov-ered in the bile in free and conjugated form within 48h was 11% for the silybin-phos-phatidylcholine and 3% for silymarin *(Schandalik R, Gatti G, Perucca E. Pharmacoki-netics of silybin in bile following administration of silipide and silymarin in cholecys-tectomy patients. Arzneim Forsch 42(7):964-8, 1992).*

Experimental Study: In order to assess the pharmacokinetic profile in man, plasma silybin levels were determined after administration of single oral doses of a silybin-phosphatidylcholine complex (IdB 1016) and silymarin (equivalent to 360 mg silybin) to 9 healthy volunteers. Although absorption was rapid with both preparations, the bioavailability of the silibin-phosphatidylcholine complex was much greater than that of silymarin, as indicated by higher plasma silybin levels at all sampling times after intake of the complex. Regardless of the preparation used, the terminal half-life was relatively short (generally less than 4 h). In a subsequent study, 9 healthy volunteers received IdB 1016 (120 mg twice daily, expressed as silybin equivalents) for 8 conse-cutive days. The plasma silybin level profiles and kinetic parameters on day 1 were similar to those determined on day 8. Most of the silybin present in the systemic circu-lation was in conjugated form. Less than 3% of the administered dose was accounted for by urinary recovery of free plus conjugated silybin, a significant proportion of the dose probably being excreted in the bile. It is concluded that complexation with phos-phatidylcholine in IdB 1016 greatly increases the oral bioavailability of silybin, prob-ably by facilitating its passage across the gastrointestinal mucosa *(Barzaghi N et al.*

Pharmacokinetic studies on IdB 1016, a silybin-phosphatidylcholine complex, in healthy human subjects. Eur J Drug Metab Pharmacokinet 15(4):333-8, 1990).

_ _

COMBINATION TREATMENT

Padma 28:

Padma 28 is a commercial product based on an ancient Tibetan (lamaistic) formula. It contains a mixture of 28 different herbs.

> **Experimental Study:** 34 pts. with chronic active hepatitis B (CAH-B) were treated with Padma 28 (3 tablets bid 30 min. before meals) for 1 year. 26 of 34 pts. (76.5%) improved or normalized in biochemical parameters as well as in CD3 and CD4/CD8 index. An improvement in histology was seen in 19 pts. (56%); 6 pts. (17.6%) eliminated HBeAg and HBV-DNA and 8 seroconverted to anti-HBE; and 8 pts. with persistent HBs and HBe-antigenemia had a decreased titre of HBsAg and HBeAg. In 8 pts. (23.5%) no influence of Padma 28 was observed. These observations indicate that treatment with Padma 28 can influence the activity of genes of HBV and stops the progression of liver inflammation (*Gladysz A, Juszczyk J, Brzosko WJ. Influence of Padma 28 on patients with chronic active hepatitis B. Phytother Res 7:244-7, 1993*).

Shosaikoto:

Bupleuri root or Chinese thoroughwax (*Bupleurum falcatum*) is the major component of Shosaikoto, one of the most famous Chinese medicines. The other 6 components of Shosaikoto are: licorice root (*Glycyrrhiza glabra*), jujube fruit (*Zizyphus jujuba*), ginger root (*Zingiber officinalis*), Panax ginseng root, Chinese skullcap root (*Scutellaria baicalensis*), and half summer root (*Pinellia ternata*). All of the individual components have exerted anti-inflammatory activity (*Cyong J. A pharmacological study of the anti-inflammatory activity of Chinese herbs. A review. Int J Acupuncture Electro-Ther Res 7:173-202, 1982*).

Administration of Shosaikoto may be effective for infectious hepatitis.

> **Experimental Study:** 7 of 14 children with chronic hepatitis B virus (HBV) infection treated with Shosaikoto became HBeAg negative in the average observation period of 0.47 years(0.2-0.9 years). 4 of these pts. developed anti-HBe. The annual sero-conversion rate in the Shosaikoto treated gp. was apparently higher than the natural annual sero-conversion rate (22.7%) of 22 untreated pts. retrospectively reviewed from the onset of hepatitis. Shosaikoto seemed to promote clearance of HBeAg in children with chronic HBV infection and with sustained liver disease (*Tajiri H et al. Effect of shosaiko-to (xiao-chai-hu-tang) on HBeAg clearance in children with chronic hepatitis B virus infection and with sustained liver disease. Am J Chin Med 19(2):121-9, 1991*).

> **Experimental Double-blind Study:** The efficacy of Shosaikoto (SST) on 222 pts. with chronic active hepatitis was studied in a double-blind multicenter clinical study. 116 pts. received SST in a daily oral dose of 5.4 g for 12 weeks, followed by the same dose for a further 12 weeks. 106 pts. received a placebo containing 0.5 g of SST for 12 weeks, followed by a cross-over to SST for a further 12 weeks. Among the liver tests, serum AST and ALT values decreased significantly with the administration of SST. The difference of the mean value between the SST gp. and the placebo gp. was signifi-

cant after 12 weeks. In pts. with chronic active type B hepatitis, a tendency towards a decrease of HBeAg and an increase of Anti-HBe antibodies was also observed. No remarkable side effects were noticed *(Okumura M et al. A multicenter randomized controlled clinical trial of Sho-saiko-to in chronic active hepatitis. Gastroenterol Jpn 24(6):715-9, 1989).*

Although all of the components of Shosaikoto have exerted anti-inflammatory actions in animal studies, the main action of the formula has been primarily attributed to Bupleuri root's steroid-like molecules known as saikosaponins. However, no pharmacological activity of the roots of B. falcatum can be explained by the actions of the saikosaponins alone. In addition, other components of Shosaikoto have shown beneficial effects in hepatitis *(see 'Licorice Root' above).*

Saikosaponins may protect the liver and exert anti-inflammatory effects.

Animal Experimental Study: Saikosaponin-d showed protection against the CCl4-hepatotoxicity enhanced by phenobarbitone. It also inhibited increases in the content of cytochrome P450 and NADPH-cytochrome c reductase activity, which are induced by the phenobarbitone treatment, but the spectral characteristics of P450 were not altered. The rate of microsomal lipid peroxidation by NADPH and CCl4 was significantly lowered in vitro in rats pretreated with phenobarbitone and saikosaponin-d compared with those pretreated with phenobarbitone alone *(Abe H et al. Effects of saikosaponin-d on enhanced CCl4-hepatotoxicity by phenobarbitone. J Pharm Pharmacol 37(8):555-9, 1985).*

HYPERTENSION

See Also: PREGNANCY-RELATED ILLNESS

<u>Abana</u>:

Abana is an Ayurvedic herbomineral medicinal preparation. A 400 mg capsule of Abana contains: 30 mg *Terminalia arjuna*; 20 mg *Withania somnifera*; 20 mg *Tinospora cordifolia*; 10 mg *Boerhaavia diffusa*, and 10 mg *Nardostachys jatamansi*.

Administration may be beneficial.

Experimental Double-blind Study: 43 Indian men and women suffering from hypertension to evaluate the antihypertensive effect of Abana and compare it with that of methyldopa (M-DOPA). 21 pts. received 800 mg tds of Abana and 22 pts. received 250 mg tds of M-DOPA for 4 weeks. In pts. treated with Abana, there was a significant fall both in systolic BP (from 167 to 145 mm Hg) and in diastolic BP (from 110 to 91 mm Hg) at the end of 4 weeks. Similarly, in pts. treated with M-DOPA, systolic BP was significantly reduced from 165 to 146 mm Hg and diastolic BP was reduced from 106 to 96 mm Hg after 4 weeks. The onset of the antihypertensive effect was earlier and there was a higher percentage of responders (80%) in the Abana-treated group. None of the pts. had clinically or biochemically significant side effects. Results suggest that Abana may be highly effective (*Dadkar VN, Tahiliani RR, Jaguste VS, et al. Double blind comparative trial of Abana and methyldopa for monotherapy of hypertension in Indian patients. <u>Jpn Heart J</u> 31(2):193-9, 1990*).

Experimental Double-blind Study: 25 pts. with ischemic heart disease (IHD) and 25 pts. with IHD and mild hypertension (HTN) received either Abana or a placebo. The effect of Abana was evaluated by means of LV apex cardiogram (ACG), phonocardiogram and carotid pulse tracing and ECG before and at the end of 8 weeks of treatment. As compared to placebo, Abana significantly reduced the frequency and severity of anginal episodes, as judged by clinical improvement and nitrate consumption. Significant improvement in ventricular function was observed as reflected by a decrease in ACG A amplitude and A wave duration, along with a significant increase in LV ejection fraction and VCF. The decrease in double and triple products reflected decreased MVO_2. A significant fall in diastolic blood pressure was noted in pts. with mild hypertension. Abana seems to reduce preload and afterload and improve diastolic function and pump function, which may be responsible for the beneficial effects of Abana in ischemic heart disease (*Antani JA et al. Effect of Abana on ventricular function in ischemic heart disease. <u>Jpn Heart J</u> 31(6):829-35, 1990*).

Coleus forskohlii:

The root of *Coleus forskohlii*, an herb used in Ayurvedic medicine, contains a diterpene molecule known as forskolin which is a powerful activator of adenylate cyclase in various tissue leading to elevations of cAMP. In the artery, this causes relaxation and a resultant lowering of blood pressure.

The forskolin content of Coleus root is typically 0.2-0.3%, therefore the forskolin content of Coleus products may not be sufficient to produce a pharmacological effect. Therefore, it is best to use standardized extracts which have concentrated the forskolin content. The dosage of the extract should provide a daily intake of 5-10 mg of forskolin. (*See: 'CONGESTIVE HEART FAILURE'*)

Administration may be beneficial.

> **Animal Experimental Study:**   The main pharmacological action of coleonol (forskolin) in animals is a blood pressure-lowering effect due to relaxation of the vascular smooth muscle. In small doses it has a positive inotropic effect on isolated rabbit heart as well as on cat heart *in vivo* (*Dubey MP et al. Pharmacological studies on coleonol, a hypotensive diterpene from Coleus forskohlii. J Ethnopharmacol 3:1-13, 1981*).

> **Animal Experimental Study:** Forskolin exerts positive inotropic effects which are not blocked by beta-blockers. Forskolin also lowers blood pressure in dogs, cats, spontaneously hypertensive rats, and renal hypertensive rats (*Lindner E, Dohadwalla AN, Bhattacharya BK. Positive inotropic and blood pressure lowering activity of a diterpene derivative from Coleus forskohli: Forskolin. Arzneim Forsch 28(2):284-9, 1978*).

Garlic (*Allium sativum*) or
Onion (*Allium cepa*):

Administration may be beneficial.

> **Experimental Double-blind Crossover Study:** 20 normal volunteers (mean BP range from 88-108 mm Hg) were randomly divided into 2 gps., each of which rotated for 4-wk. periods through 2 different sequences during which they received 18 mg of garlic oil (extracted from 9 gms of fresh garlic) and placebo laced with garlic oil. During garlic administration, mean BP decreased significantly (<0.009) (*Barrie SA et al. Effects of garlic oil on platelet aggregation, serum lipids and blood pressure in humans. J Orthomol Med 2(1):15-21, 1987*).

> **Experimental Study:** Crude onion oil was given to 34 pts. with moderate hypertension or hypercholesterolemia, or both at a dose of 1 tbsp. 2-3 times daily. In 13/20 pts. with hypertension, there was a clear BP reduction of an average 25 mm Hg for the systolic and/or 15 mm Hg for the diastolic. In 9/18 pts. with hypercholesterolemia, total cholesterol levels fell between 7% and 33% (*Louria DB et al. Onion extract in treatment of hypertension and hyperlipidemia: A preliminary communication. Curr Ther Res 37(1):127-31, 1985*).

> **Animal Experimental Study:** Spontaneously hypertensive rats received 0.5 mg/kg of garlic oil. BP decreased to normal and was sustained at that level for up to 24 hrs.

(Foushee DB et al. Garlic as a natural agent for the treatment of hypertension: A preliminary report. Cytobios 34:145-52, 1982).

See Also:

> Rashid A, Khan AA. The mechanism of hypotensive effect of garlic extract. *J Pakistan Med Assoc 35:357, 1985*
>
> Ruffin J, Hunter SA. An evaluation of the side effects of garlic as an antihypertensive agent. *Cytobios 37(146):85-9, 1983*
>
> Malik SA, Siddiqui S. Hypotensive effect of freeze-dried garlic sap in dogs. *J Pakistan Med Assoc 31:12, 1981*

Hawthorn *(Crataegus oxyacantha and C. monogyna)*:

Extracts of hawthorn berry, leaves, and flowering tops extracts are widely used by physicians in Europe for their cardiotonic effects. The beneficial effects of hawthorn extracts are due to the presence of proyanidin flavonoids. Standardized extracts, similar to those used in the clinical studies cited below are the preferred form. The dosage for hawthorn extracts standardized to contain 1.8% vitexin-4[1]-rhamnoside or 10% procyanidins is 120-240 mg three times daily; for extracts standardized to contain 18% procyanidolic oligomers, the dosage is 240 to 480 mg daily. *(See: 'ATHEROSCLEROSIS'; 'CARDIAC ARRHYTHMIA'; 'CONGESTIVE HEART FAILURE')*

Procyanidins and procyanidolic oligomers inhibit angiotensin converting enzymes *(Uchida S, Ikari N, Ohta H, et al. Inhibitory effects of condensed tannins on angiotensin converting enzyme. Jap J Pharmacol 43:242-5, 1987).*

Administration may be effective in mild to moderate hypertension.

> **Review Article:** From experiments with animals, preparations of Crataegus exhibited decreased arterial BP as well as increased coronary artery and peripheral blood flow, decreased heart rate, and improved contractility of the heart muscle. Crataegus preparations are extremely well-tolerated. The acute oral toxicity (LD50) of Crataegus preparations and constituents was found to be in the range of 6 g/kg *(Ammon HPT, Handel M. [Crataegus, toxicology and pharmacology, Part I: Toxicity]. Planta Med 43(2):105-20, 1981; Part II: Pharmacodynamics. Planta Med 43(3):209-39, 1981; Part III: Pharmacodynamics and pharmacokinetics. Planta Med 43(4):313-22, 1981) (in German).*

- -

COMBINATION TREATMENT

Chinese Herbal Drugs:

In general, Chinese herbal drugs have not shown benefit in controlled trials.

> **Experimental Study:** The effects of the traditional Chinese herbal drugs, Daisaikoto (D) and Saikokaryukotsuboreito (S) on blood pressure and pulse rates in 30 pts. with mild to moderate hypertension were studied in an open, randomized trial. After the drug treatment, BP remained unchanged, but pulse rates declined significantly after 3

months in the S treated group (*Saku K et al. Effects of Chinese herbal drugs on serum lipids, lipoproteins and apolipoproteins in mild to moderate essential hypertensive patients. J Hum Hypertens 6(5):393-5, 1992*).

Experimental Study: 45 pts. with diastolic BP greater than or equal to 105 mm Hg were randomly assigned to receive Western (gp. 1, n = 21) or a classical Chinese herbal preparation (gp. 2, n = 24) to treat their hypertension. All remained hypertensive after 4 days in the hospital without treatment. Except for baseline Na^+ excretion (higher in gp. 1) and somewhat more evidence of end organ damage in gp. 1, the pt. groups were comparable. Those in gp. 1 were given a thiazide diuretic and propranolol if needed, and those in gp. 2, a mixture of 12 herbs. Pts. on active therapy in gp. 1 had a drop in BP from 172.6/107.4 to 141.2/89.6 mm Hg, whereas those in gp. 2 had no change in BP, 168.8/107.7 mm Hg to 165.7/106.0 mm Hg. Although 66% of pts. in gp. 1 had a diastolic BP under 90 mm Hg by discharge, only 8% of those in gp. 2 did. Except for a fall in serum K^+ in gp. 1, there were no significant biochemical or clinical problems in either gp. (*Black HR et al. A comparison of the treatment of hypertension with Chinese herbal and Western medication. J Clin Hypertens 2(4):371-8, 1986*).

IMMUNODEPRESSION

See Also: **AIDS**
CANCER
CANDIDIASIS
INFECTION

Aloe vera:

Acemannan, a water-soluble, long-chain polydispersed beta-(1,4)-linked mannan polymer interspersed with O-acetyl groups, found in Aloe vera is a potent immunostimulant. _(See: 'ACQUIRED IMMUNODEFICIENCY SYNDROME')_

In vitro Study: Acemannan incubation with monocytes permitted monocyte driven signals to enhance T-cell response to lectin. Acemannan increases lymphocyte response to alloantigen by enhancing the monocyte release of interleukin-I _(Womble D, Helderman JH. Enhancement of allo-responsiveness of human lymphocytes by acemannan (Carrisyn). Int J Immunopharmacol 10(8):967-74, 1988)._

Astragalus membranaceus:

A traditional Chinese medicinal herb historically used in viral infections.

Administration may enhance T-lymphocyte function.

Animal Experimental Study: _Astragalus membranaceus_ extracts injected into normal mice or mice immunodepressed by cyclophosphamide or radiation treatment or by aging are able to enhance the antibody response to a T-dependent antigen. Enhancement of the antibody response was associated with increase of T cell activity in normal and immunodepressed mice _(Zhao KS, Mancini C, Doria G. Enhancement of the immune response in mice by Astragalus membranaceus extracts. Immunopharmacol 20(3):225-33, 1990)._

In vitro Experimental Study: The immunopotentiating activity of 2 fractions extracted from _A. membranaceus_ was capable of fully correcting _in vitro_ T-cell function deficiency found in cancer patients _(Chu D-T et al. Immunotherapy with Chinese medicinal herbs. I. Immune restoration of local xenogeneic graft-versus-host reaction in cancer patients by fractionated Astragalus membranaceus in vitro. J Clin Lab Immunol 25:119-23, 1988)._

See Also:

Animal Experimental Study: _Chu DT et al. Immunotherapy with Chinese medicinal herbs. II. reversal of cyclophosphamide-induced immune suppression by_ *administration of fractionated Astragalus membranaceus in vivo. J Clin Lab Immunol 25:125-9, 1988*

Sun Y et al. Preliminary observations on the effects of the Chinese medical herbs Astragalus membranaceus and Ligustrum lucidum on lymphocyte blastogenic responses. J Biol Resp Modif 2:227-37, 1983

Administration may enhance macrophage phagocytic function.

In vitro Study: Chemiluminescent oxidative bursts were used as an indicator of phagocytic function in a murine macrophage cell line. Following incubation with the aqueous herbal extract of *Astragalus membranaceus*, significant dose-related augmentation of chemiluminescence occurred (*Lau BHS et al. Macrophage chemiluminescence modulated by Chinese herbs Astragalus membranaceus and Lingustrum lucidum. Phytotherapy Res 3(4):148-53, 1989*).

Echinacea spp.:

Echinacea species, primarily *E. angustifolia, E. purpurea*, and *E. pallida*, have historically been used in infections and as 'blood purifiers'. Echinacea was used for more ailments than any other plant by Native Americans of the Plains tribes.

Currently more than 300 echinacea-containing products are sold worldwide as non-specific immunostimulants.

The important chemicals, from a pharmacological perspective, of Echinacea can be divided into the following categories: (1) polysachharides; (2) flavonoids, (3) caffeic acid derivatives; (4) essential oils; (5) polyacetylenes; and (6) alkylamides. Extracts of these these various components have all demonstrated immune-enhancing effects.

Review Article: The chemistry, pharmacology and clinical applications of Echinacea has been the subject of over 350 scientific studies. Echinacea possesses a broad-spectrum of effects on the immune system as a result of its content of a broad-range of active components affecting diffferent aspects of immune function including activation of complement, thus promoting chemotaxis of neutrophils, monocytes, and eosinophils; solubilization of immune complexes; neutralization of viruses; and bacteriolysis. The high-molecular weight heteroglycan polysaccharide components of Echinacea have profound immunostimulatory effects. The majority of these effects appear to be mediated by the binding of active Echinacea polysaccharides to carbohydrate receptors on the cell surface of macrophages and T-lymphocytes. Echinacea promotes nonspecific T-cell activation, i.e., transformation, production of interferon, and secretion of lymphokines. The resultant effect is enhanced T-cell mitogenesis, macrophage phagocytosis, antibody binding, and natural killer cell activity; and increased circulating PMNs. Echinacea polysaccharides have also been shown to enhance macrophage phagocytosis and stimulate macrophages to produce increased amounts of tumor-necrosis-factor (TNF), interferon, interleukin 1, and destroy tumor cells in tissue culture. Clinical studies have confirmed Echinacea's general immune-enhancing effects Numerous clinical studies have confirmed Echinacea's immune enhancing actions. Various Echinacea extracts or products have shown results in general infectious conditions, influenza, colds, upper respiratory tract infections, urogenital infections, and other infectious conditions

(*Bauer R, Wagner H. Echinacea species as potential immunostimulatory drugs. Econ Med Plant Res 5:253-321, 1991*).

See Also:

> **Review Article:** *Awang DVC, Kindack DG. Echinacea. Can Pharm J 124:512-6, 1991.*

Although many of the clinical studies have utilized injectable administration (primarily Echinacin®, a commercial product containing the juice of the aerial portion of *E. purpurea*), oral administration of Echinacin® or root extracts may yield similar or even better results.

Experimental Study: The oral administration of an *E. purpurea* root extract at a dose of 30 drops 3 times daily to healthy males for 5 consecutive days resulted in an increase of 120% in granulocytic phagocytosis (*reported in: Bauer R, Wagner H. Echinacea species as potential immunostimulatory drugs. Econ Med Plant Res 5:253-321, 1991*).

Experimental Study: Echinacin® administered IM to healthy males on 4 successive days was shown to increase granulocytic phagocytosis by nearly 50% (*Mose J. Effect of echinacin on phagocytosis and natural killer cells. Med Welt 34:1463-7, 1983*).

Water-soluble extracts of *E. angustifolia* may not be as beneficial on enhancing phagocytosis as water-soluble extracts of *E. purpurea* or ethanolic extracts.

Negative Animal Experimental Study: Experiments were performed with a water-soluble extract of *E. angustifolia* standardized on echanocoside content. Under various conditions, using the carbon clearance test, the extract failed to have an effect on immune function after IP, IV or oral administration (*Schumacher A, Friedberg KD. Analysis of the effect of Echinacea augustifolia on unspecified immunity of the mouse. Arzneim-Forsch 41:141-7, 1991*).

In vitro and Animal Experimental Study: Ethanolic extracts of *E. purpurea, E. pallida* and *E. augustifolia* roots were found to significantly enhance phagocytosis in mice. The results were confirmed *in vitro* (*Bauer VR et al. Immunological in vivo and in vitro examinations of Echinacea extracts. Arznein-Forsch 38:276-81, 1988*).

See Also:

> *Gaisbauer M et al. [The effect of Echinacea purpurea Moench on phagocytosis in granulocytes measured by chemiluminescence]. Arzneim Forsch 40(5):594-8, 1990) (in German).*

> *Wagner H, Proksch A. An immunostimulating active principle from Echinacae purpurea. Z Angew Phytother 2:166-68, 1981*

> *Kuhn D. Echinacin and its reaction with phagocytes. Arzneim-Forsch 3:194-98, 1953*

A number of immunostimulatory and mild anti-inflammatory polysaccharides have been isolated from Echinacea species. Most notable are the water soluble, acidic, branched-chain heteroglycans.

Polysaccharide extracts produced from large-scale cell cultures of *E. purpurea* may improve immune function.

Animal Experimental Study: Polysaccharides purified from large-scale cell cultures of *Echinacea purpurea* (EP) were effective in activating peritoneal macrophages isolated from animals after administration of cyclophosphamide (CP) or cyclosporin A (CsA). Treated macrophages exhibited increased production of tumor necrosis factor-alpha (TNF) and enhanced cytotoxicity against tumor target WEHI 164 as well as against the intracellular parasite Leishmania enrietti. After a CP-mediated reduction of leukocytes in the peripheral blood, the polysaccharides induced an earlier influx of neutrophil granulocytes as compared to controls. EP treatment of mice, immunosuppressed with CP or CsA, restored their resistance against lethal infections with the predominantly macrophage-dependent pathogen Listeria monocytogenes and predominantly granulocyte-dependent Candida albicans *(Steinmuller C et al. Polysaccharides isolated from plant cell cultures of Echinacea purpurea enhance the resistance of immunosuppressed mice against systemic infections with Candida albicans and Listeria monocytogenes. Int J Immunopharmacol 15(5):605-14, 1993).*

Experimental Study: Polysaccharides purified from large-scale cell cultures of *Echinacea purpurea* were given by intravenous application to test subjects. Upon administration, an immediate fall in the number of PMN in the peripheral blood, indicating activation of adherence to endothelial cells, occurred. This fall was followed by a leukocytosis due to an increase in the number of PMN and a lesser increase of monocytes. The appearance of stab cells and some juvenile forms and even myelocytes indicated the migration of cells from the bone marrow into the peripheral blood. The acute phase C-reactive protein (CRP) was induced, probably due to activation of monocytes and macrophages to produce IL-6 *(Roesler J et al. Application of purified polysaccharides from cell cultures of the plant Echinacea purpurea to test subjects mediates activation of the phagocyte system. Int J Immunopharmacol 13(7):931-41, 1991).*

In vitro Study: Acidic arabinogalactan, a highly purified polysaccharide from *Echinacea purpurea*, was effective in activating macrophages to cytotoxicity against micro-organisms. Furthermore, it induced macrophages to produce tumor necrosis factor, interleukin-1, and interferon-beta 2. It also stimulated macrophages when injected IP *(Luettig B et al. Macrophage activation by the polysaccharide arabinogalactan isolated from plant cell cultures of Echinacea purpurea. J Natl Cancer Inst 81(9):669-75, 1989).*

See Also:

Animal Experimental Study: *Roesler J et al. Application of purified polysaccharides from cell cultures of the plant Echinacea purpurea to mice mediates protection against systemic infections with Listeria monocytogenes and Candida albicans. Int J Immunopharmacol 13(1):27-37, 1991*

Garlic (*Allium sativum*):

Garlic possesses significant anti-infective and immune enhancing properties. (*See: 'AC-QUIRED IMMUNODEFICIENCY SYNDROME'; 'CANCER'; 'INFECTION'*)

While fresh garlic, and commercial products containing alliin or allicin may be useful, an aged garlic preparation (Kyolic®) has also demonstrated immune-enhancing effects.

Administration may enhance T-lymphocyte and macrophage function.

In vitro Study: An aqueous aged garlic extract (Kyolic®) and a protein fraction isolated from the extract enhanced T-lymphocyte and macrophage activity. A significant dose-related augmentation of oxidative burst was observed and the protein fraction also enhanced the T-lymphocyte blastogenesis (*Lau BH, Yamasaki T, Gridley DS. Garlic compounds modulate macrophage and T-lymphocyte functions. Mol Biother 3(2):103-7, 1991*).

Administration may increase interleukin-1 levels.

In vitro Study: Fraction 4 (F4), a protein fraction isolated from aged garlic extract (Kyolic®), enhanced cytotoxicity of human peripheral blood lymphocytes (PBL) against leukemia and melanoma cell lines. Although F4 treatment alone increased cytotoxicity, such effect was more remarkable together with suboptimal doses of interleukin-2 (IL-2). The enhancement of cytotoxicity both by F4 alone and by F4 plus IL-2 was abolished by anti-IL-2 antibody. F4 also enhanced concanavalin A (Con A)-induced proliferation of PBL. Radiolabeled Con A binding assays revealed that F4 treatment greatly augmented the affinity and slightly increased the number of Con A binding sites in PBL. F4 also enhanced Con A-induced Tac expression and IL-2 production of PBL. Anti-IL-2 antibody inhibited the effect of F4 on Con A-induced proliferation of PBL. These data suggest that IL-2 is involved in the augmentative effects of F4 (*Morioka N, Morton DL, Irie RF. A protein fraction from aged garlic extract enhances cytotoxicity and proliferation of human lymphocytes mediated by interleukin-2 and concanavalin A. Proc Annu Meet Am Assoc Cancer 34:A3297, 1993*).

Administration may increase natural killer cell activity.

In vitro Study: 3 healthy volunteers ate the equivalent of 2 bulbs (0.5 gm/kg) of garlic daily, while 3 took the equivalent dose in the form of 1800 mg of a cold-aged, odorless garlic capsule (Kyolic®) and 3 served as controls. After 3 wks., natural killer (NK) cells from the subjects ingesting raw garlic killed 140% more lymphoma cells in culture than NK cells from the controls, while NK cells from the subjects ingesting garlic capsules killed 156% more lymphoma cells than controls (*Kandil OM et al. Garlic and the immune system in humans: Its effect on natural killer cells. Fed Proc 46(3):441, 1987*).

Administration may enhance phagocytic cell function.

Animal Experimental Study: Mice received either 0.1 ml of a 1:2 dilution of aged garlic extract (Kyolic®) injected subcutaneously into the local inguinal site, 0.1 ml of diluted Kyolic® injected systemically into the peritoneal cavity, or served as controls. Four days later, leukocytes were obtained from the peritoneal cavity, spleen, and inguinal lymph notes. For the mice who received garlic locally, compared to controls, only slightly increased activity was noted with leukocytes from the peritoneal cavity and spleen, but a very significant increase in phagocytic activity (p<0.001) was noted with leukocytes from the inguinal lymph nodes. For the mice who received systemic garlic, a significant increase of phagocytic activity (p<0.001) was noted with leukocytes from all 3 sites, but the effect on leukocytes from both the peritoneal cavity and the spleen was clearly greater than on those from the inguinal lymph nodes (*Lau BHS. Detoxifying, radioprotective and phagocyte-enhancing effects of garlic. Int Clin Nutr Rev 9(1):27-31, 1989*).

See Also:

> *Hirao Y et al. Activation of immunoresponder cells by the protein fraction from aged garlic extract. Phytotherapy Res 1:161-4, 1987*

Lentinus edodes (Shiitake mushroom):

Administration of lentinan (preferably IM or IV), a glucan extract, may be beneficial. (*See: 'CANCER'*)

Review Article: Lentinan appears to be a T-cell oriented adjuvant. It triggers the increased production of various bioactive serum factors associated with immunity and inflammation (such as IL-1, CSF, IL-3, vascular dilation inducer, and acute-phase protein inducer) by the direct impact of macrophages or indirectly via lentinan-stimulated T cells. Toxic side effects are minimal (*Chihara G et al. Antitumor and metastasis-inhibitory activities of lentinan as an immunomodulator: An overview. Cancer Detect Prev Suppl 1:423-43, 1987*).

Experimental Study: 7 male and 16 female pts. aged 14-77 with low natural killer syndrome (lowered NK cell activity against K562 target cells in association with remittent fever and uncomfortable fatigue for over 6 months) responded well to the administration of lentinan despite no responses to conventional fever treatments such as antipyretics or antibiotics (*Aoki T et al. Low natural killer syndrome: Clinical and immunologic features. Nat Immunol Cell Growth Regul 6(3):116-28, 1987*).

In vitro Animal Study: Polyclonal antibody response induced by pokeweed mitogen against sheep red blood cells was augmented by an extract of cultured *Lentinus edodes* mycelia. There was evidence that interleukin-1 was produced which had caused, at least partially, the enhancement of antibody response (*Mizoguchi Y et al. Effects of extract of cultured Lentinus edodes mycelia (LEM) on polyclonal antibody response induced by pokeweed mitogen. Gastroenterol Jap 22(5):629-32, 1987*).

Panax ginseng:

Administration may be effective in improving immune function. (*See: 'CANCER'*)

Experimental Double-blind Study: 3 groups, each consisting of 20 healthy volunteers, were given capsules containing 100 mg of aqueous extract of *Panax ginseng* (gp. A), 100 mg of lactose (gp. B), or capsules containing 100 mg of standardized extract of *Panax ginseng* (gp. C). All subjects took one capsule every 12 h for 8 weeks. Blood samples were withdrawn before beginning the treatment, at week 4 and week 8. Immune parameters examined were chemotaxis of PMNs, phagocytosis index (PHI), phagocytosis fraction (PHF), intracellular killing, total lymphocytes (T3), T helper (T4) subset, suppressor cells (T8) subset, blastogenesis of circulating lymphocytes, and natural killer-cell activity (NK). Chemotaxis was already significantly enhanced at the fourth week in gp. A as well as in gp. C; the increase became even more marked at week 8 in subjects belonging to gp. C. PHI and PHF were significantly enhanced at week 8 in subjects of gp. A; these increases were significantly higher in subjects of gp. C starting at week 4. Intracellular killing was significantly increased at week 4 in gp. A and gp. C; the increase became highly significant in both groups at 8 weeks; however, a significant increase at week 8 was also noted in the placebo gp. (B). Total lymphocytes (T3) were significantly increased at week 4 in gp. A as well as in gp. C; at week 8 this enhancement became highly significant in both groups. The T4 subset was significantly increased at week 8 in gp. A; in gp. C the rise was initially seen at week 4 and became more marked at week 8. The T4/T8 ratio showed a significant enhancement in gp. C at week 4. Blastogenesis underwent significant enhancement at week 8 in gp. A and week 4 in gp. C. Stimulation of blastogenesis was highly significant in gp. C. Thus the *Panax ginseng* extract standardized for a 4% ginsenoside content was more active than the aqueous extract, probably due to higher ginsenoside levels (*Scaglione F et al. Immunomodulatory effects of two extracts of Panax ginseng C.A. Meyer. Drugs Exp Clin Res 16(10):537-42, 1990*).

Animal Experimental Study: In mice, ginsenoside Rg1 at a dose of 10 mg/kg administered for three consecutive days before immunization increased the number of spleen plaque-forming cell, the titers of sera hemagglutinins as well as the number of antigen-reactive T-cells. Ginsenoside Rg1 also increased the number of T-helper cells with respect to the whole T- cell number and the splenocyte natural killer activity. Ginsenoside Rg1 induced an augmentation of the production of IL-1 by macrophages and exerted a direct mitogenic effect on microcultured thymus cells. Ginsenoside Rg1 also partly restored the impaired immune reactivity by cyclophosphamide treatment (*Kenarova B et al. Immunomodulating activity of ginsenoside Rg1 from Panax ginseng. Jpn J Pharmacol 54(4):447-54, 1990*).

In vivo and In vitro Study: An aqueous extract of *Panax ginseng* was administered orally to mice for 5 to 6 days at the daily dose of 10, 50 and 250 mg/kg or was added to cultures of mouse spleen cells at concentrations varying between 0.25 and 8 mg/ml. Treated mice responded with enhanced antibody formation to either a primary or a secondary challenge with sheep red cells. The effects were dose-dependent. At the highest dose regimen, the primary IgM response was increased by 50% and the secondary IgG and IgM responses were increased by 50 and 100%, respectively. An even more pronounced effect was obtained with natural killer cell activity which was enhanced between 44 and 150% depending on the effector-to-target cell ratios used in the assay. *In vitro*, ginseng showed two main effects, an inhibition of stimulated and spontaneous lymphocyte proliferation at high, but not cytotoxic concentrations and an enhancement of interferon production particularly in non-stimulated spleen cells. The immunostimulating effects obtained *in vivo* are in agreement with the stimulation of interferon production observed *in vitro*. The inhibition of lymphocyte proliferation, however, cannot be reconciled with the immunostimulatory action of *P. ginseng* observed *in vivo* (*Jie YH, Cammisuli S, Baggiolini M. Immunomodulatory effects of Panax Ginseng C.A. Meyer in the mouse. Agents Actions 15(3-4):386-91, 1984*).

See Also:

In vitro Study: *Tomoda M et al. Characterization of two acidic polysaccharides having immunological activities from the root of Panax ginseng. Biol Pharm Bull 16(1):22-5, 1993*

Siberian Ginseng (*Elutherococcus senticosus*):

Administration may improve immune function.

Experimental Double-blind Study: 36 healthy volunteers received 10 ml of a standardized ethanolic preparation of *Elutherococcus senticosus* or ethanol placebo 3 times daily. After 4 wks., the study gp. showed a drastic increase in the absolute number of immunocompetent cells, with an especially pronounced effect on T lymphocytes, predominantly helper/inducers, but also cytotoxic and natural killer cells. In addition, there was a general enhancement of T lymphocyte activation. No side effects were observed during a 6-month observation period (*Bohn B, Nebe CT, Birr C. Flow-cytometric studies with Eleutherococcus senticosus extract as an immunomodulatory agent. Arzneim-Forsch 37(10):1193-6, 1987*).

Silymarin:

The flavonolignan complex of milk thistle (*Silybum marianum*), silymarin is a potent antioxidant that is concentrated within hepatic tissue.

Administration may enhance immune function.

Experimental Double-blind Study: The effects of the hepatoprotective antioxidant drug silymarin (Legalon) on some cellular immune parameters of pts. with histologically proven chronic alcoholic liver disease were studied in a 6-mo. double-blind study. The lectin-induced proliferative activity of the lymphocytes was enhanced, the originally low T cell percentage and the originally high CD8+ cell percentage normalized, and the antibody-dependent and natural cytotoxicity of the lymphocytes decreased during silymarin therapy. All these changes were significant, while in the placebo gp. no significant changes occurred, except for a moderate elevation of the T cell percentage. The immunomodulatory activity of silymarin might be involved in the hepatoprotective action of the drug and improves the depressed immunoreactivity of the pts. (*Deak G et al. [Immunomodulator effect of silymarin therapy in chronic alcoholic liver diseases.] Orv Hetil 131(24):1291-2, 1295-6, 1990*) (*in Hungarian*).

Tinospora cordifola:

Tinospora cordifola is an Ayurvedic herb used historically in infections and fever. It may be effective in improving survival rates after high risk surgeries by enhancing the immune system.

Experimental Controlled Study: Immunosuppression associated with deranged hepatic function and sepsis results in poor surgical outcome in extrahepatic obstructive jaundice. The effect of *Tinospora cordifolia*, which has been shown to have hepatoprotective and immunomodulatory properties, on surgical outcome in pts. with malignant obstructive jaundice was evaluated. 30 pts. were randomly divided into two groups, matched with respect to clinical features, impairment of hepatic function (as judged by liver function tests including antipyrine elimination) and immunosuppression (phagocytic and killing capacities of neutrophils). Gp. 1 received conventional management, i.e. vitamin K, antibiotics and biliary drainage; gp. 2 received *Tinospora cordifolia* (16 mg/kg/day orally) in addition, during the period of biliary drainage. Hepatic function remained comparable in the two groups after drainage. However, the phagocytic and killing capacities of neutrophils normalized only in pts. receiving *Tinospora cordifolia* (28.2 ± 5.5% and 29.47 ± 6.5% respectively). Post-drainage bactobilia was observed in 8 pts. in gp. 1 and 7 in gp. 2, but clinical evidence of septicemia was observed in 50% of patients in gp. 1 as against none in gp. 2 (p). Post-operative survival in gp. 1 and gp. 2 was 40% and 92.4% respectively (p) (*Rege N et al. Immunotherapy with Tinospora cordifolia: a new lead in the management of obstructive jaundice. Indian J Gastroenterol 12(1):5-8, 1993*).

Tolpa Torf Preparation:

Tolpa Torf Preparation (TTP) is a natural immunomodulating drug registered in Poland for human use. It is the immunoactive fraction with strictly defined biological properties of an extract from crude peat. TTP is produced in a quality controlled, patented method.

Experimental Double-blind Study: TTP was administered orally at 5 mg daily for 3 weeks. At 3 month and 6 month follow-up, favorable results of treatment were obtained in 14/20 and 9/20 TTP treated pts. and in 8/19 and 4/19 placebo pts., respectively. The phagocytic activity of granulocytes was significantly stimulated with TTP, but not with placebo (*Jankowski A et al. A randomized, double-blind study of the efficacy of Tolpa Torf Preparation (TTP) in the treatment of recurrent respiratory tract infections. Archiv Immunol Ther Experimental 41:95-7, 1993*).

Experimental Study: TTP administered orally at 5 mg daily for 3 one-week on, one-week off, courses to healthy volunteers induced hyporeactivity to interferon and tumor necrosis factor in peripheral bloood leukocytes cultures indicative of *in vivo* interferon and TNF induction (*Inglott AD et al. A method to assess the immunnomodulating effects of the Tolpa Torf Preparation (TTP) by measuring the hyporeactivity to interferon inductions and tumor necrosis factor response. Archiv Immunol Ther Experimental 41:87-93, 1993*).

See Also:

In vitro Study: *Inglott AD et al. Tolpa Torf Preparation (TTP) induces interferon and tumor necrosis factor production in human peripheral blood leukocytes. Archiv Immunol Ther Experimental 41:73-80, 1993*

– –

COMBINATION TREATMENT

Shosaikoto:

Bupleuri root or Chinese thoroughwax (*Bupleurum falcatum*) is the major component of Shosaikoto, one of the most famous Chinese medicines. The other 6 components of Shosaikoto are: licorice root (*Glycyrrhiza glabra*), jujube fruit (*Zizyphus jujuba*), ginger root (*Zingiber officinalis*), *Panax ginseng* root, Chinese skullcap root (*Scutellaria baicalensis*), and half summer root (*Pinellia ternata*). All of the individual components have exerted anti-inflammatory activity (*Cyong J. A pharmacological study of the anti-inflammatory activity of Chinese herbs. A review. Int J Acupuncture Electro-Ther Res 7:173-202, 1982*).

Saikosaponins may enhance immune function.

Animal Experimental Study: Treatment with saikosaponin increased the antibody response in plaque-forming cell numbers after *in vivo* immunization with sheep red blood cells (SRBC) and an augmentation of spleen cell proliferation responses to stimulation with T- or B-cell mitogens both before and after immunization. Furthermore, after SRBC immunization, the macrophages from mice treated with saikosaponin-d revealed significant increases in spreading activity and lysosomal enzyme activity (*Ushio Y, Oda Y, Abe H. Effect of saikosaponin on the immune responses in mice. Int J Immunopharmacol 13(5):501-8, 1991*).

In vitro Study: Macrophages from saikosaponin-d-treated mice showed a significant increase in spreading activity followed by an increase in phagocytic activity. An intense distribution of microfilaments and microtubules was also observed in these macrophages by immunofluorescence microscopy (*Ushio Y, Abe H. Effects of saikosaponin-d on the functions and morphology of macrophages. Int J Immunopharmacol 13(5):493-9, 1991*).

See also:

In vitro Study: *Ushio Y, Abe H. The effects of saikosaponin on macrophage functions and lymphocyte proliferation. Planta Med 57(6):511-4, 1991.*

In vitro Study: *Kumazawa Y et al. Activation of murine peritoneal macrophages by saikosaponin a, saikosaponin d and saikogenin d. Int J Immunopharmacol 11(1):21-8, 1989.*

Saikosaponins (steroid-like molecules in Bupleuri root) and Shosaikoto may enhance cortisol or protect against adrenal atrophy induced by corticosteroids.

Animal Experimental Study: Intraperitoneal administration of various saikosaponins and their intestinal metabolites showed corticosterone secretion-inducing activity (*Nose M, Amagaya S, Ogihara Y. Corticosterone secretion-inducing activity of saikosaponin metabolites formed in the alimentary tract. Chem Pharm Bull 37(10):2736-40, 1989*).

Animal Experimental Study: The oral administration of Shosaikoto (1.1 g/kg) corresponding to 10 times the usual human dose was compared to prednisolone alone and in combination with Shosaikoto in experimental models of inflammation. Shosaikoto showed mild anti-inflammatory action on its own, but significantly increased the anti-inflammatory effect of prednisolone. The blood prednisolone level was about 2 times as high when it was combined with Shosaikoto and when Shosaikoto was given alone it significantly increased the blood cortisol level (*Shimizu K et al. Combination effects of Shosaikoto (Chinese traditinal medicine) and prednisolone on the anti-inflammatory action. J Pharm Dyn 7:891-9, 1984*).

Animal Experimental Study: Saikosaponin d (0.1 mg/kg/day x 4 days) and dexamethasone (0.1 mg/kg/day x 4 days) reduced the weight of cotton-induced granuloma to 89.58% and 88.54% of the control, respectively. These antigranulomatous actions failed to show a significant difference from the control. However, the combined administration of saikosaponin d and dexamethasone produced a significant antigranulomatous action, namely, the decrease in the weight of granuloma to 62.5% of the control. While the combination of saikosaponin d and dexamethasone showed an inhibitory trend against the increase in serum triglyceride as induced by dexamethasone, the cholesterol level was elevated by the combination. The body weight was significantly reduced by the combined administration as compared with the gp. treated with dexamethasone alone, but no apparent difference existed in the adrenal and thymus weights between them (*Abe H, Sakaguchi M, Arichi S. [Pharmacological studies on a prescription containing Bupleuri Radix (IV). Effectsof saikosaponin on the anti-inflammatory action of glucocorticoid]. Nippon Yakurigaku Zasshi 80(2):155-61, 1982*) (*in Japanese*).

Animal Experimental Study: A single dose of saikosaponin-a significantly increased plasma ACTH and corticosterone levels 30 and 60 minutes after treatment (*Hiai S et al. Stimulation of the pituitary-adrenocortical axis by saikosaponin of Bupleuri radix. Chem Pharm Bull 29(2):495-9, 1981*).

IMPOTENCE

The term 'impotence' has historically been used to signify the inability of the male to attain and maintain erection of the penis sufficient to permit satisfactory sexual intercourse. Impotence, in most circumstances, is more precisely referred to as erectile dysfunction as this term differentiates itself from loss of libido, premature ejaculation, or inability to achieve orgasm (*Lerner SE et al. A review of erectile dysfunction: New insights and more questions. J Urol 149:1246-55, 1993*).

CAUSES OF ERECTILE DYSFUNCTION

ORGANIC (85%)
  Drugs
    Alcohol
    Antihistamines
    Antihypertensives
    Anticholinergics
    Antidepressants
    Antipsychotics
    Tobacco
    Tranquilizers
  Endocrine disorders
    Diabetes
    Hypothyroidism
    Reduced male sex hormones
    Elevated prolactin levels
    Elevated estrogen levels
    Diseases of or trauma to male sexual organs
  Neurological disorders
    Multiple sclerosis
  Other
    Atherosclerosis
    Pelvic surgery
    Pelvic trauma
    Vascular insufficiency
    Venous shunting
PSYCHOLOGICAL (10%)
  Depression
  Performance anxiety
  Stress
UNKNOWN (5%)

Atherosclerosis of the penile artery is the primary cause of impotence in nearly half the men over the age of 50 that have erectile dysfunction (*NIH Consensus Conference Panel on Impotence. Impotence. JAMA 270:83-90, 1993*)

The diagnosis of erectile dysfunction due to atherosclerosis can be made with the aid of ultrasound techniques. Another popular method of diagnosis involves the injection of papaverine, a drug which causes the arteries to dilate thus delivering more blood to erectile tissues. If the erectile dysfunction is due to arterial insufficiency the penis will become erect and will be sustained after papaverine injection. But, if the erection cannot be maintained it is a sign of venous leakage. This form of erectile dysfunction is much more difficult to treat and may require surgery.

— —

Ginkgo biloba:

Extracts of _Ginkgo biloba_ leaves standardized to contain 24% ginkgoflavonglycosides may be effective in cases of erectile dysfunction due to arterial insufficiency. (_See: 'PERIPHERAL VASCULAR DISEASE'_)

Experimental Study: 60 pts. with proven arterial erectile dysfunction who had not reacted to papaverine injections up to 50 mg, were treated with 60 mg per day of _Ginkgo biloba_ extract for 12 to 18 months. The penile arterial blood flow was re-evaluated by duplex sonography every 4 weeks. The first signs of improved blood supply were seen after 6 to 8 weeks. After 6 months of therapy, 50% of the patients had regained potency; 20% responded to a new trial of papaverine; 25% showed improved arterial inflow, but still did not respond to papaverine; and the remaining 5% were unchanged (_Sikora R et al. Ginkgo biloba extract in the therapy of erectile dysfunction. J Urol 141:188A, 1989_).

Note: The standard dose of Ginkgo biloba extract (24% ginkgoflavonglycosides) is 120 mg/d (40 mg t.i.d.). Using this dosage may produce better results than the 60 mg/d dose used in the study above.

Muira Puama or Potency Wood (_Ptychopetalum olacoides_):

Muira puama, also known as potency wood, is native to Brazil and has long been used as a powerful aphrodisiac and nerve stimulant in South American folk medicine.

May be effective in restoring libido and treating erectile dysfunction.

Experimental Study: 262 pts. complaining of lack of sexual desire and the inability to attain or maintain an erection were given Muira puama extract. Within 2 wks. at a daily dose of 1 to 1.5 grams of the extract, 62% of pts. with loss of libido claimed that the treatment had dynamic effect while 51% of pts. with 'erection failures' felt that Muira puama was of benefit. Although the mechanism of action of Muira puama is unknown, it appears that it works on enhancing both psychological and physical aspects of sexual function (_Waynberg J. Aphrodisiacs: Contribution to the clinical validation of the traditional use of Ptychopetalum guyanna. Presented at The First International Congress on Ethnopharmacology, Strasbourg, France, June 5-9, 1990_).

Yohimbine:

Yohimbine is an alpha-adrenergic blocker originally isolated from yohimbe bark (_Pausinystalia johimbe_) and is currently (1993) the only drug approved by the U.S. Food and Drug Administration for erectile dysfunction.

When used alone, yohimbine is successful in 34-43% of cases of either organic or pschogenic erectile dysfunction. However, side effects often make yohimbine difficult to utilize.

> WARNING: May induce anxiety, panic attacks, and hallucinations in some individuals. Other side effects include elevations in blood pressure and heart rate, dizziness, headache, and skin flushing. Yohimbine should not be used in individuals with kidney disease, women, and individuals with psychological disturbances.

The standard dose of yohimbine is 15-20 mg per day. Higher doses, up to 42 mg of yohimbine, may prove to be more effective. Clinical effectiveness of yohimbe bark is dependent upon yohimbine content of yohimbe bark.

Experimental Double-blind Study: 82 men with erectile dysfunction underwent a multifactorial evaluation, including determination of penile brachial blood pressure index, cavernosography, sacral evoked response, testosterone and prolactin determination, Derogatis sexual dysfunction inventory and daytime arousal test. After 1 month of treatment with a maximum of 42.0 mg. oral yohimbine hydrochloride daily 14% of the pts. experienced restoration of full and sustained erections, 20% reported a partial response to the therapy and 65% reported no improvement. 3 pts. reported a positive placebo effect. Maximum effect takes 2 to 3 weeks to manifest itself. Yohimbine was active in some pts. with arterial insufficiency and a unilateral sacral reflex arc lesion, and in 1 with low serum testosterone levels. The 34% response is encouraging, particularly in a U.S. Veterans Administration population presenting with a high incidence of diabetes and vascular pathological conditions not found in regular office patients. Only few and benign side effects were recorded (*Susset JG et al. Effect of yohimbine hydrochloride on erectile impotence: a double-blind study. J Urol 141(6):1360-3, 1989*).

Experimental Double-blind Study: 100 men with organic erectile dysfunction participated in the study. The first phase of the study showed a positive response in 42.6% of the pts. receiving yohimbine versus 27.6% in the placebo group. Although favorable to the test medication these values did not reach statistical significance (P=0.42). A similar pattern was noted in the second phase of the study. The over-all response rate of 43.5% was consistent with a previous noncontrolled trial but it was much lower than previous studies. The response rate of organically impotent pts. to yohimbine is at best marginal. Owing to its ease of administration, safety and modest effect it still is used in those pts. who do not accept more invasive methods. Adrenoceptors are involved in the erectile process, although other neurotransmitter systems also are putative modulators of penile erection, including cholinergic, dopaminergic and vasoactive intestinal polypeptide pathways. It is beyond reasonable expectation that a single agent be of value for all cases of organic impotence. However, yohimbine has shown modest effectiveness at the doses used in this trial (18 mg. per day). Higher doses or a different route of administration may produce different effects (*Morales A et al. Is yohimbine effective in the treatment of organic impotence? Results of a controlled trial. J Urol 137(6):1168-72, 1987*)

Experimental Double-blind Crossover Study: 48 men meeting strict diagnostic criteria for psychogenic impotence took part in a 10 week placebo-controlled, double-blind, partial crossover trial of yohimbine (18 mg daily) for restoring erectile function. At the end of the first arm of the trial 62% of the yohimbine group and 16% of the placebo group reported some improvement in sexual function (chi 2 = 10.41, df = 2, p<0.05).

21% of the originally placebo-treated group noticed some improvement over pre-treatment levels when they were put on yohimbine in the second arm of the trial. Overall 46% of those who received yohimbine reported a positive response to the drug. Response to yohimbine thus seemed to be unrelated to current groupings of the cause of impotence. Results suggest that yohimbine is a safe treatment for psychogenic impotence that may be as effective as sexual and marital therapy for restoring satisfactory sexual functioning (*Reid K et al. Double-blind trial of yohimbine in treatment of psychogenic impotence. Lancet ii:421-3, 1987*).

INFECTION

See Also: CANDIDIASIS
IMMUNODEPRESSION
PROSTATITIS

Astragalus membranaceus:

A Chinese herb historically used in <u>viral</u> infections. *(See: 'IMMUNODEPRESSION')*

Experimental Controlled Study: 10 pts. suffering from Coxsackie B viral myocarditis with depressed natural killer (NK) activity were treated with *Astagalus membranaceus* intramuscularly for 3-4 months. After the treatment, the NK activity increased significantly from 11.5% to 44.9%. The NK activity of the control gp. of 6 pts. receiving conventional therapy remained unchanged. The general condition and symptoms improved in all pts. given Astragalus and their alpha- and gamma-interferon levels were increased *(Yang YZ et al. Effect of Astragalus membranaceus on natural killer cell activity and induction with coxsakie B viral myocarditis. Chin Med J 103(4):304-7, 1990).*

Berberine:

Berberine is an alkaloid extracted from the roots and bark of various plants such as goldenseal *(Hydrastis canadensis)*, barberry root bark *(Berberis vulgaris)*, and Oregon grape root *(Berberis aquifolium).*

Berberine possesses antibacterial, antifungal, and antiprotozoal activities *(Amin AH, Subbaiah TV, Abbasi KM. Berberine sulfate: antimicrobial activity, bioassay, and mode of action. Can J Microbiol 15(9):1067-76, 1969).*

Bacteria

In vitro Study: Most studies have focused on the bacteriostatic or bactericidal activities of this compound. Berberine sulfate is bacteriostatic for streptococci and that submean inhibitory concentrations (MIC) of berberine blocked the adherence of streptococci to host cells, immobilized fibronectin, and hexadecane. Concentrations of berberine below its MIC caused an eightfold increase in release of lipoteichoic acid from streptococci. Higher concentrations of berberine directly interfered with the adherence of streptococi to host cells either by preventing the complexing of lipoteichoic acid with fibronectin or by dissolution of such complexes once they were formed. Thus, berberine sulfate interferes with the adherence of group A streptococci by two distinct mechanisms: one by releasing the adhesin lipoteichoic acid from the streptococcal cell surface and another by directly preventing or dissolving lipoteichoic acid-fibronectin complexes *(Sun D, Courtney HS, Beachey EH. Berberine sulfate blocks adherence of*

Streptococcus pyogenes to epithelial cells, fibronectin, and hexadecane. Antimicrob Agents Chemother 32:1370-4, 1988).

See Also:

> *Mohan M, Pant CR, Angra SK, Mahajan VM. Berberine in trachoma. (A clinical trial). Indian J Ophthalmol 30(2):69-75, 1982*

> *Sabir M, Mahajan VM, Mohapatra LN, Bhide NK. Experimental study of the anti-trachoma action of berberine. Indian J Med Res 64(8):1160-7, 1976*

Fungi

In vitro Study: Berberine sulfate inhibited the growth of 11/13 fungi (*Mahajan VM, Sharma A, Rattan A. Antimycotic activity of berberine sulfate: An alkaloid from an Indian medicinal herb. Sabouraudia 20:79-81, 1982*).

Parasites

Experimental Controlled Study: Pediatric pts. aged 5 mo. to 14 yrs. with giardiasis received berberine 10 mg/kg daily while controls received established antigiardial drugs. After 10 days, 90% of the berberine gp. (38 pts.) had negative stool cultures compared to 95% of the metronidazole group. At 1 mo. follow-up, 83% of berberine gp. continued to have negative stool cultures compared to 90% of the metronidazole group. Berberine-treated pts. had no side effects (*Gupte S. Use of berberine in the treatment of giardiasis. Am J Dis Child 129:866, 1975*).

See Also:

> *Kaneda Y, Torii M, et al. In vitro effects of berberine sulfate on the growth of Entamoeba histolytica, Giardia lamblia an Trichimonas vaginalis. Ann Trop Med Parasitol 85:417-25, 1991*

> *Kaneda Y et al. Effect of berberine: a plant alkaloid on the growth of anaerobic protozoa in axenic culture. Tokai J Exp Clin Med 15(6):417-23, 1990*

> *Ghosh AK, Bhattacharyya FK, Ghosh DK. Leishmania donovani: amastigote inhibition and mode of action of berberine. Exp Parasitol 60(3):404-13, 1985*

> *Subbaiah TV, Amin AH. Effect of berberine sulfate on Entamoeba histolytica. Nature 215(100):527-8, 1967*

Bromelain:

A mixture of sulfur-containing proteolytic enzymes or proteases derived from the stem of the pineapple plant (*Ananas comosus*).

Administration may combat infection.

Experimental Double-blind Study: 48 pts. with moderately severe to severe acute sinusitis were placed on standard therapy and then received a 6 day supply of either bromelain (Ananase®, Rorer) 2 tabs 4 times daily or placebo and were reassessed 9 days later. General improvement was reported for more pts. receiving bromelain than for controls. For example, 83% of pts. receiving bromelain had complete resolution of nasal mucosal inflammation compared to 52% of controls (p>0.02). Of the pts. not receiving antibiotics, 85% of treated pts. compared to 40% of controls showed complete resolution of inflammation of the nasal mucosa (p>0.02). With respect to ease of breathing, the percentage incidence was 85% vs. 53% (p>0.10) (*Ryan RE. A double-blind clinical evaluation of bromelains in the treatment of acute sinusitis. Headache 7(1):13-17, 1967*).

Experimental Double-blind Study: Between the third and sixth days of treatment with bromelain, the majority of 60 pts. with chronic sinusitis had observable marked improvement in inflammation, nasal discharge, breathing and headache (*Taub SJ. The use of bromelains in sinusitis: A double-blind clinical evaluation. Eye Ear Nose Throat Mon 46(3):361-62 passim, 1967*).

See Also:

Experimental Double-blind Study: *Mori S et al. The clinical effect of proteolytic enzyme containing bromelain and trypsin on urinary tract infection evaluated by double blind method. Acta Obstet Gynaecol Jpn 19(3):147-53, 1972*

Experimental Double-blind Study: *Weiss S, Scherrer M. [Crossed double-blind trial of potassium iodide and bromelain (Traumanase) in chronic bronchitis.] Schweiz Rundsch Med Prax 61(43);1331-3, 1972*

Administration may potentiate antibiotics due to both its anti-inflammatory effects and its ability to improve absorption and tissue penetration of antibiotics.

Experimental Controlled Study: Serum, uterine, ovarian tube and ovarian levels of amoxycillin and tetracycline were higher in pts. treated with bromelain in addition to these antibiotics than in pts. treated with the antibiotics alone, suggesting that bromelain favors the absorption and tissue penetration of antibiotics by mechanisms that are not shared by other anti-inflammatory drugs (*Lucerti M, Vignali M. Influence of bromelain on penetration of antibiotics in uterus, salpinx and ovary. Drugs Exp Clin Res 4 (1):45-8, 1978*).

Experimental Controlled Study: Concentrations of amoxycillin in gallbladder, bile, appendix and skin were higher in pts. treated with bromelain concomitantly with the antibiotic than in pts. treated with antibiotic alone or associated with indomethacin (*Tinozzi S, Venegoni A. Drugs Exp Clin Res 4(1):39-44, 1978*).

Experimental Controlled Study: Bromelain (Ananase®, Rorer), two 20 mg enteric-coated tablets 4 times daily, appeared as effective as antibiotics in treating a variety of infectious processes, including pneumonia, skin staph infections, kidney infections and bronchitis. 53 pts. were treated with bromelain plus antibiotics and were compared with 56 pts. treated with antibiotics alone. Morbidity, judged by the ave. number of days required for successful treatment, was reduced by >1/3 when antibiotics were supplemented with bromelain. 23 of the pts. had previously failed to respond to antibiotics, but improved almost immediately when bromelain was added. Results with another gp. of 106 cases treated with bromelain alone were comparable to those treated with antibiotics alone. It is suggested that bromelain be used to potentiate antibiotics (*Neubauer R. A plant protease for the potentiation of and possible replacement of antibiotics. Exp Med Surg 19:143-60, 1961*).

See Also:

> Takahashi K. [Experimental study on the combined therapy of antibiotics and bromelain. *Shigaku* 65(5):874-904, 1978 (in Japanese)

Cranberry (*Vaccinium macrocarpon*):

Administration of cranberry juice or extracts may be beneficial in treating urinary tract infections.

Experimental Double-blind Study: 153 elderly women (mean age, 78.5 yrs.) randomly received either 300 mL daily of a commercial cranberry beverage or a specially prepared synthetic placebo drink that was indistinguishable. For the 6 mo. study, a baseline urine sample and 6 clean-voided urine samples were collected at about 1-mo. intervals. Treated subjects had odds of bacteriuria (organisms numbering $\geq 10^5$/ml) with pyuria that were only 42% of the odds in the control gp. (p=0.004). Their odds of remaining bacteriuirc-pyuric, given that they were bacteriuric-pyuric in the previous month, were only 27% of the odds in the control gp. (p=0.006). Results suggest that the use of a cranberry beverage reduces the frequency of bacteriuria with pyuria in older women (*Avorn J, Monane M, Gurwitz JH, et al. Reduction of bacteriuria and pyuria after ingestion of cranberry juice. JAMA 271:751-4, 1994*).

Experimental Study: In a nursing home population, 4-6 oz/d of commericial cranberry juice significantly prevented urinary tract infections (*Kilbourne JP. Cranberry juice in urinary tract infection. J Naturopathic Med 2(1):45-7, 1991*).

Experimental Study: 53% of 44 female and 16 male pts. with acute urinary tract infections received 480 mL (16 oz) of cranberry juice for 21 days. 53% had a positive clinical response, while an additional 20% noted moderate improvement. Six wks. after the juice was discontinued, 27 of the pts. had persistent or recurrent infection which was asymptomatic in 8 of them, while 17 pts. were asymptomatic and had negative urine cultures (*Papas PN, Brusch CA, Ceresia GC. Cranberry juice in the treatment of urinary tract infections. Southwest Med 47(1):17-20, 1966*).

Experimental Study: 12 oz of cranberry juice daily relieved urinary symptoms of pts. with chronic urethritis, with or without caruncle formation, or with trigonitis (*Moen DV. Wisconsin Med J 61:282, 1962*).

Administration may increase the acidity of the urine.

> *Note: Other studies have yielded conflicting results (Fellers CR, Redmon BC, Parrott EM. The effect of cranberries on urinary acidity and blood alkali reserve. J Nutr 6:455-63, 1933; McLeod DC, Nahata MC. Methenamine therapy and urine acidification with ascorbic acid cranberry juice. Am J Hosp Pharm 35:654, 1978; Nickey KE. Urine pH: effect of prescribed regimens of cranberry juice and ascorbic acid. Arch Phys Med Rehab 55:556, 1975).*

Experimental Study: 4 healthy male volunteers with noninfected urine received 1500-4000 ml of standard cranberry juice cocktail. Three demonstrated a transient decrease in pH and increase in titratable acidity while, in the fourth, similar changes occurred which lasted for one wk. (*Kahn DH, Panariello V, Saeli J, et al. Effect of cranberry juice on urine. J Am Diet Assoc 51:251, 1967*).

See Also:

> *Schultz AS. Efficacy of cranberry juice on urinary pH. J Community Health Nursing 1:155-69, 1984*

> *Kinney AB, Blount M. Effect of cranberry juice on urinary pH. Nursing Res 28:287-90, 1979*

> *Moen DV. Observations on the effectiveness of cranberry juice in urinary infections. Wis Med J 61:282-3, 1962*

Cranberry components may prevent the adherence of bacteria to fimbriae. (Fimbriae are specialized structures on the surface of bacteria which bind selectively to certain complex carbohydrates on the surface of bladder endothelial cells to form a tight linkage between the host bladder cells and the bacteria.)

In vitro Study: Cranberry juice inhibited the adherence of urinary *E. coli* isolates expressing type I fimbriae and type P fimbriae, but had no effect on a diarrheal isolate expressing a CFA/I adhesion. Because increased adherence of bacteria to bladder cells is involved in the pathogenesis of urinary tract infections, these findings may have relevance for prevention and treatment (*Zafriri D, Ofek I, Adar R, et al. Inhibitory activity of cranberry juice on adherence of type I and type P fimbriated Escherichia coli to eucaryotic cells. Antimicrob Agents Chemother 33(1):92-8, 1989*).

In vitro Study: Both cranberry juice and the urine produced by mice fed cranberry beverage inhibited adherence of *E. coli* to uroepithelial cells by about 80%. Similar anti-adherence activity was also found in human urine (*Schmidt D, Sobota A. An examination of the anti-adherence activity of cranberry juice on urinary and nonurinary bacterial isolates. Microbios 55:173-81, 1988; Sobota AE. Inhibition of bacterial adherence by cranberry juice: Potential use for the treatment of urinary tract infection. J Urol 131:1013-16, 1984*).

Blueberry juice may be equally effective.

In vitro Study: Of 7 juices studied (cranberry, blueberry, grapefruit, guava, mango, orange, and pineapple) only cranberry and blueberry contained anti-*Escherichia coli* adhesin activity. Blueberry juice may prove to be a suitable alternative to cranberry juice in bladder infections (*Ofek I, Goldhar J, Zafriri D, et al. Anti-escherichia adhesin activity of cranberry and blueberry juices. New Engl J Med 324:1599, 1991*).

Echinacea spp.:

Echinacea species, primarily *E. angustifolia*, *E. purpurea*, and *E. pallida*, have historically been used in infections and as 'blood purifiers'. Echinacea was used for more ailments than any other plant by Native Americans of the Plains tribes.

Currently more than 300 Echinacea-containing products are sold worldwide as non-specific immunostimulants. (*See: 'IMMUNODEPRESSION'*)

Review Article: The chemistry, pharmacology and clinical applications of Echinacea has been the subject of over 350 scientific studies. Echinacea possesses a broad-spectrum of effects on the immune system as a result of its content of a broad-range of active components affecting diffferent aspects of immune function including activation of complement, thus promoting: chemotaxis of neutrophils, monocytes, and eosinophils; solubilization of immune complexes; neutralization of viruses; and bacteriolysis. The high-molecular weight heteroglycan polysaccharide components of Echinacea have profound immunostimulatory effect. The majority of these effects appear to be mediated by the binding of active Echinacea polysaccharides to carbohydrate receptors on the cell surface of macrophages and T-lymphocytes. Echinacea promotes nonspecific T-cell activation, i.e., transformation, production of interferon, and secretion of lymphokines. The resultant effect is enhanced T-cell mitogenesis, macrophage phagocytosis, antibody binding, and natural killer cell activity; and increased circulating PMNs. Echinacea polysaccharides have also been shown to enhance macrophage phagocytosis and stimulate macrophages to produce increased amounts of tumor-necrosis-factor (TNF), interferon, and interleukin 1, and destroy tumor cells in tissue culture. Numerous clinical studies have confirmed Echinacea's immune enhancing actions. Various Echinacea extracts or products have shown results in general infectious conditions, influenza, colds, upper respiratory tract infections, urogenital infections, and other infectious conditions (*Bauer R, Wagner H. Echinacea species as potential immunostimulatory drugs.* Econ Med Plant Res *5:253-321, 1991*).

See Also:

> **Review Article:** *Awang DVC, Kindack DG. Echinacea.* Can Pharm J *124:512-6, 1991*

Administration may inhibit hyaluronidase activity and activate fibroblasts to produce hyaluronic acid (*Busing KH. [Inhibition of hyaluronidase by Echinacin.]* Arzneimittelforsch *2:467-72, 1952 (in German); Bonadeo I et al. [Echinacin B: Active polysaccharide from Echinacea.* Riv Ita. Essenze Profumi Piante *53:281-95, 1971) (in Italian).*

> *Note: Hyaluronic acid helps to bind cells together; hyaluronidase is often produced by pathogens to facilitate their spread.*

Administration may enhance phagocytosis (*Kuhn D.[Echinacin and its reaction with phagocytes.]* Arzneimittelforsch *3:194-98, 1953; Quadripur SA. [Drug modification of the phagocytic capacity of granulocytes.]* Ther Ggw *115 (6):1072-78, 1976).*

In vitro studies suggest that administration may have antiviral activity (*Kelling CL et al. Effects of crude extracts of various plants on infectious rhinotracheitis virus-plaque production.* Am J Vet Res *37:215-20, 1976; Orinda D et al. [Antiviral activity of constituents of the compositae purpurea.]* Arzneimittelforsch *23:1119-20, 1973 (in German).*

Administration may be effective.

Influenza

Experimental Double-blind Study: 180 pts. with influenza aged 18-60 were given either *Echinacea purpurea* extract (Echinacin) at a dose of 450 mg, *E. purpurea* at a dose of 900 mg, or a placebo. The 450 mg dose was found to be no more effective than a placebo, however the gp. taking the 900 mg dose showed significant reduction of flu symptoms (*Braunig B et al. [Echinacea purpurea radix for strengthening the immune response in flu-like infections.] Z Phytother 13:7-13, 1992*) (*in German*).

Skin Infections

Case Report: A male with recurrent genital herpes for 12 yrs. took powdered *Echinacea purpurea* (Phytokold; Arkopharma) at the listed dosage. He found that, if he began treatment within 1-2 hrs. of the onset of the prodromal neuralgia, pain subsided within 6 hrs. and the outbreak was aborted. Moreover, recurrences have become less and less frequent. While, previously, he had never been able to prevent an outbreak once the neuralgia began, he has not had a single eruption since starting Echinacea (*Br J Phytotherapy 2(2), 1991*).

Experimental Study: Pts. with various skin infections had rapid and complete healing of the lesions after administration of Echinacea (*Quadripur SA. [Drug modification of the phagocytic capacity of granulocytes.] Ther Ggw 115 (6):1072-78, 1976*) (*in German*).

Upper Respiratory Infections (common cold)

Experimental Double-blind Study: 108 pts. with colds received either an extract of the fresh juice of *Echinacea purpurea*, Echinacin, (4 ml twice daily) or placebo for 8 weeks. The number of pts. remaining healthy: Echinacin 35.2%, placebo 25.9%). Length of time between infections: Echinacin 40 days days, placebo 25 days. When infections did occur in pts. receiving Echinacin, they were less severe and resolved quicker. Pts. showing evidence of a weakened immune system (CD4/CD8-ratio <1.5) benefitted the most from Echinacea (*Schoneberger D. [The influence of immune-stimulating effects of pressed juice from Echinacea purpurea on the course and severity of colds. Results of a double-blind study.] Forum Immunologie 8:2-12, 1992*) (*in German*).

Garlic (*Allium sativum*):

Consumption or administration may be beneficial in fighting a broad range of infectious agents, including viruses, fungi, protozoa, parasites and bacteria (*Koch HP. Garlicin - Fact or fiction? Phytother Res 7:278-80, 1993; Hughes BG, Lawson L. Antimicrobial effects of Allium sativum L. (Garlic), Allium ampeloprasum L. (elephant garlic, and Allium cepa L. (onion), garlic compounds and commercial garlic supplement products. Phytother Res 5:154-8, 1991*).

Administration may be effective against pathogenic fungi.

Experimental Study: Of 21 cases of cryptococcal meningitis encountered in a 5-year period, 16 were treated with garlic alone and 5 were treated with garlic and other drugs. The usual oral dosage was either 1-2 bulbs were ingested with each meal or 10-20 ml 3 times daily of a raw garlic preparation made by mixing 20-30 g of garlic with 100 ml H_2O. 11 of the 16 pts. (68.75%) treated successfully with garlic alone. In pts. who responded to garlic, headache, vomiting, and neurological signs gradually subsided and body temperatures returned to normal within 3-4 days of treatment. In the gp. treated with garlic plus antifungal drugs (amphotericin B or clotrimazole), 4 pts. (80%) were treated successfully (*Hunan Medical College. Garlic in Cryptococcal meningitis: A preliminary report of 21 cases. Chinese Med. J. 93:123, 1980*).

In vitro Study: Garlic demonstrated a broad spectrum of activity against 17 strains of fungi and was more effective than nystatin against pathogenic yeasts (*Adetumbi MA, Lau BH. Allium sativum (garlic): A natural antibiotic. Med. Hypotheses 12(3):227-37, 1983*).

See Also:

> *Caporaso N et al. Antifungal activity in human urine and serum after ingestion of garlic. Antimicrob Agents Chemother 23(5):700-2, 1983*

> *Amer M et al. The effect of aqueous garlic extract on the growth of dermatophytes. Int J.Dermatol 19:285, 1980*

Administration may be effective in viral infections.

In vitro Study: The *in vitro* virucidal effects of fresh garlic, diallyl thiosulfinate (allicin), allyl methyl thiosulfinate, ajoene, alliin, deoxyalliin, diallyl disulfide, and diallyl trisulfide were determined against herpes simplex type 1 and 2, parainfluenza virus type 3, vaccinia virus, vesicular stomatitis virus, and human rhinovirus type 2. The order for virucidal activity was: ajoene allicin allyl methyl thiosulfinate methyl allyl thiosulfinate. Ajoene was found in oil-macerates of garlic, but not in fresh garlic extracts. No activity was found for alliin, deoxyalliin, diallyl disulfide, or diallyl trisulfide. Fresh garlic extract was virucidal against all viruses tested. Virucidal activity of commercial products were dependent upon their preparation processes. Those products producing the highest level of allicin and other thiosulfinates had the best virucidal activity (*Weber ND et al. In vitro virucidal effects of Allium sativum (Garlic) extract and compounds. Planta Med 58:417-23, 1992*).

Animal Experimental Study: Garlic administration protected mice against intranasal inoculation with influenza viruses and enhanced the production of neutralizing antibodies when they were given the vaccine (*Nagai K. Experimental studies on the preventive effect of garlic extract against infection with influenza virus. Jpn J Infect Dis 47:321, 1973*).

See Also:

> *Weber N et al. Antiviral activity of Allium sativum (garlic). Abstract. Ann Mtg Am Soc Microbiol 88:22, 1988*

Tsai Y et al. Antiviral properties of garlic: In vitro effects on influenza B, herpes simplex and coxsackie viruses. Planta Medica 5:460-61, 1985

Elnima EI et al. The antimicrobial activity of garlic and onion extracts. Pharmazie 38(11):747-48, 1983

Grapefruit seed:

Administration of the extract may inhibit intestinal pathogens.

Experimental Study: 15 pts. with atopic eczema, which has demonstrated a high correlation with increased facal pathogens, received oral grapefruit seed extract 150 mg 3 times daily. After 1 mo., the extract proved to be most effective against Candida and Geotrichum sp. and hemolytic coliforms. Slight inhibition occurred of Staphylococcus aureus and aerobic spore formers and no inhibition was demonstrated against Klebsiella species. Normal fecal organisms were largely unaffected and there were no side effects. All pts. noted improvement in constipation, flatulence and abdominal discomfort (*Ionescu G et al. Oral citrus seed extract in atopic eczema: In vitro and in vivo studies on intestinal microflora. J Orthomol Med 5:155-7, 1990*).

Tea tree oil:

Tea tree (*Melaleuca alternifolia*) is a small tree native to only one area of the world - the northeast coastal region of New South Wales, Australia. The oil is exrtacted from the leaves. (*See: 'WOUND HEALING'*)

Administration may be effective.

Case Report: A 40-year-old woman with non-specific vaginitis used a 5-day course of tea tree oil vaginal pessaries, each of which contained 200 mg of oil distilled from the tea tree in a vegetable oil base. At follow-up 1 mo. later, the abnormal bacteria were replaced exclusively by gram-positive bacilli (*Blackwell AL. Tea tree oil and anaerobic (bacterial) vaginosis. Letter. Lancet 337:300, 1991*).

Review Article: Tea tree oil possesses significant antiseptic properties and is regarded by many as the ideal skin disinfectant. Reasons for this claim include that it is active against a wide range of organisms, possesses good penetration, and is non-irritating to the skin. Tea tree oil has been used in the following conditions: acne, aphthous stomatitis (canker sores), athlete's foot, boils, burns, carbuncles, corns, empyema, gingivitis, herpes, impetigo, infections of the nail bed, insect bites, lice, mouth ulcers, psoriasis, root canal treatment, ringworm, sinus infections, sore throat, skin and vaginal infections, tinea, thrush, and tonsilitis (*Altman PM. Australian tea tree oil. Australian J Pharmacy 69:276-8, 1988*).

See Also:

Belaiche P. Treatment of skin infection with the essential oil of Melaleuca alternifolia. Phytotherapie 15:9-12, 1985

Belaiche P. Treatment of vaginal infections of Candida albicans with the essential oil of Melaleuca alternifolia. Phytotherapie vol. 15, 1985

Pena EO. Melaleuca alternifolia oil. Uses for trichomonal vaginitis and other vaginal infections. Obstet Gynecol June, 1962

Tolpa Torf Preparation:

Tolpa Torf Preparation (TTP) is a natural immunomodulating drug registered in Poland for human use. It is the immunoactive fraction with strictly defined biological properties of an extract from crude peat. TTP is produced by a quality controlled, patented method. *(See: 'IMMUNODEPRESSION')*

Administration of TTP may help prevent recurrent upper respiratory tract infections.

Experimental Double-blind Study: TTP was administered orally at 5 mg daily for 3 weeks. At 3 month and 6 month follow-up, favorable results of treatment were obtained in 14/20 and 9/20 TTP treated pts. and in 8/19 and 4/19 placebo pts., respectively. The phagocytic activity of granulocytes was significantly stimulated with TTP, but not with placebo *(Jankowski A et al. A randomized, double-blind study of the efficacy of Tolpa Torf Preparation (TTP) in the treatment of recurrent respiratory tract infections. Archiv Immunol Ther Experimental 41:95-7, 1993).*

Valerian spp.:

Administration of Valerian species such as *Valeriana officinalis* may be effective in viral gastroenteritis.

Experimental Study: 74 pts. with rotavirus enteritis were randomly divided into 3 groups: Gp. A (n=46) received a dosage of 5 ml of Valerian extract every 6 hrs for pts. under 1 year and 10 ml every 6 hrs to pts. over 1 year; Gp. B (n=12) received a solution of B vitamins and vitamin C; and Gp. C (n=16) were treated with gentamycin or SMZ. Groups A and C also received the same vitamin solution as Gp. B. Pts. with fluid and electrolyte disturbances received appropriate therapy. Within 72 hours of medication, the rate of cessation of diarrhea was 74% in Gp. A, 42% in Gp. B, and 56% in Gp. C. Percentages of pts. whose temperature returned to normal after treatment in Groups A, B, and C were 91%, 60%, and 92%, respectively *(Shide C et al. Infantile rotavirus enteritis treated with herbal Valiriana jatamansi (VJ). J Tradit Chin Med 4(4):297-300, 1984).*

- -

COMBINATION TREATMENT

Flower Pollen extract:

Administration of standardized mixed plant pollen extracts may be effective in reducing illness due to upper respiratory tract infections as well as chronic infections of the prostate. *(See: 'PROSTATITIS')*

Experimental Double-blind Study: The effects of a 6-week course of a plant pollen extract administration to a gp. of 20 adolescent swimmers was studied. The number of training days missed due to upper respiratory tract infections was much less in the pollen treatment gp. (4 days) than in the placebo gp. (27 days)   (*Maughan RJ, Evans SP. Effects of pollen extract upon adolescent swimmers. Br J Sports Med 16(3):142-5, 1982*).

INFLAMMATION

See Also: ALLERGY

Bilberry (*Vaccinium myrtillus*):

Bilberry or European blueberry contains flavonoid compounds known as anthocyanosides. Bilberry anthocyanosides are potent antioxidants that may also reduce inflammation. (*See: 'VASCULAR FRAGILITY'; 'MACULAR DEGENERATION'*).

The standard dose for *Vaccinium myrtillus* extract (VME) is based on its anthocyanoside content, as calculated by its anthocyanidin percentage. Most studies have used a bilberry extract standardized for an anthocyanidin content of 25% at a dosage of 160 mg to 480 mg daily.

Administration of an anthocyanoside extract may reduce inflammation.

> **Animal Experimental Study:** Oral administration of VME to rats inhibited carrageenin-induced paw edema, showing a dose-response relationship (*Lietti A et al. Studies on Vaccinium myrtillus anthocyanosides. I. Vasoprotective and anti-inflammatory activity. Arzneim Forsch 26(5):829-32, 1976*).

Bromelain:

Bromelain refers to the mixture of sulfur containing proteolytic enzymes or proteases obtained from the stem of the pineapple plant (*Ananas comosus*).

The standard dosage of bromelain (1,800-2,000 m.c.u.) is 125-450 mg 3 times daily on an empty stomach.

> **Review Article:** Bromelain was introduced as a medicinal agent in 1957, and since that time over 400 scientific papers on its therapeutic applications have appeared in medical literature. Bromelain has been reported in these scientific studies to exert a wide variety of beneficial effects, including reducing inflammation in cases of arthritis, sports injury or trauma and prevention of swelling after trauma or surgery (*Taussig S, Batkin S. Bromelain, the enzyme complex of pineapple (Ananas comosus) and its clinical application. An update. J Ethnopharmacol 22:191-203, 1988*).

Although most of the early clinical trials used an enteric-coated bromelain product (Ananase®, 20 mg bromelain per tablet), enteric coating may not be necessary. The failure of some of the early clinical studies to demonstate effectiveness may have been a result of the enteric coating or inadequate dosages (*Taussig S, et al. Bromelain, a proteolytic enzyme and its clinical application. A review. Hiroshima J Med Sci 24:185-93, 1975*).

Proposed mechanisms of action:

A. Promotes fibrinolysis by activating the production of plasmin from plasminogen (*Ako H et al. Arch Int Pharmacodyn 254:157-67, 1981; Felton GE. Fibrinolytic and antithrombotic action of bromelain may eliminate thrombosis in heart patients. Med Hypotheses 6:1123-33, 1980; Tausig SJ. The mechanism of the physiological action of bromelain. Med Hypotheses 6:99-104, 1980*).

B. Selectively stimulates the production of anti-inflammatory prostaglandin E_1, possibly due to the formation of active peptides formed from fibrinolysis (*Tausig SJ. The mechanism of the physiological action of bromelain. Med Hypotheses 6:99-104, 1980*) or due to factor XII activation of low levels of thrombin (*Felton GE. Fibrinolytic and antithrombotic action of bromelain may eliminate thrombosis in heart patients. Med Hypotheses 6:1123-33, 1980*).

C. Inhibits the synthesis of pro-inflammatory prostaglandin E_2.

> **Animal Experimental Study:** There was a direct relationship between bromelain dose and inhibition of biosynthesis of prostaglandin E_2 in rats. Prednisone produced the same anti-inflammatory effect, but at 10 times higher dosage (*Vellini M et al. Possible involvement of eicosanoids in the pharmacological action of bromelain. Arzneimittelforschung 36:110-12, 1986*).

D. Reduces edema and inflammation by inhibiting kinin formation.

> **Animal Experimental Study:** Bromelain educed symptoms of inflammation, lowered kininogen and bradykinin levels by up to 60%, and decreased prostaglandin E_2 and thromboxane B_2 levels (*Lotz-Winter H. On the pharmacology of bromelain: An update with special regard to animal studies and dose-dependent effects. Planta Med 56:249-53, 1990*).

Administration may be beneficial.

Animal Experimental Study: The anti-inflammatory effect of 9 drugs (including aspirin) was compared in the treatment of experimentally induced edema in rats. Bromelain was found to be the most potent agent (*Uhlig G. Schwellungsprophylaxe nach Exogenem Trauma. Zeitschrift fuer Allgemeine Medizin 57:127-31, 1981*) (*in German*).

Animal Experimental Study: Intraduodenal bromelain significantly reduced post-traumatic swelling in the hindlegs of rats, while parenteral application had only a minimal therapeutic effect; results support the observation that enzymes can be absorbed by the gut without losing their biological properties (*Uhlig G, Seifert J. Efficacy of proteolytic enzymes traumanase (Bromelain) on post traumatic edema. Fortschr Med 99(15):554-6, 1981*) (*in German*).

Animal Experimental Study: Bromelain's anti-inflammatory properties in rabbits were equal or superior to those of indomethacin and salicylates following certain chemical assaults (ex. carrageenan), although it showed little anti-inflammatory activity with other chemicals where salicylates are effective (ex. mustard), suggesting that its mode of act on is through increasing vascular permeability to reduce edema and facilitate WBC mobility (*Ito C et al. Anti-inflammatory actions of proteases, bromelain, trypsin and their mixed preparations. Folia Pharmachol. Japan 75:227-37, 1979*).

Animal Experimental Studies: Bromelain reduced paw edema induced by egg white, carrageenin, dextran, serotonin, bradykinin, and yeast as well as reducing the increased permeability induced by histamine, bradykinin and serotonin (*Pirotta F, De Giuli-Morghen C. Drugs Exp Clin Res 4(1):1-20, 1978; Hiramatso Y. Chem Abstracts 72:11264b, 1970*).

Clinical Observations: 1.) 219 pts. with inflammation and edema associated with traumatic injuries, postoperative tissue reactions, cellulitis, and certain types of ulceration were given 400,000 Rorer units of bromelains (Ananase®) daily in the form of enteric-coated tablets (2 tabs 4 times daily) in addition to standard treatment. 75% of the pts. were rated as showing excellent or good responses (substantially better than expected based on previous experience with similar cases). There were no undesirable effects. 2.) The median time from admission to discharge for 150 pts. treated with bromelains was 8 days compared to 100 pts. with similar diagnoses not given bromelains whose median time was 16 days. 3.) 62.5% of 339 adult pts. for whom bromelains was added due to poor responses to conventional treatments were judged to have made accelerated recoveries (*Cirelli MG. Five years of clinical experience with bromelains in therapy of edema and inflammation in postoperative tissue reaction, skin infections and trauma. Clin Med 74(6):55-9, 1967*).

Experimental Double-blind Crossover Study: 16 pts. with multiple tooth impactions were randomly provided with either bromelain (Ananase®, Rorer, 20 mg tabs) or placebo 2 tabs 4 times daily starting 72 hrs. prior to the first surgical procedure. Following recovery, they were crossed over for their second surgical procedure. 24 hrs. after surgery, 12/16 (75%) of pts. on bromelain had mild or no inflammation compared to 3/16 (19%) pts. on placebo. 72 hrs. after surgery, 14/16 (85%) pts. on bromelain compared to 7/16 (44%) were considered to have mild or no swelling. Similar results were found in regard to post-surgical pain. In addition, pain and swelling were present for a longer period of time in the cases receiving placebo (*Tassman G et al. A double-blind crossover study of a plant proteolytic enzyme in oral surgery. J Dent Med 20:51-4, 1965*).

See Also:

> Bucci E et al. [Clinico-pharmacological comparison between enzyme-type anti-inflammatory agents postoperatively in oral surgery.] Minerva Stomatol 35(5):503-6, 1986

Curcumin:

Curcumin is the yellow pigment and active component of turmeric (*Curcuma longa*). *Curcuma longa* has been used in Ayurvedic medicine, the indigenous systems of medicine of India, both locally and internally, in the treatment of sprains and inflammation.

The recommended dosage for curcumin as an anti-inflammatory is 400 to 600 mg 3 times daily. To achieve a similar amount of curcumin using turmeric would require a dosage of 8,000 to 60,000 mg.

Curcumin exhibits many direct anti-inflammatory effects including: inhibiting leukotriene formation, inhibiting platelet aggregation, promotion of fibrinolysis, and inhibition of neutrophil response to various stimuli involved in the inflammatory process (*Srivastava R. Inhibition of neutrophil response by curcumin. Agents Actions 28:298-303, 1989; Flynn DL, Rafferty MF. Inhibition of 5-hydroxy-eicosatetraenoic acid (5-HETE) formation in intact human neutrophils by naturally-occurring diarylheptanoids: Inhibitory activities of curcuminoids and yakuchinones. Prost Leukotri Med 22:357-60, 1986*). It also appears to exert some indirect anti-inflammatory effects. In models of chronic inflammation, curcumin is much less active in adrenalectomized animals. Possible mechanisms of action include: (1) stimulation of the release of adrenal corticosteroids; (2) 'sensitizing' or priming cortisol receptor sites, thereby potentiating cortisol action; and (3) increasing the half-life of endogenous cortisol through alteration of hepatic degradation.

Animal Experimental Study: Curcumin was found to be more potent than ibuprofen as a stabilizer of lysosomal membranes and an uncoupler of oxidative phosphorylation. At higher doses, curcumin was shown to act by stimulation of the adrenals resulting in the release of endogenous cortisone. Curcumin also inhibited prostaglandin synthesis, but was weaker than ibuprofen in this respect (*Srivastava R, Srimal RC. Modification of certain inflammation-induced biochemical changes by curcumin. Indian J Med Res 81:215-23, 1985*).

Animal Experimental Study: Curcumin is as effective as cortisone or phenylbutazone in models of acute inflammation, but only half as effective in chronic models. However, while phenylbutazone and cortisone are associated with significant toxicity, curcumin displays virtually no toxicity (*Srimal R and Dhawan B. Pharmacology of diferuloyl methane (curcumin), a non-steroidal anti-inflammatory agent. J Pharm Pharmac 25:447-52, 1973*)

See Also:

> **Animal Experimental Study:** *Ghatak N and Basu N: Sodium curcuminate as an effective anti-inflammatory agent. Ind J Exp Biol 10:235-6, 1972.*

> **Animal Experimental Study:** *Arora R, Basu N, Kapoor V and Jain A: Anti-inflammatory studies on curcuma longa (turmeric). Ind J Med Res 59:1289-95, 1971.*

Administration may be beneficial.

Experimental Double-blind Study: A new human model for evaluating NSAIDs, the postoperative inflammation model, was used to evaluate the anti-inflammatory action of curcumin compared to phenylbutazone. 45 pts. having inguinal hernia and/or hydrocele surgery received either curcumin 400 mg, placebo, or phenylbutazone 100 mg 3 times daily for a period of 5 days form the first postoperative day. Pts. receiving both curcumin and phenylbutazone exhibited better anti-inflammatory response than placebo, but only curcumin reduced cord edema and tenderness significantly compared to placebo and phenylbutazone (*Satoskar RR, Shah SJ, Shenoy SG. Evaluation of anti-inflammatory property of curcumin (diferuloyl methane) in patients with postoperative inflammation. Int J Clin Pharmacol Ther Toxicol 24:651-4, 1986*).

Topical application may also be effective, possibly due to its counterirritant effect. Capsaicin, a similar pungent principle from *Capsicum frutescens*, has been shown to be effective as a topical pain reliever in cases of post-herpetic neuralgia and arthritis. Both capsaicin and curcumin deplete nerve endings of the neurotransmitter of pain, substance P (*Patacchini R, Maggi CA, Meli A. Capsaicin-like activity of some natural pungent substances on peripheral ending of visceral primary afferents. Arch Pharmacol 342:72-7, 1990*).

See Also:

> **Animal Experimental Study:** *Mukhopadhyay A et al. Anti-inflammatory and irritant activities of curcumin analogues in rats. Agents Actions 12:508-15, 1982*

Devil's Claw (*Harpagophytum procumbens*):

Devil's claw is an herb native to Africa that has a long history of use in the treatment of arthritis. (*See: 'OSTEOARTHRITIS' ; 'RHEUMATOID ARTHRITIS'*)

The equivocal anti-inflammatory effects of Devil's claw in experimental models may reflect: a mechanism of action that is inconsistent with current anti-inflammatory drugs, a lack of quality control (standardization) of the Devil's claw preparations used, or inactivation of inflammatory principles during the process of digestion.

> **Animal Experimental Study:** An aqueous extract of *Harpagophytum procumbens* exhibited significant and dose-dependent anti-inflammatory effects. However, the anti-inflammatory effect of *H. procumbens* could be eliminated after an acid treatment similar to the physiochemical conditions found in the stomach. The main iridoid glycoside, harpagoside, exerted no anti-inflammatory effect (*Lanhers MC et al. Anti-inflammatory and analgesic effects of an aqueous extract of Harpagophytum procumbens. Planta Med 58:117-23, 1992*).

> **Negative Experimental Study:** Healthy volunteers took 4 capsules of 500 mg *H. procumbens* daily for 21 days. No biochemical effects on arachidonic acid or eicosanoid metabolism were noted (*Moussard C et al. A drug used in traditional medicine, Harpagophytum procumbens: No evidence for NSAID-like effect on whole blood eicosanoid production in humans. Prostaglan Leukotri Essent Fatty Acids 46:283-6, 1992*).

> **Negative Animal Experimental Study:** At doses 100 times or greater than the recommended daily dose for humans, *H. procumbens* was completely ineffective in reducing rat hind foot edema. *H. procumbens* was also ineffective in inhibiting prostaglandin synthesis *in vitro* (*Whitehouse LW, Znamirowski M, Paul CJ. Devil's claw (Harpagophytum procumbens): no evidence for anti-inflammatory activity in the treatment of arthritic disease. Can Med Assoc J 129:249-51, 1983*).

> **Negative Animal Experimental Study:** No anti-inflammatory effect was noted for *H. procumbens* (*McLeod DW, Revell P, Robinson BV. Investigations of Harpagophytum procumbens (Devil's claw) in the treatment of experimental inflammation and arthritis in the rat. Br J Pharmacol 66:140P-141P, 1979*).

Feverfew (*Tanacetum parthenium*):

A medicinal herb whose active component (parthenolide) inhibits the secretory action of polymorphonuclear leukocytes involved in the production of cytotoxic and chemotaxic compounds and appears to inhibit the synthesis of prostaglandins PGE2, thromboxane, and leukotrienes that are involved in the inflammatory and pain process (*Heptinstall S et al. Extracts of fevewfew inhibit granule secretion in blood platelets and polymorphonuclear leucocytes. Lancet i:1071-4, 1985*).

> **In vitro Study:** Feverfew was found to contain a factor that inhibits prostaglandin synthesis, but differs from salicylates by not inhibiting cyclo-oxygenase by prostaglandin (PG) synthase. "The ability of feverfew to inhibit PG production may account for its effectiveness as a herbal remedy in conditions responding to acetylsalicylate and like-acting drugs" (*Collier HOJ, Butt NM, McDonald-Gibson WJ, Saeed SA. Extract of feverfew inhibits prostaglandin biosynthesis. Letter. Lancet October 25, 1980*).

> > *Note: The efficacy of feverfew is dependent upon adequate levels of parthenolide, the active ingredient. (The preparations used in successful clinical trials have a parthenolide content of 0.4-0.66%.)*

> > **Animal Ex vivo Study:** Extracts of fresh feverfew caused a dose- and time-dependent, irreversible inhibition of the contractile response of rabbit aortic rings to all receptor-acting agonists tested. The presence of potentially SH reacting parthenolide and other sesquiterpene alpha-methylenebutyrolactones in these extracts, and the close parellelism of pure parthenolide, suggest that the inhibitory effects are due to these compounds. Extracts of the dry leaves were not inhibitory and actually caused potent and sustained contractions of aortic smooth muscle; these extracts were found to be devoid or parthenolide or butyrolactones (*Barsby RWJ, Salan U, Knight BW, Hoult JRS. Feverfew and vascular smooth muscle: Extracts from fresh and dried plants show opposing pharmacological profiles, dependent upon sesquiterpene lactone content. Planta Medica 59:20-5, 1993*).

> > **Chemical Analysis:** The parthenolide content of over 35 different commercial preparations of feverfew was determined by bioassay, 2 HPLC methods, and NMR. The results indicate a wide variation in the amts. of parthenolide in commercial preparations. The majority of products contained no parthenolide or only traces (*Heptinstall S et al. Parthenolide content and bioactivity of feverfew (Tanacetum parthenium (L.) Schultz-Bip.). Estimation of commercial and authenticated feverfew products. J Pharm Pharmacol 44:391-5, 1992*).

> WARNING: No long-term toxicity studies have been conducted. While feverfew is extremely well-tolerated and no serious side effects have ever been reported, chewing the leaves can result in small ulcerations in the mouth and swelling of the lips and tongue in about 10% of users (*Awang DVC. Feverfew. Can Pharm J 122:266-70, 1989*).

See Also:

Berry MI. Feverfew faces the future. Pharm J 611-14, May, 1984

Makheja AN, Bailey JM. A platelet phospholipase inhibitor from the medicinal herb feverfew. Prostaglan Leukotri Med 8:653-60, 1982

Makheja AN, Bailey JM. The active principle in feverfew. Lancet ii:1054, 1981

Collier HO et al. Extract of feverfew inhibits prostaglandin biosynthesis. Lancet ii:1054, 1981

Licorice root (*Glycyrrhiza glabra*):

Licorice root contains about 6% glycyrrhizin, which in the body is cleaved to form glycyrrhetinic acid. Glycyrrhetinic acid exhibits profound pharmacological activity including anti-inflammatory properties. It is capable of binding to cortisol receptors, but its major effect is thought to be preventing the degradation, and extending the half-life, of endogenous cortisol.

> WARNING: If ingested regularly, licorice root (>3 g/d for more than 6 weeks) or glycyrrhizin (>100 mg/d) may cause sodium and water retention, hypertension, hypokalemia, and suppression of the renin-aldosterone system through a pseudo-aldosterone action of glycyrrhetinic acid. Monitoring of BP and electrolytes and increasing potassium intake is suggested (*Farese RV et al. Licorice-induced hypermineralocorticoidism. N Engl J Med 325(17):1223-7, 1991; MacKenzie MA et al. The influence of glycyrrhetinic acid on plasma cortisol and cortisone in healthy young volunteers. J Clin Endocrinol Metab 70:1637-43, 1990*).

Glycyrrhizin inhibits prostaglandin synthesis in a manner similar to cortisone (*Okimasa E et al. Inhibition of phospholipase A2 by glycyrrhizin, an anti-inflammatory drug. Acta Med Okayama 37:385-91, 1983; Ohuchi K et al. Glycyrrhizin inhibits prostaglandin E2 formation by activated peritoneal macrophages from rats. Prostagland Med 7:457-63, 1981*).

Administration may be effective when given alone or as an as an adjunct to corticosteroid treatment.

> **Experimental Controlled Study:** Each subject (n=6) received an IV dose of prednisolone (PSL) with or without 200 mg glycyrrhizin (GL). GL was found to increase significantly the concentration of total PSL and free PSL by inhibiting the breakdown of PSL. The effects of PSL are potentiated by GL (*Chen MF et al. Effect of glycyrrhizin on the pharmacokinetics of prednisolone following low dosage of prednisolone hemisuccinate. Endocrinol Japan 37(3):331-41, 1990*).

Onion (*Allium cepa*):

Administration may have an anti-inflammatory effect.

> **In vitro Study:** Onion extracts inhibited *in vitro* chemically-induced chemotaxis of human granulocytes in a dose-dependent manner and were more active than prednisolone. Results suggest that the anti-inflammatory properties of these extracts are related, at least partly, to the inhibition of inflammatory cell influx by thiosulfinates and

cepanes (*Dorsch W, Schneider E, et al. Anti-inflammatory effects of onions: Inhibition of chemotaxis of human polymorphonuclear leukocytes by thiosulfinates and cepanes. Int Arch Allergy Appl Immunol 92:39-42, 1990*).

See Also:

> **In vitro Study:** *Bayer T, Wagner H, Wray V, Dorsch W. Inhibitors of cyclo-oxygenase and lipoxygenase in onions. Letter. Lancet ii:906, 1988*

- -

COMBINATION TREATMENT

<u>Shosaikoto</u>:

Bupleuri root or Chinese thoroughwax (*Bupleurum falcatum*) is the major component of Shosaikoto, one of the most famous Chinese medicines. The other 6 components of Shosaikoto are: licorice root (*Glycyrrhiza glabra*), jujube fruit (*Zizyphus jujuba*), ginger root (*Zingiber officinalis*), *Panax ginseng* root, Chinese skullcap root (*Scutellaria baicalensis*), and half summer root (*Pinellia ternata*). All of the individual components have exerted anti-inflammatory activity (*Cyong J. A pharmacological study of the anti-inflammatory activity of Chinese herbs. A review. Int J Acupuncture Electro-Ther Res 7:173-202, 1982*).

The main anti-inflammatory action of Shosaikoto has been primarily attributed to Bupleuri root's steroid-like molecules known as saikosaponins. Saikosaponins exhibit potent anti-inflammatory action as well as prevent adrenal atrophy caused by repeated administration of corticosteroids.

Extracts of *Bupleurum falcatum* or Shosaikoto may be effective on their own as an anti-inflammatory agent or as an adjunct to corticosteroid therapy.

> **Animal Experimental Study:** Intraperitoneal administration of various saikosaponins and their intestinal metabolites showed corticosterone secretion-inducing activity (*Nose M, Amagaya S, Ogihara Y. Corticosterone secretion-inducing activity of saikosaponin metabolites formed in the alimentary tract. Chem Pharm Bull 37(10):2736-40, 1989*).

> **Animal Experimental Study:** The oral administration of Shosaikoto (1.1 g/kg) corresponding to 10 times the usual human dose was compared to prednisolone alone and in combination with Shosaikoto in experimental models of inflammation. Shosaikoto showed mild anti-inflammatory action on its own, but significantly increased the anti-inflammatory effect of prednisolone. The blood prednisolone level was about 2 times as high when it was combined with Shosaikoto. When Shosaikoto was given alone, it significantly increased the blood cortisol level (*Shimizu K et al. Combination effects of Shosaikoto (Chinese traditional medicine) and prednisolone on the anti-inflammatory action. J Pharm Dyn 7:891-9, 1984*).

> **Animal Experimental Study:** Saikosaponins inhibited the synthesis, release, and action of inflammatory mediators including histamine, prostaglandin E_2, and leukotrienes (*Zhongchu A, Guizhi W, Junling M. The anti-allergic inflammation action of saikosaponins. J Tradit Chin Med 3(2):103-12, 1983*).

Animal Experimental Study: Saikosaponin d (0.1 mg/kg/day x 4 days) and dexamethasone (0.1 mg/kg/day x 4 days) reduced the weight of cotton-induced granuloma to 89.58% and 88.54% of the control, respectively (results not significant). The combined administration of saikosaponin d and dexamethasone produced a significant anti-granulomatous action, namely, the decrease in the weight of granuloma to 62.5% of the control. While the combination of saikosaponin d and dexamethasone showed an inhibitory trend against the increase in serum triglyceride induced by dexamethasone, the cholesterol level was elevated by the combination. Body weight was significantly reduced by the combined administration as compared with the group treated with dexamethasone alone, but no apparent difference existed in the adrenal and thymus weights between them (*Abe H, Sakaguchi M, Arichi S. [Pharmacological studies on a prescription containing Bupleuri Radix (IV). Effects of saikosaponin on the anti-inflammatory action of glucocorticoid]. Nippon Yakurigaku Zasshi 80(2):155-61, 1982) (in Japanese).*

Animal Experimental Study: A single dose of saikosaponin-a significantly increased plasma ACTH and corticosterone levels 30 and 60 minutes after treatment (*Hiai S et al. Stimulation of the pituitary-adrenocortical axis by saikosaponin of Bupleuri radix. Chem Pharm Bull 29(2):495-9, 1981).*

Animal Experimental Study: The anti-inflammatory actions of saikosaponins were demonstrated in experimental models. The oral administration of saikosaponins in 10 times the dosage of IM injection showed almost the same effect. Among saikosaponins isolated from *Bupleurum falcatum*, saikosaponins a and d, but not c, were demonstrated to have anti-inflammatory action (*Yamamoto M, Kumagai A, Yamamura Y. Structure and actions of saikosaponins isolated from Bupleurum falcatum L. I. Anti-inflammatory action of saikosaponins. Arzneim Forsch 25(7):1021-3, 1975).*

INNER EAR DYSFUNCTION
(including HEARING LOSS, TINNITUS and VERTIGO)

See Also: CEREBROVASCULAR DISEASE
NAUSEA AND VOMITING

<u>Ginger</u> (<u>*Zingiber officinale*</u>):

Administration of ginger root may reduce <u>vertigo</u> caused by vestibular stimulation.

Experimental Double-blind Study: 80 naval cadets unaccustomed to sailing in heavy seas were studied during voyages on the high seas. Each randomly received either 1 gm of powered ginger root or a placebo and symptoms of seasickness were recorded each hour for 4 hours. Ginger was significantly better than placebo in reducing the frequency of vomiting (72% reduction) and cold sweats (p<0.05). Cadets receiving ginger also indicated a reduction in nausea and vertigo compared to controls; however, the reduction failed to reach statistical significance. Overall, symptoms were 38% less in the ginger gp. than in the controls (*Grontved A et al. Ginger root against seasickness. A controlled trial on the open sea <u>Acta Otolaryngol</u> 105 (1-2):45-9, 1988*).

Experimental Double-blind Crossover Study: 18 healthy volunteers received either 1 gm of ginger root or a lactose placebo 1 hr. prior to caloric stimulation of the vestibular system. Compared to controls, ginger root significantly reduced vertigo scores; however, it failed to affect nystagmus as measured by electronystagmograms (*Grontved A, Hentzer E. Vertigo-reducing effect of ginger root. A controlled clinical study. <u>ORL J Otorhinolaryngol Relat Spec</u> 48(5):282-6, 1986*).

Experimental Double-blind Study: 18 male and 18 female pts. with a history of extreme susceptibility to motion sickness randomly received a placebo, dimenhydrinate 100 mg or powdered ginger 940 mg. 25 min later they were blindfolded and spun in a mechanical rotating chair. The test was stopped when either the subject vomited or asked that it be stopped. Subjects who received ginger remained in the chair an ave. of 5.5 min., compared with an ave. of 3.5 min for the dimenhydrinate gp. and 1.5 min. for the placebo group. Once nausea began, however, sensations of nausea and vomiting progressed at the same rate in all groups. More than 90% of pts. with motion sickness who took 2-4 caps of ginger root prior to traveling, and took 2 more approximately every hr. or whenever they felt slightly nauseated, reported excellent results. Ginger root was found to be equally effective for automobile, airplane, train or boat trips (*Mowrey DB, Clayson DE. Motion sickness, ginger and psychophysics. <u>Lancet</u> i:655-7, 1982*).

The efficacy of ginger root appears to be due to anticholinergic and antihistaminic actions.

Animal Experimental Studies: Results of studies with rabbits, isolated rat fundus strip preparations and guinea-pig isolated ileum suggest that the pungent consituents of ginger release substance P from sensory fibers which either stimulates cholinergic and histaminic neurons to release acetylcholine and histamine, respectively, or produces direct smooth muscle contraction by activating M and H_1 receptors correspondingly. It is proposed that after being excited by substance P, M and H_1 receptors are inactive temporarily and unable to be excited by agonists; therefore ginger juice exhibits anti-cholinergic and antihistamine actions (*Qian DS, Liu ZS. [Pharmacologic studies of antimotion sickness actions of ginger.] Chung Kuo Chung Hsi I Chieh Ho Tsa Chih 12(2):95-8, 70, 1992) (in Chinese).*

Experimental Double-blind Study: In order to determine whether the nystagmus response to optokinetic or vestibular stimuli might be altered by some agent in powdered ginger root, normal subjects were examined after administration of ginger root, dimen-hyrinate and placebo. Eye movements were recorded using standard EMG equipment and evaluation was performed by automatic nystagmus analysis. Ginger root had no effect on experimentally-induced nystagmus, while demenhydrinate caused a reduction in the nystagmus response to caloric, rotatory and optokinetic stimuli. Results suggest that neither the vestibular nor the oculomotor system are influenced by ginger, and thus a central nervous system mechanism, which is characteristic of conventional anti-motion sickness drugs, can be excluded. It is likely that any reduction of motion-sickness symptoms derives from the influence of ginger root agents on the gastric system (*Holt-mann S, Clarke AH, Scherer H, Hohn M. The anti-motion sickness mechanism of ginger. A comparative study with placebo and dimenhydrinate. Acta Otolaryngol (Stockh) 108(3-4):168-74, 1989).*

Experimental Double-blind Crossover Study: 18 healthy volunteers received either 1 gm of ginger root or a lactose placebo 1 hr. prior to caloric stimulation of the vestibular system. Compared to controls, ginger root failed to affect nystagmus as measured by electronystagmograms (*Grontved A, Hentzer E. Vertigo-reducing effect of ginger root. A controlled clinical study. ORL J Otorhinolaryngol Relat Spec 48(5):282-6, 1986).*

Theoretical Discussion: Unlike dimenhydrinate, which works in the central nervous sytem, ginger appears to work in the gastrointestinal tract by slowing the feedback interaction between the stomach and the nausea center in the brain by absorbing and neutralizing gastrointestinal toxins and acid (*Mowrey DB, Clayson DE. Motion sickness, ginger and psychophysics. Lancet i:655-7, 1982).*

Ginkgo biloba:

Extracts of *Ginkgo biloba* leaves standardized to contain 24% ginkgoflavonglycosides may be beneficial, especially if the condition is due to cerebrovascular insufficiency. (*See: 'CEREBROVASCULAR DISEASE'*)

The standard dose of *Ginkgo biloba* extract (GBE) is 40 mg 3 times daily.

Administration may be beneficial in <u>vertiginous syndromes</u>.

Experimental Double-blind Study: 70 pts. with vertiginous syndromes of recent onset and undetermined origin received either *Ginkgo biloba* extract or placebo in a double-blind manner. After 3 mo., the effectiveness of *Ginkgo biloba* on the intensity, frequency and duration of the disorder was statistically significant. 47% of treated pts.

became symptom-free vs. 18% of controls (*Haguenauer JP et al. [Treatment of equilibrium disorders with Ginkgo biloba extract. A multicenter double-blind drug vs. placebo study.] Presse Med 15(31):1569-72, 1986*) (*in French*).

Experimental Double-blind Study: Craniocorpography, a method of objectively recording nystagmus and oscillation of the head and body, was used instead of the subjective symptoms of vertigo or dizziness and nausea in order to assess the outcome of a double-blind study of Ginkgo biloba extract in vertiginous syndromes with no obvious anatomical localization. In this study, cranicorpography demonstrated the beneficial effects of *Ginkgo biloba* as compared to placebo (*Claussen CF. [Diagnostic and practical value of craniocorpography in vertiginous syndromes.] Presse Med 15(31):1565-8, 1986*) (*in French*).

Administration may be beneficial in tinnitus.

Negative Experimental Study: 21 pts. with tinnitus (18 with 3 yrs. onset) took GBE for 12 weeks. 11 reported no change, 4 slight to very slight improvement, and 5 reported their tinnitus was worse (*Coles R. Trial of an extract of Ginkgo biloba (EGB) for tinnitus and hearing loss. Clin Otolaryngol 13:501-4, 1988*).

Experimental Double-blind Study: 103 pts. with recent onset tinnitus were given either GBE or placebo. The overall evolution of tinnitus, time before disappearance, evolution of intensity, and decrease in impairment showed a significant difference in favor of the GBE (*Meyer B. A multicenter randomized double-blind study of Ginkgo biloba extract versus placebo in the treatment of tinnitus, in EW Funfgeld, Ed. Rokan (Ginkgo Biloba) Recent Results in Pharmacology and Clinic. New York, Springer-Verlag, 1988:245-50*).

Experimental Study: GBE was given to 62 pts. with inner ear difficulties in an open 9-week trial. 12/33 tinnitus pts. had complete remission and 5 had reductions (*Sprenger FH. Gute therapie ergebnissemit Ginkgo biloba. Arztlich Praxis 12:938-40, 1986*) (*in German*).

See Also:

> **Experimental Double-blind Study:** *Meyer B. [A multicenter randomized double-blind drug vs. placebo study of ginkgo biloba extract in the treatment of tinnitus.] Presse Med 15(31):1562-4, 1986 (in French)*

Administration may be beneficial in acute cochlear deafness.

Experimental Double-blind Study: GBE was compared under double-blind conditions to a standard alpha blocker (nicergoline) in the treatment of acute cochlear deafness, an illness whose pathogenetic mechanism appears to be ischemia and the metabolic disorder it entails, regardless of the triggering process. A significant recovery was observed in both therapeutic gps.; however, improvement was distinctly better in the GBE group (*Dubreuil C. [Therapeutic trial in acute cochlear deafness. A comparative study of Ginkgo biloba extract and nicergoline. Presse Med 15(31):1559-61, 1986*) (*in French*).

INSOMNIA

Passion flower (_Passiflora incarnata_):

Passion flower was widely used by the Aztecs as a diaphoretic, a sedative, and and analgesic.

As a mild sedative, passion flower may be taken at the following dose 30 to 45 minutes before retiring:

>   Dried plant (or as tea) - 1-2 grams
>   Tincture (1:5) - 4-6 ml
>   Fluid extract (1:1)- 1-2 ml
>   Solid (dry powdered) extract (5:1) - 200-400 mg

Administration may be beneficial.

>   **Animal Experimental Study:** Rats given an oral Passiflora extract for 3 weeks demonstrated a diminished general activity indicative of sedative effects despite surface and deep EEG recordings showing 'normal' electric activity (_Sopranzi N et al. [Biological and electroencephalographic parameters in rats in relation to Passiflora incarnata L.] Clin Ter 132(5):329-33, 1990) (in Italian)._

>   **Animal Experimental Study:** The fluid extract of Passiflora given orally and intraperitoneally to rats raised the nociceptive threshold in the tail-flick and hot-plate tests, but not in the voculization test; prolonged sleeping time; provided protection against the convulsive effects of pentylenetetrazole; and reduced locomotor activity (_Speroni E, Minghetti A. Neuropharmacological activity of extracts from Passiflora incarnata. Planta Med 54(6):488-91, 1988)._

>   See Also:

>>   **Animal Experimental Study:** _Oga S et al. Pharmacological trials of crude extract of Passiflora alata. Planta Med 50(4):303-6, 1984_

Valerian (_Valeriana officinalis_):

Valerian is a perennial plant native to North America and Europe that has a long history of use as a sedative.

As a mild sedative, Valerian may be taken at the following dose 30-45 minutes before retiring:

Dried root (or as tea) - 1-2 grams
Tincture (1:5) - 4-6 ml
Fluid extract (1:1)- 1-2 ml
Solid (dry powdered) extract (1.0-1.5% valtrate or 0.8% valeric acid) - 150-300 mg.

If morning sleepiness does occur, reduce dosage. If dosage was not effective be sure to eliminate those factors that disrupt sleep, such as caffeine and alcohol, before increasing dosage.

Valerian is generally regarded as safe and is approved for food use by the US Food and Drug Administration.

Originally it was thought the active constituents of Valerian were the valepotriates (fat-soluble), but recent research has focused primarily on the water-soluble components.

> *Note: The safety of valepotriates was questioned after studies demonstrated mutagenicity (von der Hude W, Scheutwinkel-Reich M, Braun R. Bacterial mutagenicity of the tranquilizing constituents of Valerianaceae roots. Mut Research 169:23-7, 1986; von der Hude W, et al. In vitro mutagenicity of valepotriates. Arch Toxicol 56:267-71, 1985), although there is also evidence that they possess cytotoxic and antitumor effects (Bounthanh C et al. Valepotriates, a new class of cytotoxic and antitumor agents. Planta Med 41:21-8, 1981).*

Review Article: A comprehensive review of the constituents of Valerianaceae with particular reference to the sedative activity of the valepotriates present and to a lesser extent the sesquiterpene constituents of the volatile oils. Recent research into the activity of the water-soluble components as well as the toxicology of the valepotriates is also reviewed (*Houghton PJ. The biological activity of Valerian and related plants. J Ethnopharmacol 22(2):121-42, 1988*).

Valerian components may interact with various brain receptor cites to promote sedation.

In vitro Study: Both hydroalcoholic and aqeuous extracts of valerian showed affinity for GABA receptors. The chemical nature of the compounds are not consistent with sesquiterpenes or valepotriates. The lipophilic fraction of the hydroalcoholic extract and dihydrovaltrate, a valepotriate, showed affinity for barbiturate receptors and a mild affinity for benzodiazepine receptors (*Mennini T et al. In vitro study on the interaction of extracts and pure compounds from Valeriana officinalis roots with GABA, benzodiazepine and barbiturate receptors in rat brain. Fitoterapia 54(4):291-300, 1993*).

Administration may be beneficial.

Experimental Double-blind Study: Insomniacs received either a Valerian preparation (Valerina Natt) containing primarily sesquiterpenes or placebo. Compared to placebo, it showed a significant effect on poor sleep ($p < 0.001$). 44% reported perfect sleep and 89% reported improved sleep. No side effects were observed (*Lindahl O, Lindwall L. Double blind study of a valerian preparation. Pharmacol Biochem Behav 32(4):1065-6, 1989*).

Experimental Double-blind Study: 8 mild insomniacs received 450 mg or 900 mg of an aqueous extract of Valerian root or placebo. Using the first period of 5 consecutive minutes without movement as a criterian of sleep onset, there was a significant decrease in sleep latency with 450 mg Valerian compared to placebo (p<0.01); the higher dosage of valerian produced no further improvement (*Leathwood PD, Chauffard F. Aqueous extract of valerian reduces tendency to fall asleep in man. Planta Medica 54:144-8, 1985*).

Experimental Study: The effect of an aqueous extract of Valerian root on sleep was studied in two groups of healthy, young subjects. One group (n=10) slept at home, the other (N = 8) in the sleep laboratory. Sleep was evaluated on the basis of questionnaires, self-rating scales and night-time motor activity. In addition, polygraphic sleep recordings and spectral analysis of the sleep EEG was performed in the laboratory group. Under home conditions, both doses of Valerian extract (450 and 900 mg) reduced perceived sleep latency and wake time after sleep onset. Night-time motor activity was enhanced in the middle third of the night and reduced in the last third. The data suggest a dose-dependent effect. In the sleep laboratory, where only the higher dose of Valerian was tested, no significant differences from placebo were obtained. However, the direction of the changes in the subjective and objective measures of sleep latency and wake time after sleep onset, as well as in night-time motor activity, corresponded to that observed under home conditions. There was no evidence for a change in sleep stages and EEG spectra. The results indicate that the aqueous Valerian extract exerts a mild hypnotic action (*Balderer G, Borbely AA. Effect of valerian on human sleep. Psychopharmacol 87(4):406-9, 1985*).

Experimental Double-blind Study: 128 subjects received 3 samples containing 400 mg Valerian extract, 3 containing a proprietary over-the-counter Valerian preparation, and 3 containing placebo. Samples were presented in random order and were taken on non-consecutive nights. Valerian produced a significant decrease in subjectively evaluated sleep latency scores. It also produced a significant improvement in sleep quality - especially among people who considered themselves poor or irregular sleepers, smokers, and people who thought they had long sleep latencies. Night awakenings, dream recall and somnolence the next morning were relatively unaffected. The proprietary preparation only produced a significant increase in reports of feeling more sleepy than normal the next morning (*Leathwood PD et al. Aqueous extract of valerian root (Valeriana officinalis L.) improves sleep quality in man. Pharmacol Biochem Behav 17(1):65-71, 1982*).

- with *Melissa officinalis*:

Experimental Placebo-controlled Study: 20 volunteers received either a combination of Valerian root 160 mg and *Melissa officinalis* 80 mg., triazolam 0.125 or placebo. In the insomniac gp., the herbal preparation showed an effect comparable to that of the benzodiazopine as well as an increase in deep sleep stages 3 and 4. The herbal preparation did not cause daytime sedation or rebound phrenomena and there was no evidence of diminished concentration based on the Concentration Performance Test or impairment of physical performance based on the Labyrinth Test (*Dressing H, Riemann D, et al. Insomnia: Are Valerian/Melissa combinations of equal value to benzodiazepine? Therapiewoche 42:726-36, 1992*) (*in German*).

COMBINATION TREATMENT

Suanzaorentang:

Suanzaorentang is an ancient Chinese remedy composed of five herbs: zizyphi seed (*Zizyphus jujuba*), poria (*Poria cocos*), ligustrum root (*Ligustrum lucidum*), bunge root (*Anemarrhea asphodeloides*) and licorice root (*Glycyrrhiza glabra*). Pharmacological studies have shown two components (zizyphi and ligustrum) exert anti-anxiety and sedative effects; however, these effects are not nearly as strong as that of Suanzaorentang.

Administration may be beneficial.

Experimental Double-Blind Study: Suanzaorentang (250 mg t.i.d.) and diazepam (2 mg t.i.d.) had almost the same anxiolytic effect in patients with anxiety, weakness, irritability, and insomnia. However, Suanzaorentang, but not diazepam, improved psychomotor performance during the daytime. No side effects were observed during the treatment with Suanzaorentang *(Chen HC, Hsieh MT, Shibuya TK. Suanzaorentang versus diazepam: a controlled double-blind study in anxiety. Int J Clin Pharmacol Ther Toxicol 24(12)646-50, 1986).*

Experimental Double-blind Crossover Study: 60 pts. with insomnia received 1 g of Suanzaorentang or placebo 30 minutes before bedtime for 1 week and then crossed over. During the week Suanzaorentang was given, all sleep measures were significantly improved including insomnia. One week after the active compound was withdrawn, all sleep measures deteriorated significantly. While on Suanzaorentang, pts. noted increased feelings of daytime well-being and improvements in many of the accompanying symptoms of insomnia including palpitations, neck stiffness, perspiration, nervousness, restlessness, and lower back pain. No side effects were reported *(Chen MC, Hsieh MT. Clinical trial of Suanzaorentang in the treatment of insomnia. Clin Ther 7(3):224-7, 1985).*

IRRITABLE BOWEL SYNDROME

See Also: CONSTIPATION
DIARRHEA

<u>Peppermint Oil</u>: 1-2 enteric-coated capsules (0.2 ml/cap) 3 times daily between meals
(capsules must be enteric-coated to prevent premature oil release)

Peppermint oil relaxes gastrointestinal smooth muscle by reducing calcium influx   (*Hills JM, Aaronson PI. The mechanism of action of peppermint oil in gastrointestinal smooth muscle. <u>Gastroenterology</u> 101:55-65, 1991; Hawthorne M et al. The actions of peppermint oil and menthol on calcium channel dependent processes in intestinal, neuronal, and cardiac preparations. <u>J Aliment Pharmacol Therap</u> 2:101-8, 1988*).

Experimental Double-blind Study: Pts. who took 3-6 caps (0.2 ml/cap) of peppermint oil daily were relieved of their symptoms, while the number of daily bowel movements was unaffected (*Dew MJ, Evans BK, Rhodes J. Peppermint oil for the irritable bowel syndrome: a multicentre trial. <u>Br J Clin Pract</u> 38:394-8, 1984*).

Experimental Double-blind Crossover Study: Capsules of enteric-coated peppermint oil significantly reduced abdominal symptoms (*Rees WD, Evans BK, Rhodes J. Treating irritable bowel syndrome with peppermint oil. <u>Br Med J</u> 2(6194):835-6, 1979*).

See Also:

Negative Experimental Double-blind Study: *Nash P, Gould SR, Bernardo DE. Peppermint oil does not relieve the pain of irritable bowel syndrome. <u>Br J Clin Pract</u> 40(7):292-3, 1986*

Pharmacokinetic Study: *Somerville KW, Richmond Cr, Bell GD. Delayed release peppermint oil capsules (Colpermin) for the spastic colon syndrome: A pharmacokinetic study. <u>Br J Clin Pharmacol</u> 18(4):638-40, 1984*

<u>Psylllium</u> (<u>Ispaglula</u>; *Plantago ovata*): (*See: '<u>CONSTIPATION</u>'*)

Available as whole or powdered seeds (which are rich in mucilage, a hemicellulose) and as a refined hydrophilic colloid obtained from the seeds.

Administration may be effective.

Experimental Study: 20 pts., 14 of whom had pain and constipation and 6 of whom had pain and diarrhea, received *Plantago ovata* fiber. Pain decreased or disappeared in 16/20; constipation decreased or disappeared in 11/14 and diarrhea decreased or disappeared in 5/6. There was a significant increase in fecal weight without changes in the dry residue. Using radio-opaque markers, there was evidence of an acceleration of colonic transit (fewer retained markers) in pts. with constipation and a slowing of colonic transit (more retained markers) in pts. with diarrhea, suggesting that *Plantago ovata* fiber regulates or moderates colonic motility and enables a physiologic balance of colonic transit (*Soifer LO, De Paula JA, Caruso P. [Effects of medicinal fiber on colic transit in patients with irritable colon syndrome.] <u>Acta Gastroenterol Latinoam</u> 17(4):317-23, 1987*) (*in Spanish*).

See Also:

Experimental Double-blind Study: *Arthurs Y, Fielding JF. Double blind trial of ispaglula/poloxamer in the irritable bowel syndrome. <u>Ir Med J</u> 76(5):253, 1983*

KIDNEY STONES
(CALCIUM OXALATE)

<u>Cranberry</u> (<u>*Vaccinnium macrocarpon*</u>):

Cranberry juice or extracts may reduce urinary ionized calcium.

Experimental Study: In 10 pts. with calcium-containing renal stones, the urinary ion-ized calcium was reduced following cranberry juice ingestion by an ave. of 50% (p<0.001). There was no consistent change in total or ionized calcium excretion in normals by the administration of as much as 5 pts. of cranberry juice *(Light I et al. Urinary ionized calcium in urolithiasis. <u>Urology</u> 1(1):67-70, 1973).*

<u>*Desmodium styracifolium*</u>:

Desmodium styracifolium is a Chinese herb with a long history of use in treating kidney stones.

Administration may be beneficial.

Animal Experimental Study: The effect of *Desmodium styracifolium*-triterpenoid (Ds-t) on the formation of calcium oxalate renal stones induced experimentally by eth-ylene glycol (EG) and 1-alpha(OH)D3 in rats was studied. The incidence of urinary stone formation was 81% in the control group, which received EG and D3, and 29% in the Ds-t group, which received EG and 1 alpha(OH)D3 supplemented by Ds-t. The serum calcium concentration in the Ds-t group was significantly elevated and urinary calcium excretion was markedly reduced. Urinary excretion of citrate, a factor that prevents stone formation, was significantly increased in the Ds-t group. Excretion of urinary phosphorus, which was elevated to a significantly greater extent in the controls than in the Ds-t group, was increased in both groups. The increase in urine volume in the Ds-t group was significantly greater than in the control group. The 24-h creatinine clearance rate was significantly lower in the controls. These findings suggest that Ds-t inhibits the formation of calcium oxalate stones in rat kidneys by increasing the output of urine, decreasing the excretion of calcium and increasing the urinary excretion of citrate *(Hirayama H et al. Effect of Desmodium styracifolium-triterpenoid on calcium oxalate renal stones. <u>Br J Urol</u> 71(2):143-7, 1993).*

<u>Rose hips</u> (<u>*Rosa canina*</u>):

Rose hips tea may be beneficial.

Animal Experimental Study: Calciuria decreased and citriuria increased when rats were given an infusion of rose hips tea   (*Grases F et al. Effect of "Rosa canina" infusion and magnesium on the urinary risk factors of calcium oxalate urolithiasis.* *Planta Med* 58:509-12, 1992).

LUPUS

<u>Alfalfa</u>:

WARNING: Canavanine may produce a lupus-like syndrome or aggravate SLE. Canavanine is found in alfalfa seeds and sprouts, but not the mature tops.

Animal Experimental Study: Hematologic and serologic abnormalities similar to those observed in human systemic lupus erythematosus developed in monkeys fed alfalfa sprouts. L-canavanine sulfate, a constituent, was incorporated into the diet and reactivated the syndrome (*Malonow MR et al. Systemic lupus erythematosus-like syndrome in monkeys fed alfalfa sprouts: Role of a nonprotein amino acid. <u>Science</u> 216:415-17, 1982*).

See Also:

Case Report: *Roberts JL, Hayashi JA. Exacerbation of SLE associated with alfalfa ingestion. Letter. <u>N Engl J Med</u> 308(22):1361, 1983*

<u>*Tripterygium wilfordi*</u>:

The root of *Tripterygium wilfordi* may be beneficial.

WARNING: Use with caution in children as well as in adults in their reproductive years as it may lead to impaired spermatogenesis or amenorrhea. Both of these side effects may eventually disappear following discontinuation.

Several components exert anti-inflammatory action, but immunomodulation is thought to be the major mechanism of action. In the case of autoimmune disorders, *Tripterygium wilfordi* appears to act as an immunosuppressor, although its results come much quicker than with other disease-modifying or immunosuppressive drugs. (*See: '<u>RHEUMATOID ARTHRITIS</u>'*)

The glycoside extract of the decorticated root is regarded as being better tolerated and less harmful to reproductive function compared to crude *Tripterygium wilfordi* preparations.

Experimental Study: 26 pts. with discoid lupus erythematosus were treated with *Tripterygium wilfordi*. The roots and stems were used without the cortex. The daily dose was 30-60 gm in divided doses and course of treatment was 14 days. 24/26 (92.3%) showed various degrees of improvement. The criteria of therapeutic results were: 'clinical cure' meant all skin lesions resolved (8 pts.); 'marked improvement' meant that over 50% of lesions regressed (10 pts.); and 'effective' meant that some lesions regressed (6 pts.). Beneficial results were observed within 2-4 weeks in 21 cases. All pts. were followed up for a minimum of 5 months. Gastrointestinal discomfort and mild abdominal pain were experienced early in treatment in 3 pts. Hyperpigmentation of face, dizziness, anorexia, and menstrual disturbance occurred in only 2 cases. Side effects usually subsided spontaneously and were not serious enough to affect treatment (*Wanzhang Q et al. Clinical observations on Tripterygium wilfordi in treatment of 26 cases of discoid erythematosus. J Trad Chin Med 3(2):131-2, 1983*).

Experimental Study: 103 pts. with systemic lupus erythematosus treated with *Tripterygium wilfordi*. The roots and stems of were used without the cortex. The daily dose was 30-45 gm in divided doses and a course of treatment was 1 month. 94/103 (91.2%) showed various degrees of improvement with 56 (54.3%) experiencing marked improvement. The criteria of effectiveness were: 'markedly improved' if clinical signs and symptoms markedly improved or disappeared, if laboratory findings markedly improved or became normal, corticosteroids decreased in amount or stopped, or pts. returned to work or engaged in normal activity; 'improved' if symptoms, signs, and laboratory finding improved or if the dosage of corticosteroids decreased; and 'ineffective' if the disease did not improve after more than 2 weeks of treatment. There was amelioration of signs and symptoms, including relief of malaise, joint pain, lumbago, Raynaud's phenomena, and skin rash. After treatment, LE cells became negative in 23 cases and RF negative in 75.9%. Among 66 cases with positive antinuclear antibodies before treatment, the titer decreased in 29. In 19 of 21 cases who had lowered complement at pretreatment, the level elevated and most returned to normal range. In most cases, effectiveness was observed within the first 2 months. Side effects were common. Amenorrhea occurred in 32 (33.3%) women of child-bearing age. In 14 menstruation reappeared 2-6 months after termination of treatment. The other side effects were gastrointestinal discomfort, nausea, and mild abdominal pain. These side effects occurred early on in treatment and disappeared spontaneously after a few days (*Wanzhang Q et al. Tripterygium wilfordii hook F. in systemic lupus erythematosus. Report of 103 cases. Chin Med J 94:827-34, 1981*).

MENOPAUSAL SYMPTOMS

Black Cohosh (*Cimicifuga racemosa*):

Black cohosh was widely used by native Americans and later by American colonists for the relief of menstrual cramps and menopause.

Administration may be beneficial due to its estrogenic effects.

Experimental Study: 110 menopausal women were treated with an ethanolic extract of the rhizome of Cimicifuga (Remifemin) at a dose of 8 mg/d or a placebo. After 8 weeks of treatment, LH but not FSH levels were significantly reduced in pts. receiving the Cimicifuga extract, thus implying a significant estrogenic effect. (*Duker EM et al. Effects of extracts from Cimicifuga racemosa on gonadotropin release in menopausal women and ovariectomized rats. Planta Med 57(5):420-4, 1991*).

Animal and in Vitro Experimental Study: A lipophilic extract of Cimicifuga was prepared and subjected to Sephadex chromatography. Fractions obtained were tested for their ability to reduce LH secretion in ovariectomized rats and to compete *in vitro* with 17 beta-estradiol for estrogen receptor binding sites. Three types of endocrinologically active compounds were obtained: (1) Constituents which were not ligands for the estrogen receptor but suppress LH release after chronic treatment, (2) constituents binding to the estrogen receptor and also suppressing LH release, and (3) compounds which are ligands for the estrogen receptor but without an effect of LH release. It is concluded that the LH suppressive effect of Cimicifuga extracts is caused by at least three different synergistically acting compounds (*Duker EM et al. Effects of extracts from Cimicifuga racemosa on gonadotropin release in menopausal women and ovariectomized rats. Planta Med 57(5):420-4, 1991*).

Dong Quai (*Angelica sinensis*):

In Asia, dong quai's reputation is perhaps second only to ginseng. Predominantly regarded as a 'female' remedy, angelica has been used in menopausal symptoms (especially hot flashes) and other female complaints. (*See: 'DYSMENORRHEA'*)

Its efficacy in hot flashes may be due to a combination of its mild estrogenic effects coupled with other components acting to stabilize blood vessels (*Zhy DPQ. Dong quai. Am J Chin Med 15(3-4):117-25, 1987*).

Licorice Root (*Glycyrrhiza glabra*):

The medicinal use of licorice in both Western and Eastern cultures dates back several thousand years. Historically, one of its primary uses was in treating female disorders.

Administration may be beneficial due to its estrogenic effects (*Costello CH, Lynn EV. Estrogenic substances from plants: I. Glycyrrhiza. J Am Pharm Soc 39:177-80, 1950; Kumagai A, Nishino K, Shimomura A, Kin T, Yamamura Y. Effect of glycyrrhizin on estrogen action. Endocrinol Japon 14:34-8, 1967*).

Panax ginseng:

Also known as Chinese or Korean ginseng, *Panax ginseng* is perhaps the most famous medicinal plant of China. Although often viewed as a 'male tonic', *Panax ginseng* can exert estrogenic activity.

> WARNING: Due to its estrogen-like effect on genital tissues, topical or systemic administration may induce postmenopausal bleeding (*Hopkins MP et al. Ginseng face cream and unexplained vaginal bleeding. Am J Obstet Gynecol 159(5):1121-2, 1988*).

The estrogen-like action on the vaginal epithelium may prevent atrophic vaginitis.

> **Case Report:** A vaginal smear from a 62 year-old woman who had undergone a hysterectomy and bilateral ovarectomy 14 yrs. earlier showed a strong estrogenic effect which was found to be due to ingestion of Rumanian ginseng for the previous year. The vaginal and cervical epithelium were normal, and there were no atrophic changes. The spinbarkeit was about 5 cm and there was no arborization. While the ginseng tablets contained no estrogen, a crude menthanolic extract competed very strongly with 17-estradiol and R5020 for estrogen and progesterone binding sites in the human myometrial cytosol (*Punnonen R, Lukola A. Oestrogen-like effect of ginseng. Br Med J 281:1110, 1980*).

Phytoestrogens:

Phytoestrogens (usually isoflavones, phytosterols, saponins, or lignans) are compounds in plants that are capable of exerting mild estrogenic effects (usually about 2% as strong as estrogen). However, at high enough levels, phytoestrogens are capable of exerting significant estrogenic effects. The high intake of dietary phytoestrogens is thought to explain why hot flashes and other menopausal symptoms rarely occur in cultures consuming predominantly a plant-based diet (*Kaldas RS, Hughes CL. Reproductive and general metabolic effects of phytoestrogens in mammals. Reprod Toxicol 3:81-9, 1989*).

Dietary phytoestrogens and phytoestrogen-containing herbs may offer significant advantages over the use of estrogens in the treatment of menopausal symptoms. While both synthetic and natural estrogens may pose significant health risks, including increasing the risk of cancer, gallbladder disease, and thrombo-embolic disease (strokes, heart attacks, etc.), phytoestrogens have not been associated with these side effects. Experimental studies in animals have demonstrated phytoestrogens are extremely effective in inhibiting mammary tumors not only because they occupy estrogen receptors, but also by other unrelated anticancer mechanisms (*Rose DP. Dietary fiber, phytoestrogens, and breast cancer. Nutrition 8:47-51, 1992*).

Some specific foods that are high in phytoestrogens include: soy; fennel, celery, and parsley; clover sprouts; high-lignan flaxseed oil; and nuts and seeds.

Dietary phytoestrogens may be beneficial.

> *Note: The four most popular phytoestrogen-containing herbs in the treatment of hot flashes are: black cohosh (Cimicifuga racemosa), Dong quai (Angelica sinensis), licorice root (Glycyrrhiza glabra), and Panax ginseng. Each is discussed in this chapter.*

Experimental Study: One cup of soybeans provides approximately 300 mg. of isoflavone. This level would be the equivalent to about 0.45 mg of conjugated estrogens or one tablet of Premarin. In a study of postmenopausal women, those women consuming enough soyfoods to provide about 200 mg. of isoflavone demonstrated signs of estrogenic activity when compared to a control group. Specifically, the women consuming the soyfoods demonstrated an increase in the number of superficial cells which line the vagina. This increase results in offsetting the vaginal drying and irritation that is common in postmenopausal women *(reported in Messina M, Barnes S. The roles of soy products in reducing risk of cancer. <u>J Natl Cancer Inst</u> 83:541-6, 1991).*

Experimental Study: After a 14 day baseline, 25 post-menopausal women aged 51-70 who were not on drugs known to affect estrogen status supplemented their diets with soy flour (45 g/d), red clover sprouts (10 g dry seed/d), and linseed (25 g/d), each for 2 weeks. After 6 weeks, there were significant increases in vaginal cell maturation which persisted for 2 weeks after supplementation was stopped, but had disappeared after 8 weeks. There was a significant cumulative effect on serum concentrations of follicle sitmulating hormone, but not on leutinizing hormone, over the 6-week supplementation period. Up to half of the diet of some populations may comprise foods containing phytoestrogens, while in this study such foods comprised only 10% of energy intake for a fairly short time *(Wilcox G et al. Oestrogenic effects of plant foods in postmenopausal women. <u>Br Med J</u> 301:905-6, 1990).*

MULTIPLE SCLEROSIS

<u>*Ginkgo biloba*</u>:

Ginkgo biloba contains several unique terpene molecules known collectively as ginkgolides that antagonize platelet activating factor (PAF), a key chemical mediator in many inflammatory and allergic processes including multiple sclerosis. (*See:* '<u>*ALLERGIES*</u>')

Pure ginkgolide B, mixtures of ginkgolides (BN 52063), as well as the *Ginkgo biloba* extract standardized to contain 24% ginkgoflavonglycosides, may be beneficial.

Experimental Study: 10 pts. with relapsing-remitting multiple sclerosis in acute relapse were treated with a five-day course of intravenous ginkgolide B, a specific inhibitor of PAF-acether. 8 pts. had improvement of their neurological score, beginning 2 to 6 days after the initiation of therapy. This improvement was sustained in 5 pts. and only transient in 3 pts. 2/3 pts. with secondary failure and the other 2 pts. who did not respond to ginkgolide therapy, received IV methylprednisolone. 3 pts. experienced mild side effects under ginkgolide therapy but none of the pts. had any serious adverse effect (*Brochet B et al. [Pilot study of Ginkgolide B, a PAF-acether specific inhibitor in the treatment of acute outbreaks of multiple sclerosis.]* <u>*Rev Neurol*</u> *(Paris) 148(4):299-301, 1992*) (*in French*).

- -

COMBINATION TREATMENT

<u>Padma 28</u>:

Padma 28 is a commercial product based on an ancient Tibetan (lamaistic) formula. It contains a mixture of 28 different herbs.

Experimental Study: 100 pts. suffering from a chronic progressive form of multiple sclerosis received either Padma 28, 2 tabs 3 times daily or only symptomatic treatment for 1 year. A positive effect of Padma 28 was observed in 44% of pts. in the form of improvement of their general condition, increase of muscle strength, and decrease or disappearance of affected sphincters. In 41% of patients with initially an abnormal tracing of visual evoked potentials, an improvement or normalization was achieved. Of pts. who did not receive Padma 28, none felt better and 40% of them showed a deterioration (*Korwin-Piotrowska T et al. Experience of Padma 28 in multiple sclerosis.* <u>*Phytother Res*</u> *6:133-6, 1992*).

NAUSEA AND VOMITING
(including MOTION SICKNESS)

See Also: INNER EAR DYSFUNCTION

Ginger (*Zingiber officinale*):

Administration may be effective. (*See:* '*PREGNANCY-RELATED ILLNESS*')

> WARNING: Although it appears to be non-toxic, ginger is a very powerful thromboxane synthetase inhibitor and prostacyclin agonist; thus it may be wise to follow bleeding times in patients receiving treatment for post-operative emesis (*Backon J. Ginger as an antiemetic: possible side effects due to its thromboxane synthetase activity. Letter. <u>Anaesthesia</u> 46(8):669-71, 1991*).

Experimental Double-blind Study: 60 women who had major gynecological surgery randomly received ginger root, metoclopramide or placebo. There were statistically significantly fewer incidences of nausea in the gp. that received ginger compared to placebo (p<0.05). The number of incidences of nausea in the gps. that received either ginger root or metoclopramide were similar. Also, the administration of an antiemetic after surgery was significantly more frequent in the placebo gp. as compared to the other 2 gps. (p<0.05) (*Bone ME, Wilkinson DJ, Young JR, et al. Ginger root — a new antiemetic. The effect of ginger root on postoperative nausea and vomiting after major gynaecological surgery. <u>Anaesthesia</u> 45(8):669-71, 1990*).

Experimental Double-blind Study: 80 naval cadets unaccustomed to sailing in heavy seas were studied during voyages on the high seas. Each randomly received either 1 gm of powered ginger root or a placebo and symptoms of seasickness were recorded each hour for 4 hours. Ginger was significantly better than placebo in reducing the frequency of vomiting (72% reduction) and cold sweats (p<0.05). Cadets receiving ginger also indicated a reduction in nausea and vertigo compared to controls; however, the reduction failed to reach statistical significance. Overall, symptoms were 38% less in the ginger gp. than in the controls (*Grontved A et al. Ginger root against seasickness. A controlled trial on the open sea <u>Acta Otolaryngol</u> 105 (1-2):45-9, 1988*).

Experimental Double-blind Study: 18 male and 18 female volunteers who had previously indicated an extreme susceptibility to motion sickness were randomly divided into 3 groups. The first gp. received a placebo, the second 100 mg dimenhydrinate, and the third 940 mg of powdered ginger root 25 min. before testing. The subjects were then blindfolded, led to a concealed mechanical rotating chair, spun around, and asked to report their feelings of nausea every 15 seconds while they performed mental tasks. The test was stopped when either the subject vomited or asked that it be stopped. Subjects who received ginger remained in the chair an ave. of 5.5 min., compared with an ave. of 3.5 min. for the dimenhydrinate gp. and 1.5 min. for the placebo group.

Once nausea began, however, sensations of nausea and vomiting progressed at the same rate in all groups. More than 90% of pts. with motion sickness who took 2-4 caps of ginger root prior to traveling, and took 2 more approximately every hr. or whenever they felt slightly nauseated, reported excellent results. Ginger root was found to be equally effective for automobile, airplane, train or boat trips. It is hypothesized that, unlike dimenhydrinate that works on the central nervous system, ginger affects the gastrointestinal tract and slows the feedback interaction between the stomach and the nausea center in the brain by absorbing and neutralizing GI toxins and acids (*Mowrey DB, Clayson DE. Motion sickness, ginger, and psychophysics. Lancet i:655-7, 1982*).

The efficacy of ginger root appears to be due to anticholinergic and antihistaminic actions.

Animal Experimental Studies: Results of studies with rabbits, isolated rat fundus strip preparations and guinea-pig isolated ileum suggest that the pungent consituents of ginger release substance P from sensory fibers which either stimulates cholinergic and histaminic neurons to release acetylcholine and histamine, respectively, or produces direct smooth muscle contraction by activating M and H_1 receptors correspondingly. It is proposed that after being excited by substance P, M and H_1 receptors are inactive temporarily and unable to be excited by agonists; therefore ginger juice exhibits anticholinergic and antihistamine actions (*Qian DS, Liu ZS. [Pharmacologic studies of antimotion sickness actions of ginger.] Chung Kuo Chung Hsi I Chieh Ho Tsa Chih 12(2):95-8, 70, 1992*) (*in Chinese*).

Experimental Double-blind Study: In order to determine whether the nystagmus response to optokinetic or vestibular stimuli might be altered by some agent in powdered ginger root, normal subjects were examined after administration of ginger root, dimenhyrinate and placebo. Eye movements were recorded using standard EMG equipment and evaluation was performed by automatic nystagmus analysis. Ginger root had no effect on experimentally-induced nystagmus, while demenhydrinate caused a reduction in the nystagmus response to caloric, rotatory and optokinetic stimuli. Results suggest that neither the vestibular nor the oculomotor system are influenced by ginger, and thus a central nervous system mechanism, which is characteristic of conventional anti-motion sickness drugs, can be excluded. It is likely that any reduction of motion-sickness symptoms derives from the influence of ginger root agents on the gastric system (*Holtmann S, Clarke AH, Scherer H, Hohn M. The anti-motion sickness mechanism of ginger. A comparative study with placebo and dimenhydrinate. Acta Otolaryngol (Stockh) 108(3-4):168-74, 1989*).

Experimental Double-blind Crossover Study: 18 healthy volunteers received either 1 gm of ginger root or a lactose placebo 1 hr. prior to caloric stimulation of the vestibular system. Compared to controls, ginger root failed to affect nystagmus as measured by electronystagmograms (*Grontved A, Hentzer E. Vertigo-reducing effect of ginger root. A controlled clinical study. ORL J Otorhinolaryngol Relat Spec 48(5):282-6, 1986*).

Theoretical Discussion: Unlike dimenhydrinate, which works in the central nervous sytem, ginger appears to work in the gastrointestinal tract by slowing the feedback interaction between the stomach and the nausea center in the brain by absorbing and neutralizing gastrointestinal toxins and acid (*Mowrey DB, Clayson DE. Motion sickness, ginger and psychophysics. Lancet i:655-7, 1982*).

NEURALGIA AND NEUROPATHY

See Also: DIABETES MELLITUS

Bilberry:

Bilberry or European blueberry contains flavonoid compounds known as anthocyanosides. Bilberry anthocyanosides are potent antioxidants that improve the microcirculation and protect the vascular endothelium. (*See: 'PERIPHERAL VASCULAR DISEASE'; 'VASCULAR FRAGILITY'*)

The standard dose for *Vaccinium myrtillus* extract (VME) is based on its anthocyanoside content, as calculated by its anthocyanidin percentage. Most studies have used a bilberry extract standardized for an anthocyanidin content of 25% at a dosage of 160 mg to 480 mg daily.

Administration may be effective in polyneuritis.

> **Experimental Study:** 15 pts. with polyneuritis due to peripheral vascular insufficiency were given VME (480 mg/d). Significant improvements were noted due to improved microcirculatory function as demonstrated by capillographic examinations of the ungual bed by plethysmography and thermographic techniques (*Pennarola R et al. The therapeutic action of the anthocyanosides in microcirculatory changes due to adhesive-induced polyneuritis. Gazz Med Ital 139:485-91, 1980*).

Capsaicin:

Capsaicin is the active component of cayenne pepper (*Capsicum frutescens*). When topically applied, capsaicin is known to stimulate and then block small-diameter pain fibers by depleting them of the neurotransmitter substance P. Substance P is thought to be the principle chemomediator of pain impulses from the periphery.

Commercial ointments containing 0.025% or 0.075% capsaicin are available over-the-counter.

> **Review Article:** A brief overview of the chemical history, analysis, nomenclature, biology, pharmacology, and pharmacotherapy of capsaicin is presented including a review of clinical studies in the treatment of rheumatoid arthritis, osteoarthritis, and peripheral neuropathies (*Cordell GA, Araujo OE. Capsaicin: Identification, nomenclature, and pharmacotherapy. Ann Pharmacother 27:330-6, 1993*).

Topically applied capsaicin may be effective in relieving the pain of post-herpetic neuralgia.

Experimental Study: 39 pts. with chronic post-herpetic neuralgia (PHN), median duration 24 months, were treated with 0.025% capsaicin cream for 8 weeks. During therapy the pts. rated their pain on a visual analogue scale (VAS) and a verbal outcome scale. A follow-up investigation was performed 10-12 months after study onset on the pts. who had improved. Nineteen pts. (48.7%) substantially improved after the 8-week trial; 5 (12.8%) discontinued therapy due to side-effects such as intolerable capsaicin-induced burning sensations (4) or mastitis (1); 15 (38.5%) reported no benefit. The decrease in VAS ratings was significant after 2 weeks of continuous application. Of the responders 72.2% were still improved at the follow-up; only one-third of them had continued application irregularly. Treatment effect was not dependent on patient's age, duration or localization of PHN (trigeminal involvement was excluded), sensory disturbance or pain character. Treatment response was not correlated with the incidence, time-course or severity of capsaicin-induced burning (*Peikert A et al. Topical 0.025% capsaicin in chronic post-herpetic neuralgia: efficacy, predictors of response and long-term course. J Neurol 238(8):452-6, 1991*).

Experimental Study: Sensory and pain thresholds to cutaneous argon laser stimulation were significantly elevated on the affected side compared to the contralateral normal area at baseline. After 1 wk. of capsaicin treatment both thresholds were significantly increased compared to the pre-treatment values, and subjective pain relief on a visual analog scale (VAS) was 24%. More than a 10% decrease in VAS pain score was obtained by 62.5% of patients. Allodynia to laser stimulations changed during treatment towards normal (*Bjerring P et al. Argon laser induced cutaneous sensory and pain thresholds in post-herpetic neuralgia. Quantitative modulation by topical capsaicin. Acta Derm Venereol (Stockh) 70(2):121-5, 1990*).

Experimental Double-blind Study: Over half the pts. using capsaicin cream obtained substantial pain relief compared with <10% with a placebo cream (*Bernstein JE et al. Topical capsaicin treatment of chronic postherpetic neuralgia. J Am Acad Dermatol 21(2 Pt 1):265-70, 1989*).

Experimental study: Pts. with post-herpetic neuralgia of greater than 3 months duration were treated topically with 0.025% capsaicin (Zostrix®, Genderm, US) applied 4 times daily. 39% of the 33 pts. who entered the trial achieved a good to excellent result. After 4 wks., 56% of the 23 pts. who completed the trial had at least a good response and 78% were improved. Post-capsaicin burning was a common untoward effect in most pts., and was so unbearable in about 1/3 that treatment was terminated prematurely (*Watson CP et al. Post-herpetic neuralgia and topical capsaicin. Pain 33(3):333-40, 1988*).

> *Note: Burning may be reduced in some patients by the application of 5% lidocaine ointment prior to application of capsaicin, by covering smaller skin areas and by analgesics. In addition, it becomes less of a problem with continued usage (Watson CPN et al. Post-herpetic neuralgia: 208 cases. Pain 35:289-97, 1988).*

Experimental Study: 12 pts. with postherpetic neuralgia completed a study in which capsaicin was applied topically. After 4 wks., 9/12 (75%) experienced substantial relief. The only adverse reaction was an intermittent, localized burning sensation experienced by 1 pt. (*Bernstein JE et al. Treatment of chronic postherpetic neuralgia with topical capsaicin. A preliminary study. J Am Acad Dermatol 17(1):93-6, 1987*).

See Also:

> **Review Article:** *Lynn B. Review article. Capsaicin: actions on nociceptive C-fibres and therapeutic potential. Pain 41:61-9, 1990*
>
> *Hawk RJ, Millikan LE. Treatment of oral postherpetic neuralgia with topical capsaicin. Int J Dermatol 27(5):336, 1988*

Topically applied capsaicin may be effective in <u>trigeminal neuralgia</u>.

> **Experimental Study:** 12 pts. were studied to determine the influence of capsaicin on idiopathic trigeminal neuralgia. These pts. were followed up for 1 yr after the topical application over the painful area of 1.0 g of capsaicin 3 times a day for several days. 6 pts. had complete and 4 pts. had partial relief of pain; the remaining 2 pts. had no relief of pain. Of the 10 pts. who were responsive to therapy, 4 had relapses of pain in 95-149 days. There were no relapses following the second therapy for the remainder of the year *(Fusco BM, Alessandri M. Analgesic effect of capsaicin in idiopathic trigeminal neuralgia. Anesth Analg 74(3):375-7, 1992).*

Topically applied capsaicin may be effective in <u>diabetic neuropathy</u>.   *(See: 'DIABETES MELLITUS')*

Ginkgo biloba:

- with <u>Folic Acid</u>:

> Combined administration may be beneficial for <u>autonomic neuropathies</u>.

> **Experimental Study:** 10 pts. with neuropathies caused by various diseases and with autonomic disregulation of the skin received intravenously 87.5 mg *Ginkgo biloba* extract standardized to 21 mg flavonglycosids and folic acid 3 mg. After 14 days, autonomic nerve function (as measured by hyperthermal laser-Doppler-Flowmetry) was significantly improved (p<0.01). Parameters for pain and sensitivity were also improved *(Költringer P et al. [Ginkgo biloba extract and folic acid in the therapy of changes caused by autonomic neuropathy.] Acta Med Austriaca 16(2):35-7, 1989).*

OBESITY

Ephedrine, found in *Ephedra sinica*, may be useful as a weight loss aid, either alone or in combination with methylxanthine containing herbs, by stimulating thermogenesis.

A certain amount of ingested food is converted immediately to heat. This is known as diet-induced thermogenesis. The activity of diet induced thermogenesis is thought to play a major role in determining whether an individual is likely to be lean or obese. In lean individuals, a meal may stimulate an up to 40% increase in thermogenesis. In contrast, obese individuals often display only a 10% or less increase in thermogenesis production. The food energy is stored versus converted to heat.

The reason for the decreased thermogenesis in obese individuals is impaired sympathetic nervous system activity. This portion of the nervous system controls many body functions including metabolism. In other words, the reason why many obese individuals have a "slow metabolism" is because of a lack of stimulation by the sympathetic nervous system. Ephedrine, as well as methylxanthines, can activate the sympathetic nervous system, thereby increasing the metabolic rate and thermogenesis.

The thermogenic effects of ephedrine can be enhanced by methylxanthines and salicylates. Herbs rich in these active ingredients can be used in a similar fashion to the isolated principles. Good methylxanthine sources include coffee (*Coffea arabica*), tea (*Camellia sinensis*), cola nut (*Cola nitida*), and guarana (*Paullinea cupana*). Natural salicylates can be found in members of the mint and oak families. The optimum dosage of the crude plant preparation or extract will depends on the content of active ingredient. Standardized preparations may produce more dependable results.

> WARNING: The U.S. Food and Drug Administration advisory review panel on nonprescription drugs has recommended that ephedrine not be taken by patients with heart disease, high blood pressure, thyroid disease, diabetes, difficulty in urination due to enlargement of the prostate gland, or those taking antihypertensive or antidepressant drugs. These warnings are appropriate for ephedra preparations as well.

Administration may promote weight loss.

> *Note: Ephedrine may not be effective in obese individuals with normal diet-induced thermogenesis.*

> **Experimental Double-blind Study:** A double-blind controlled study was performed in unselected obese outpts. to assess the effects of ephedrine on weight loss. Pts. were treated for 3 months with placebo (gp. I), 25 mg 3 times daily or 50 mg 3 times daily of ephedrine hydrochloride orally adminis-

tered (groups II and III, respectively). Dietary treatment consisted of 1000 kcal/day for females and 1200 kcal/day for males. Weight loss was similar in all groups. Pts. in gp. III (ephedrine 150 mg/day) showed significantly more side effects than the placebo group. These results do not seem to favor the hypothesis that ephedrine, a thermogenic agent, may be effective in the therapy of unselected simple obesity (*Pasquali R. A controlled trial using ephedrine in the treatment of obesity. Int J Obes 9(2):93-8, 1985*).

Experimental Double-blind Study: Ephedrine inhibited gastric emptying. This effect may account for its positive effect on satiety in weight loss (*Jonderko K, Kucio C. Effect of anti-obesity drugs promoting energy expenditure, yohimbine and ephedrine, on gastric emptying in obese patient. Aliment Pharmacol Ther 5(4):413-8, 1991*).

Experimental Double-blind Study: 10 obese women were treated with diet therapy (1000-1400 kcal/day) and either ephedrine (50 mg t.i.d.) or placebo for 2 months and then crossed-over. Weight loss was significantly greater during the ephedrine period (2.41 kg) than during the placebo period (0.64 kg). None of the pts. presented any notable side effects (*Pasquali R et al. Does ephedrine promote weight loss in low-energy-adapted obese women? Int J Obes 11(2):163-8, 1987*).

Animal Experimental Study: Ephedrine produced an anorectic effect in rats (*Zarrindast MR, Hosseini-Nia T, Farnoodi F. Anorectic effect of ephedrine. Gen Pharmacol 18(5):559-61, 1987*).

Experimental Study: The thermogenic effect of a single oral dose of ephedrine (1 mg/kg body weight) was studied by indirect calorimetry in five 14% overweight women before, during and 2 mo. after 3 mo. of chronic ephedrine treatment (20 mg, perorally, three times daily). Before treatment and 2 mo. after its cessation a similar thermogenic response to ephedrine was observed. The total extra consumption of oxygen was 1.3 before and 1.2 after cessation of the chronic treatment. After 4 and 12 wks. of treatment ephedrine elicited a more sustained response, the extra oxygen consumption in the 3 h following ephedrine intake being 7.0 and 6.9, respectively. The ratio of serum T3 to T4 increased significantly after 4 wks. of treatment (15.6 vs 19.4), but decreased below the initial value after 12 wks. of treatment. The mean body weight was significantly reduced after 4 and 12 wks. of treatment (2.5 and 5.5 kg, respectively) (*Astrup A et al. Enhanced thermogenic responsiveness during chronic ephedrine treatment in man. Am J Clin Nutr Jul 42(1):83-94, 1985*).

See Also:

> **Review Article:** *Pasquali R, Casimirri F. Clinical aspects of ephedrine in the treatment of obesity. Int J Obes 17(Suppl.1):S65-8, 1993*

> *Zgourides GD, Warren R, Englert ME. Ephedrine-induced thermogenesis as an adjunct to cognitive restructuring and covert conditioning: a proposal for treatment of obese individuals. Percept Mot Skills 69(2):563-72, 1989*

- with Methylxanthine:

> **Experimental Double-blind Study:** In a randomized, double-blind study, 180 obese pts. were treated by diet and either an ephedrine/caffeine combination

(20mg/200mg), ephedrine (20mg), caffeine (200mg) or placebo 3 times a day for 24 weeks. 141 pts. completed this part of the study. All medication was stopped between week 24-26 in order to catch any withdrawal symptoms. From week 26-50, 99 pts. completed treatment with the ephedrine/caffeine compound in an open trial design, resulting in a statistically significant (p=0.02) weight loss of 1.1 kg. Side effects were minor and transient and no withdrawal symptoms were found (*Toubro S et al. Safety and efficacy of long-term treatment with ephedrine, caffeine and an ephedrine/caffeine mixture. Int J Obes 17(Suppl.1):S69-72, 1993*).

Experimental Double-blind Study: In a randomized, double-blind 8 week study on obese subjects, a combination of ephedrine 20 mg and caffeine 200 mg showed lean body mass-conserving properties. Side effects were minor and transient and no withdrawal symptoms were found (*Toubro S et al. Safety and efficacy of long-term treatment with ephedrine, caffeine and an ephedrine/caffeine mixture. Int J Obes 17(Suppl.1):S69-72, 1993*).

Experimental Controlled Study: The thermogenic effect of ephedrine (E) and aminophylline (AP) was investigated in 27 and 20 obese adolescents by indirect calorimetry. Ten children receiving only water served as controls. Nine children from both groups had no thermic response to the drugs (NR). The responders (R) increased their fasting resting metabolic rate by 7.1% and 6.4% after E and AP administration, respectively. After one-week E treatment the thermic effect of the drug disappeared even in the R. One-week AP treatment significantly improved the thermic response in the NR and did not alter it in the R. When the combination of E and AP was given to 8 responders the thermic response was no higher than after the single drug (*Molnar D. Effects of ephedrine and aminophylline on resting energy expenditure in obese adolescents. Int J Obes 17(Suppl.1):S49-52, 1993*).

Experimental Double-blind Study: 180 obese pts. were treated by diet and either an ephedrine/caffeine combination (20mg/200mg), ephedrine (20 mg), caffeine (200 mg) or placebo three times a day for 24 weeks. Withdrawals were distributed equally in the four groups, and 141 pts. completed the trial. Mean weight losses was significantly greater with the combination than with placebo from week 8 to week 24 (ephedrine/caffeine, 16.6 kg vs. placebo, 13.2 kg; p=0.0015). Weight loss in both the ephedrine and the caffeine groups was similar to that of the placebo gp. Side effects (tremor, insomnia and dizziness) were transient and after eight weeks of treatment they had reached placebo levels. Systolic and diastolic blood pressure fell similarly in all four groups (*Astrup A et al. The effect and safety of an ephedrine/caffeine compound compared to ephedrine, caffeine and placebo in obese subjects on an energy restricted diet. A double blind trial. Int J Obes 16(4):269-77, 1992*).

Experimental Study: A daily dosage of 22 mg ephedrine, 30 mg caffeine and 50 mg theophylline was investigated in human volunteers with a predisposition to obesity and also in the lean. The ephedrine/methylxanthines mixture was twice as effective as ephedrine alone in increasing the fasting metabolic rate of both subject groups, and it normalized the reduced thermogenic response to a 1.25-MJ meal observed in those predisposed to obesity. Measurements of 24-h energy expenditure in a respirometer indicate that the mixture had no effect on the daily metabolic rate of the lean, but was effective in causing a significant 8% increase in the

24-h energy expenditure of those subjects predisposed to obesity (*Dulloo AG, Miller DS. The thermogenic properties of ephedrine/methylxanthine mixtures: human studies. Int J Obes 10(6):467-81, 1986*).

See Also:

Malecka-Tendera E. Effect of ephedrine and theophylline on weight loss, resting energy expenditure and lipoprotein lipase activity in obese over-fed rats. Int J Obes 7(6):343-7, 1993

Astrup A et al. Pharmacology of thermogenic drugs. Am J Clin Nutr 55(1 Suppl):246S-248S, 1992

Dulloo AG, Seydoux J, Girardier L. Potentiation of the thermogenic antiobesity effects of ephedrine by dietary methylxanthines: adenosine antagonism or phosphodiesterase inhibition? Metabolism 41(11):1233-41, 1992

- with <u>Aspirin</u>:

Experimental Study: The effect of ephedrine (30 mg) and aspirin (300 mg) on the acute thermogenic response to a liquid meal (250 kcal) was investigated in lean and obese women (n=10 each gp.). Resting metabolic rate (RMR) was measured prior to each of the following treatments: meal only (M), meal plus ephedrine (ME) or meal plus ephedrine and aspirin (MEA). Following the M treatment, the mean increase in metabolic rate was 0.17 and 0.13 kcal/min in the lean and obese groups respectively, with the corresponding rises being 0.21 and 0.19 kcal/min following the ME, and 0.23 and 0.23 kcal/min following the MEA. The increase in post-prandial thermogenesis with the ephedrine or ephedrine plus aspirin was significant in the obese gp. but not the lean. Furthermore, the post-treatment rise in metabolic rate, following the MEA treatment compared to the ME, was significantly greater for the obese gp. but not the lean (*Horton TJ, Geissler CA. Aspirin potentiates the effect of ephedrine on the thermogenic response to a meal in obese but not lean women. Int J Obes 15(5):359-66, 1991*).

Animal Experimental Study: Chronic administration of aspirin to obese mice had no effect on energy balance and body composition. In contrast, ephedrine increased energy expenditure by 9% and reduced body weight and body fat by 18% and 50%, respectively: obesity, however, was reduced but not reversed. In the presence of both ephedrine and aspirin, increase in energy expenditure found during treatment with ephedrine alone was doubled, and the obese gp. lost greater than 75% of body fat: obesity was reversed (*Dulloo AG, Miller DS. Aspirin as a promoter of ephedrine-induced thermogenesis: potential use in the treatment of obesity. Am J Clin Nutr 45(3):564-9, 1987*).

- with <u>Methylxanthine</u> and <u>Aspirin</u> combinations:

Experimental Double-blind Study: The safety and efficacy of a mixture of ephedrine (75-150 mg), caffeine (150 mg) and aspirin (330 mg), in divided pre-meal doses, were investigated in 24 obese humans. Energy intake was not restricted. Overall weight loss over 8 weeks was 2.2kg for ECA vs. 0.7 kg for placebo (p). 8 of 13 placebo subjects returned 5 months later and received ECA in an unblinded crossover. After 8 weeks, mean weight loss with ECA was 3.2 kg vs 1.3 kg for placebo (p=0.036). 6 subjects continued on ECA for 7 to 26 months. After 5 months on ECA, average weight loss in 5 of these was 5.2 kg compared to 0.03 kg gained during 5 months between studies with no intervention (p=0.03). The sixth subject lost 66 kg over 13 months by self-imposed caloric restriction. In all studies, no significant changes in heart rate, blood pressure, blood glucose, insulin, and cholesterol levels, and no differences in the frequency of side effects were found. ECA in these doses is thus well tolerated in otherwise healthy obese subjects, and supports modest, sustained weight loss even without prescribed caloric restriction, and may be more effective in conjunction with restriction of energy intake *(Daly PA et al. Ephedrine, caffeine and aspirin: safety and efficacy for treatment of human obesity. Int J Obes 17(Suppl 1):S73-8, 1993)*.

See Also:

> **Review Article:** *Dulloo AG. Ephedrine, xanthines and prostaglandin-inhibitors: actions and interactions in the stimulation of thermogenesis. Int J Obes 17(Suppl.1):S35-40, 1993*

Green Tea powder: 500 mg with breakfast, 750 mg with lunch and 750 mg with dinner

Administration may promote weight loss.

> **Experimental Double-blind Study:** 60 obese women aged 30-45 yrs. were placed on an 1800 calorie diet and received either green tea capsules (Arkogelules) as noted above or placebo. After 15 days, the treatment gp. had lost twice as much weight as the placebo gp. (1.7 kg vs. 0.85 kg). After 30 days, the treatment gp. had lost 3 times as much weight as the placebo gp. (2.9 kg vs. 0.935 kg). Similarly, waist measurement reduction was twice as great in the treatment gp. after 15 days and 4 times as great after 30 days. In addition, there was a significant reduction of triglycerides in the treatment gp. No side effects were reported *(Clinical study of weight loss using Arkogelules' green tea. Revue de L'association Mondiale de Phytotherapie, June, 1985)*.

- with Wall Germander:

Administration may be as effective as dexfenfluoramine, an amphetamine-like drug.

> **Experimental Double-blind Study:** 78 overweight female pts. were divided into 2 homogeneous gps. and received identical diet and menu advice. In addtion, one gp. received green tea capsules (Arkocaps) 1500 mg daily and wall germander (Arkocaps) 900 mg daily, while the other gp. received the standard dosage of dexfenfluoramine. After 45 days, the total ave. weight loss in the green tea/wall germander gp. was 10.7 lbs compared to 9.25 lbs in the drug group. While there was some insomnia and steady increase in BP in the drug gp., the green tea/wall germander gp. showed a slight decrease in systolic BP. 3 pts. discontinued dexfenfluoramine treatment due to nausea and mouth dryness, and 17 other pts. complained of side effects. No pts. discontinued treatment with the green tea/wall germander regimen; 1 pt. complained of nausea during the first 5 days *(Appetite suppressants: Herbs or amphetamines? Arkopharma's Phyto-Facts 2(1):2, 1989)*.

Malabar Tamarind (*Garcinia* spp.):

The Malabar tamarind or Brindall berry is a yellowish fruit that is about the size of an orange, with a thin skin, and deep furrows similar to an acorn squash. It is native to South India where it is dried and used extensively in curries. It has also been used historically in the Ayurvedic treatment of obesity.

The dried fruit contains 20-30% (-)-Hydroxycitric acid (HCA). Citrin®, a commercial preparation, contains about 50% HCA.

The recommended dosage of HCA is 500 mg 3 times daily with meals.

HCA inhibits lipogenesis by interfering with adenosine triphosphate (ATP) citrate lyase, the enzyme catalyzing the extra mitochondial cleavage of citrate of oxaloacetate and acetyl CoA (*Watson JA, Fang M, Lowenstein JM. Tricarbal lylate and hydroxycitrate: substrate and inhibitor of ATP citrate oxaloacetate lyase. Arch Biochem Biophys 135:209-17, 1969*). As a result it reduces the level of acetyl coenzyme A, the extramitochondrial precursor of fatty acid and cholesterol synthesis (*Watson JA, Lowenstein JM. Citrate and the conversion of carbohydrate into fat. J Biol Chem 245:599, 1970*).

HCA does not appear to inhibit brown fat formation.

> **Animal Experimental Study:** HCA did not inhibit basal rates of brown-fat lipogenesis in starved rats but suppressed the increases in lipogenesis and glucose utilization observed in response to insulin. As basal rates of lipogenesis were not inhibited by (-)hydroxycitrate, it is suggested that acetate may be a lipogenic substrate for brown fat instead of citrate (*Sugden MC et al. Brown-adipose-tissue lipogenesis in starvation: effects of insulin and (-) hydroxycitrate. Biosci Rep 2(5):289-97, 1982*).

HCA may be effective in reducing body weight.

> **Review Article:** Over 7 clinical studies with higher order animals have shown that food intake is reduced by up to 46% after an oral dosage of 3 mg/kg of HCA. No rebound eating stimuli was observed after discontinuation (*Sergio W. A natural food, the Malabar Tamarind, may be effective in the treatment of obesity. Med Hypotheses 27(1):39-40, 1988*).

> **Case Report:** The author tried eating Malabar Tamarinds. The taste was "quite delicious" and as little as 1 gm before each meal was "extremely effective" in reducing appetite. About 1 lb. of weight was lost daily without dieting and there was a sustained increase in energy (*Sergio W. A natural food, the Malabar Tamarind, may be effective in the treatment of obesity. Med Hypotheses 27(1):39-40, 1988*).

> **Animal Experimental Study:** HCA produced a significant reduction in food intake, body weight, and serum triglyceride levels in rats compared to a control gp. (*Rao RN, Sakariah KK. Lipid-lowering and antiobesity effect of (-)-hydroxycitric acid. Nutr Res 8:209-12, 1988*).

See Also:

In vitro Study: *Sener A, Malaisse WJ, Hexose metabolism in pancreatic islets. Effect of HCA upon fatty acid synthesis and insulin release in glucose-stimulated islets. Biochimie 73(10):1287-90, 1991*

In vitro Study: *Beynen AC, Geelen MJ. Effects of insulin and glucagon on fatty acid synthesis from acetate by hepatocytes incubated with (-)-hydroxycitrate. Endokrinologie 79(2):308-10, 1982*

Animal Experimental Study: *Chee H, Romsos DR, Leveille GA. Influence of (-)-hydroxycitrate on lipogenesis in chickens and rats. J Nutr 107(1):112-9, 1977*

Animal Experimental Study: *Hamilton JG et al. Hypolipidemic activity of (-)-hydroxycitrate. Lipids 12(1):1-10, 1976*

Animal Experimental Study: *Sullivan AC et al. Effect of (-)-hydroxycitrate upon the accumulation of lipid in the rat. II. Appetite. Lipids 9(2):129-34, 1974*

Animal Experimental Study: *Sullivan AC et al. Effect of (-)-hydroxycitrate upon the accumulation of lipid in the rat. I. Lipogenesis. Lipids 9(2):121-8, 1974*

In vitro Study: *Sullivan AC et al. Inhibition of lipogenesis in rat liver by (-)-hydroxycitrate. Arch Biochem Biophys 150(1):183-90, 1972*

Animal and In vitro Experimental Study: *Sullivan AC et al. Factors influencing the in vivo and in vitro rates of lipogenesis in rat liver. J Nutr 101:265-72, 1970*

HCA may not reduce the percentage of body fat.

Animal Experimental Study: Zucker lean and obese female rats were fed HCA as a dietary admixture for 39 days. In the lean rats, HCA treatment decreased body weight, food intake, percent of body fat, and fat cell size compared to a control gp. In the obese rat, food intake and body weight were reduced but the percent of body fat remained unchanged. Throughout the treatment period, obese rats maintained a fat cell size equivalent to their obese controls. Although a reduction in fat cell number in the obese rats occurred during the treatment period, marked hyperplasia was observed during the posttreatment period. The results of this study indicate that the obese rat, despite a substantial reduction in body weight produced by HCA, still defends its obese body composition (*Greenwood MR et al. Effect of (-)-hydroxycitrate on development of obesity in the Zucker obese rat. Am J Physiol 240(1):E72-8, 1981*).

OSTEOARTHRITIS

Boswellia serrata:

Boswellia serrata is a large branching tree native to India. Boswellia yields an exudative gum resin known as salai guggul. Although salai guggul has been used for centuries, newer preparations are concentrated for the active components (boswellic acids).

Boswellic acid extracts have demonstrated anti-arthritic effects in a variety of animal models. There are several mechanisms of action including inhibition of inflammatory mediators, prevention of decreased glycosaminoglycan synthesis, and improved blood supply to joint tissues (*Reddy CK, Chandrakasan G, Dhar SC. Studies on the metabolism of glycosaminoglycans under the influence of new herbal anti-inflammatory agents. <u>Biochemical Pharmacol</u> 20:3527-34, 1989; Singh GB, Atal CK. Pharmacology of an extract of salai guggal ex-Bosewellia serrata, a new non-steroidal anti-inflammatory agent. <u>Agents Action</u> 18:407-12, 1986*).

The standard dosage for boswellic acids in arthritis is 400 mg 3 times daily. No side effects due to boswellic acids have been reported.

Bromelain:

Bromelain refers to the mixture of sulfur containing proteolytic enzymes or proteases obtained from the stem of the pineapple plant (*Ananas comosus*).

The standard dosage of bromelain (1,800-2,000 m.c.u.) is 125-450 mg 3 times daily on an empty stomach.

> **Experimental Study:** 25 pts. with stages II or III RA, along with 1 pt. with both RA and osteoarthritis, 2 pts. with OA alone and 1 pt. with gout had residual joint swelling and impairment in mobility following long-term corticosteroid therapy. Their doses were tapered to small maintenance doses and they received enteric-coated bromelain 20-40 mg 3-4 times daily. In most pts. residual joint swelling was significantly reduced (p<0.01) and joint mobility was increased soon after supplementation was started. After 3 wks.- 13 mo. of observation, one of the OA pts. had good results, the other fair results. It seemed that smaller amts. of steroids were needed when bromelain was given concurrently. There were no side effects (*Cohen A, Goldman J. Bromelains therapy in rheumatoid arthritis. <u>Pennsyl Med J</u> 67:27-30, 1964*).

Capsaicin:

Capsaicin is the active component of cayenne pepper (*Capsicum frutescens*). When topically applied, capsaicin is known to stimulate and then block small-diameter pain fibers by depleting them of the neurotransmitter substance P. Substance P is thought to be the principal chemomediator of pain impulses from the periphery. In addition, substance P has been shown to activate inflammatory mediators into joint tissues in rheumatoid arthritis.

Commercial ointments containing 0.025% or 0.075% capsaicin are available over-the-counter.

Administration may be effective in relieving pain.

Experimental Double-blind Study: Twenty-one pts. with either RA (n=7) or OA (n=14) with painful involvement of the hands received applied either capsaicin 0.075% or vehicle-only cream to the hands 4 times daily. Assessments of pain (visual analog scale), functional capacity, morning stiffness, grip strength, joint swelling and tenderness (dolorimeter) were performed before randomization. Treatment was applied to each painful hand joint 4 times daily with reassessment at 1, 2 and 4 weeks after entry. Capsaicin reduced tenderness (p) and pain (p) associated with OA, but not RA as compared with placebo. A local burning sensation was the only adverse effect noted (*McCarthy GM, McCarty DJ. Effect of topical capsaicin in the therapy of painful osteoarthritis of the hands. J Rheumatol 19(4):604-7, 1992*).

Experimental Double-blind Study: 70 pts. with osteoarthritis (OA) and 31 with rheumatoid arthritis (RA) received capsaicin or placebo for four weeks. The pts. were instructed to apply 0.025% capsaicin cream or its vehicle (placebo) to painful knees four times daily. Pain relief was assessed using visual analog scales for pain and relief, a categorical pain scale, and physicians' global evaluations. Most of the pts. continued to receive concomitant arthritis medications. Significantly more relief of pain was reported by the capsaicin-treated pts. than the placebo pts. throughout the study; after four weeks of capsaicin treatment, RA and OA pts. demonstrated mean reductions in pain of 57% and 33%, respectively. These reductions in pain were statistically significant compared with those reported with placebo (p=0.003 and p=0.033, respectively). According to the global evaluations, 80% of the capsaicin-treated pts. experienced a reduction in pain after two weeks of treatment. Transient burning was felt at the sites of application by 23 of the 52 capsaicin-treated pts.; two pts. withdrew from treatment because of this side effect (*Deal CL et al. Treatment of arthritis with topical capsaicin: a double-blind trial. Clin Ther 13(3):383-95, 1991*).

Devil's Claw (*Harpagophytum procumbens*):

Devil's claw is an herb native to Africa that has a long history of use in the treatment of arthritis. (*See: 'INFLAMMATION'*)

Administration may be beneficial.

Negative Experimental Study: Human volunteers took 4 capsules of 500 mg *H. procumbens* daily for 21 days. No effects on arachidonic acid or eicosanoid metabolism were noted (*Moussard C et al. A drug used in traditional medicine, Harpagophytum procumbens: No evidence for NSAID-like effect on whole blood eicosanoid production in humans. Prostaglan Leukotri Essent Fatty Acids 46:283-6, 1992*).

Experimental Study: 43 pts. with degenerative arthritis (arthroses, poly- or periarthritis, or sequelae of surgery or trauma) received harpagophytum (Arkocaps) 1.5 gm daily. Improvement was noted by the eighth day of treatment. After 60 days, 89% reported reduced pain, 84% demonstrated increased range of motion and 86% reported reduced time for stiffness to wear off. Side effects were limited to slight digestive discomfort in 2 pts. (*Pinget M, Lecomte A. [The effects of harpagophytum capsules (Arkocaps) in degenerative rheumatology.] Médecine Actuelle 12(4):65-7, 1985*).

Negative Animal Experimental Study: At doses 100 times or greater than the recommended daily dose for humans, *H. procumbens* was completely ineffective in reducing rat hind foot edema. *H. procumbens* was also ineffective in inhibiting prostaglandin synthesis *in vitro* (*Whitehouse LW, Znamirowski M, Paul CJ. Devil's claw (Harpagophytum procumbens): no evidence for anti-inflammatory activity in the treatment of arthritic disease. Can Med Assoc J 129:249-51, 1983*).

Negative Animal Experimental Study: No anti-inflammatory effect was noted for *H. procumbens* (*McLeod DW, Revell P, Robinson BV. Investigations of Harpagophytum procumbens (Devil's claw) in the treatment of experimental inflammation and arthritis in the rat. Br J Pharmacol 66:140P-141P, 1979*).

The equivocal research results of Devil's claw in experimental models may reflect a mechanism of action that is inconsistent with current anti-inflammatory drugs, a lack of quality control (standardization) of the Devil's claw preparations used, or inactivation of inflammatory principles during the process of digestion.

Animal Experimental Study: An aqueous extract of *Harpagophytum procumbens* exhibited significant and dose dependent anti-inflammatory effects. The main iridoid glycoside, harpagoside, exerted no anti-inflammatory effect. However, the anti-inflammatory effect of *H. procumbens* could be eliminated after an acid treatment similar to the physio-chemical conditions found in the stomach (*Lanhers MC et al. Anti-inflammatory and analgesic effects of an aqueous extract of Harpagophytum procumbens. Planta Med 58:117-23, 1992*)

Ginger (*Zingiber officinale*):

Administration may be beneficial.

Experimental Study: 18 pts. with osteoarthritis who had been taking powdered ginger for periods ranging from 3 months to 2.5 years were evaluated. Based on clinical observations, it was reported that 75% of pts. experienced relief in pain or swelling. The recommended dosage was 500 to 1,000 mg per day, but many pts. took 3 to 4 times this amount. Pts. taking the higher dosages reported quicker and better relief. None reported side effects (*Srivastava KC and Mustafa T. Ginger (Zingiber officinale) in rheumatism and musculoskeletal disorders. Med Hypothesis 39:342-8, 1992*).

Yucca Saponin extract:

A saponin extract from the desert yucca plant.

Administration may be beneficial.

Experimental Double-blind Study: 149 arthritis pts., 58.9% considered to have osteoarthritis on the basis of a negative RA fixation test, were randomly given either yucca saponin extract ('Desert Pride Herbal Food Tablets') 4 daily (range of 2-8) or placebo in periods ranging from 1 wk. to 15 mo. before re-evaluation. 61% noted less swelling, pain and stiffness versus 22% on placebo. Some improved in days, some in wks., and some in 3 mo. or longer (*Bingham R et al. Yucca plant saponin in the management of arthritis. J Appl Nutr 27:45-50, 1975*).

- -

COMBINATION TREATMENT

Bostwellia serrata stem,
Curcuma longa rhizome,
Withania somnifera root and
Zinc:

Combined administration may be beneficial.

Experimental Double-blind Crossover Study: 42 pts. randomly received a combination formula (Articulin-F) (containing the stem of *Boswellia serrata* along with *Curcuma longa* rhizome, *Withania somnifera* root, and zinc) and a placebo in random order with a 15-day wash-out period between assignments. Clinical efficacy was evaluated every fortnight on the basis of pain severity, morning stiffness, Ritchie articular index, joint score, disability score, and grip strength. After 3 mo., pts. treated with the combination had a significant reduction in pain severity (p<0.001) and in disability (p<0.05) scores compared to pts. treated with placebo. Radiological assessment failed to show any signs of improvement (*Kulkarni RR, Patki PS, Jog VP, et al. Treatment of osteoarthritis with a herbomineral formulation: a double-blind, placebo-controlled, crossover study. J Ethnopharmacol 33(1-2):91-5, 1991*).

PAIN

See Also: **DYSMENORRHEA**
HEADACHE
IRRITABLE BOWEL SYNDROME
NEURALGIA AND NEUROPATHY
OSTEOARTHRITIS
RHEUMATOID ARTHRITIS

Capsaicin:

Capsaicin is the active component of cayenne pepper (*Capsicum frutescens*). When topically applied, capsaicin is known to stimulate and then block small-diameter pain fibers by depleting them of the neurotransmitter substance P. Substance P is thought to be the principal chemomediator of pain impulses from the periphery. In addition, substance P has been shown to activate inflammatory mediators into joint tissues in osteoarthritis and rheumatoid arthritis.

Commercial ointments containing 0.025% or 0.075% capsaicin are available over-the-counter.

> **Review Article:** A brief overview of the chemical history, analysis, nomenclature, biology, pharmacology, and pharmacotherapy of capsaicin is presented including a review of clinical studies in the treatment of rheumatoid arthritis, osteoarthritis, and peripheral neuropathies (*Cordell GA, Araujo OE. Capsaicin: Identification, nomenclature, and pharmacotherapy.* Ann Pharmacother *27:330-6, 1993*).

Topical application may be effective in cluster headaches. (*See: 'HEADACHE'*).

Topical application may be effective in post-herpetic neuralgia. (*See: 'HERPES ZOSTER'*).

Topical application may be effective in osteoarthritis. (*See: 'OSTEOARTHRITIS'*).

Topical application may be effective in rheumatoid arthritis. (*See: 'RHEUMATOID ARTHRITIS'*).

Topical application may be effective in trigeminal neuralgia. (*See: 'NEURALGIA AND NEUROPATHY'*).

Topical application may be effective in post-mastectomy pain.

> **Experimental Double-blind Study:** 23 pts. with postmastectomy pain syndrome (PMPS) applied either capsaicin (0.075%) or vehicle-only cream 4 times daily for 4-6 weeks. There was no significant difference in the visual analog scale (VAS) for steady

pain although a trend was present. There was a significant difference in the VAS for jabbing pain, in category pain severity scales, and in overall pain relief scales in favor of capsaicin. 5/13 pts. on capsaicin were categorized as good-to-excellent responses with 8 (62%) having 50% or greater improvement. Only 1/10 cases had a good response to vehicle with 3 rated as 50% or better (*Watson CP, Evans RJ. The postmastectomy pain syndrome and topical capsaicin: a randomized trial. Pain 51(3):375-9, 1992*).

Experimental Study: 14 pts. with post-mastectomy pain had significant pain relief following application of 0.025% capsaicin cream 4 times daily for 4-6 weeks. Unpleasant or painful sensations to light touch or pressure in the painful area (hyperaesthesia, allodynia) were also improved (*Watson CPN et al. The post-mastectomy pain syndrome and the effect of topical capsaicin. Pain 38:177-86, 1989*).

Topical application may be effective in post-amputation stump pain.

Case Report: The application of capsaicin cream (Capsig, Sigma) 4 times daily completely relieved severe stump pain in a 47 year-old diabetic female after 7 days (*Rayner HC et al. Relief of local stump pain by capsaicin cream. Letter. Lancet ii:1276-7, 1989*).

See Also:

Review Article: *Lynn B. Capsaicin: actions on nociceptive C-fibres and therapeutic potential. Pain 41(1):61-9, 1990*

Morgenlander JC et al. Capsaicin for the treatment of pain in the Guillain-Barré Syndrome. Letter. Ann Neurol 28(2):199, 1990

Curcumin:

Curcumin is the yellow pigment and active component of turmeric (*Curcuma longa*). *Curcuma longa* has been used in Ayurvedic medicine, the indigenous systems of medicine of India, both locally and internally, in the treatment of sprains and inflammation.

Topical application may be effective, possibly due to its counterirritant effect. Capsaicin, a similar pungent principle from *Capsicum frutescens*, has been shown to be effective as a topical pain reliever. Like capsaicin, curcumin depletes nerve endings of the neurotransmitter of pain, substance P (*Patacchini R, Maggi CA and Meli A. Capsaicin-like activity of some natural pungent substances on peripheral ending of visceral primary afferents. Arch Pharmacol 342:72-7, 1990*).

See Also:

Animal Experimental Study: *Mukhopadhyay A et al. Anti-inflammatory and irritant activities of curcumin analogues in rats. Agents Actions 12:508-15, 1982*

Ginger (*Zingiber officinale*):

Administration may reduce chronic muscular ('rheumatic') discomfort.

Experimental Study: 10 pts. with chronic muscular discomfort who had been taking powdered ginger for periods ranging from 3 months to 2.5 years were evaluated. Based on clinical observations, 100% of the pts. with muscular discomfort experienced relief in pain or swelling. The recommended dosage was 500 to 1,000 mg per day, but many pts. took 3 to 4 times this amount. Pts. taking the higher dosages reported quicker and better relief. None reported side effects   (*Srivastava KC and Mustafa T. Ginger (Zingiber officinale) in rheumatism and musculoskeletal disorders. Med Hypothesis 39:342-8, 1992*).

PEPTIC ULCER
(DUODENAL AND GASTRIC)

See Also: HEARTBURN

Bilberry (*Vaccinium myrtillus*):

Administration of an extract of anthocyanosides may be beneficial.

> **Animal Experimental Study:** Oral administration of *Vaccinium myrtillus* anthocyanosides to rats excerted a significant preventive and curative antiulcer activity in various experimental models of gastric ulcer without affecting gastric secretion. This activity can be attributed, at least partly, to an increase in gastric mucus (*Criston A, Magistretti MJ. Antiulcer and healing activity of Vaccinium myrtillus anthocyanosides. Il Farmaco 42(2):29-43, 1986*).

Catechin:

Catechin is a flavonoid that is found in high concentrations in *Acacia catechu* (black catechu, black cutch) and *Uncaria gambier* (pale catechu, gambier).

Isolated catechin or plant extracts concentrated for catechin may be effective.

> WARNING: Catechin can induce autoimmune hemolysis. Use with caution. (*See: 'HEPATITIS'*)

Administration may reduce gastric acid release by inhibiting the formation of histamine by histadine decarboxylase.

> **Experimental Study:** Catechin (1 g 5 X d) resulted in reduced histamine levels in the gastric tissue (determined by biopsy) of normal pts. and those with gastric and duodenal ulcers and acute gastritis. It was also demonstrated that gastric histamine levels, which significantly increase in pts. with urticaria and food allergy after the local application of the antigen to the gastric mucosa, could be decreased by the prior administration of catechin (*Wendt P et al. The use of flavonoids as inhibitors of histidine decarboxylase in gastric diseases, Experimental and clinical studies. Naunyn-Schmiedeberg's Arch Pharma Suppl.313:238, 1980*)

See Also:

> **Experimental Study:** *Parmar N, Hennings G, Gulati O. Histidine decarboxylase inhibition: a novel approach towards the development of an effective and safe anti-ulcer drug. Agents Actions 15:494-501, 1984*

Experimental Study: *Parmar N, Ghosh M. Gastric anti-ulcer activity of (+)-cya-nidanol-3, a histidine decarboxylase inhibitor. Eur J Pharmacol 69:25-32, 1981*

Administration may be effective for postoperative stress ulcers.

Note: This study used a synthetic flavonoid (meciadanol) that is very similar to catechin.

Experimental Study: 298 critically ill pts. at risk for the development of postoperative stress ulcers and bleeding were randomized into three groups. The first group comprised 85 pts. who received meciadanol, 500 mg every six hours through a nasograstric tube; the second group comprised 100 pts. who received sucralfate (crushed tablets), 1 g every six hours through a nasogastric tube, and the third group comprised 113 pts. who received an antacid (Maalox [magnesium aluminum hydroxide gel]) through a nasogastric tube at an initial dose of 15 ml every hour. The gastric pH was measured hourly and titrated to a pH greater than or equal to 4.0 in pts. in the group receiving the antacid. The gastric pH was measured every two hours in the other two groups. Bleeding in the upper part of the gastrointestinal tract was determined visually (frank blood in gastric contents) or by guaiac testing. Bleeding occurred in seven pts. receiving meciadanol, nine receiving sucralfate and six receiving the antacid. The difference in rates of bleeding was not statistically significant. Correlation between the severity of illness index and the development of bleeding was poor, at least in the low and intermediate index range. In contrast, there was a strong correlation between the age of the patient and the development of bleeding. Only one patient younger than 50 years had bleeding develop. Apparently, meciadanol exerts its action by a mechanism other than pH control. It may, therefore, fill an important gap in the ability to prevent postoperative stress ulcers and bleeding *(Kitler ME et al. Preventing postoperative acute bleeding of the upper part of the gastrointestinal tract. Surg Gynecol Obstet 171(5):366-72, 1990).*

Efficacy may be due to the binding of bile acids.

Note: This study used a synthetic flavonoid (meciadanol) that is very similar to catechin.

Experimental Study: Pts. in the surgical intensive care unit were randomized prospectively to receive nasogastric instillation of Maalox, sucralfate, or meciadanol to prevent gastrointestinal bleeding. The gastric aspirates were analyzed for bile salt concentration. The mean bile salt concentration of those treated with Maalox (0.24 mM), meciadanol (0.24 mM), or sucralfate (0.35 mM) was significantly lower than those treated with nasogastric aspiration (0.87 mM) alone *(Lipsett P, Gadacz TR. Bile salt binding by maalox, sucralfate, and meciadanol: in vitro and clinical comparisons. J Surg Res 47(5):403-6, 1989).*

In vitro Study: Sucralfate, antacid (Maalox), and meciadanol were compared with cholestyramine resin for binding bile salts. The free, glycine, and taurine conjugates of the human bile salts, cholate, chenodeoxycholate, and deoxycholate, were incubated with each of the above. Cholestyramine resin adsorbed 91-97% of all bile salts tested. Meciadanol adsorbed all of the bile salts fairly well except for the free forms of chenodeoxycholate and deoxycholate. Meciadanol (53 to 84%) adsorbed bile salts better than sucralfate (4.2 to 61%), and significantly better than Maalox (10 to 47%). Sucral-fate was not as effective in binding bile salts as previously reported (*Lipsett P, Gadacz TR. Bile salt binding by maalox, sucralfate, and meciadanol: in vitro and clinical comparisons. J Surg Res 47(5):403-6, 1989*).

Licorice Root (*Glycyrrhiza glabra*):

Licorice root contains several anti-ulcer componenents. Original research focused on glycyr-rhetinic acid until it was shown that deglycyrrhizinated licorice (DGL) root extracts were actually more effective and without side effects (*Wilson JA. A comparison of carbenox-olone sodium and deglycyrrhizinated liquorice in the treatment of gastric ulcer in the ambu-lant patient. Br J Clin Pract 26(12):563-6, 1972*).

Research is now focusing on the flavonoid derivatives of licorice contained in DGL.

Animal Experimental Study: Hydroxychalcone derivatives of licorice demonstrated impressive protection against chemically-induced ulcer formation in rats. The most ac-tive compounds, $2^1,4^1$-dihydroxychalcone, exerted a cytoprotective effect similar to PGE2 (*Yamamoto K et al. Gastric cytoprotective anti-ulcerogenic actions of hydroxy-chalcone in rats. Planta Med 58(5):389-93, 1992*).

Crude licorice root contains about 6-14% glycyrrhizin, which in the body is cleaved to form glycyrrhetinic acid.

WARNING: If ingested regularly, licorice root (>3 g/d for more than 6 weeks) or glycyrrhizin (>100 mg/d) may cause sodium and water retention, hypertension, hypokalemia, and suppression of the renin-aldosterone system through a pseudo-aldosterone action of glycyrrhetinic acid. Monitoring of BP and electrolytes and increasing potassium intake is suggested (*Farese RV et al. Licorice-induced hy-permineralocorticoidism. N Engl J Med 325(17):1223-7, 1991; MacKenzie MA et al. The influence of glycyrrhetinic acid on plasma cortisol and cortisone in healthy young volunteers. J Clin Endocrinol Metab 70:1637-43, 1990*).

Review Article: There is a great individual variation in the susceptibility to the symptom-producing effects of glycyrrhizin. Adverse effects are rarely ob-served at levels below 100 mg/day while they are quite common at levels above 400 mg/day (*Stormer FC, Reistad R, Alexander J. Glycyrrhizic acid in liqourice - Evaluation of health hazard. Fd Chem Toxicol 31(4):303-12, 1993*).

Prevention of the side effects of glycyrrhizin (pseudo-aldosteronism) may be possible by following a high-potassium, low-sodium diet. Although no formal trial of either of these guidelines has been performed, patients who normally consume high-potassium foods and restrict sodium intake, even those with hypertension and angina, have been reported to be free from the aldosterone-like side effects of glycyrrhizin (*Baron J et al. Metabolic studies, aldosterone secretion rate and plasma renin after carbenoxolone sodium as biogastrone. Br Med J 2:793-5, 1969*).

Administration of licorice root may promote healing.

Experimental Double-blind Study: 66 pts. with endoscopically proven gastric ulcer received either pirenzepine, 50 mg t.i.d. for 6 weeks, or glycyrrhetinic acid, 100 mg three times a day for one week followed by 50 mg t.i.d. for the remaining 5 weeks. At 6 weeks, the ulcers had healed in 20/34 pts. (59%) treated with pirenzepine, and in 15/29 pts. (52%) treated with glycyrrhetinic acid. Symptomatic improvement. Side effects (oedema, hypokalaemia and hypertension) occurred in approximately 30% of pts. treated with glycyrrhetinic acid (*Bianchi Porro G et al. Comparison of pirenzepine and carbenoxolone in the treatment of chronic gastric ulcer. A double-blind endoscopic trial. Hepatogastroenterol 32(6):293-5, 1985*).

Experimental Double-blind Study: The healing-rate of duodenal ulcer after short-term treatment with glycyrrhetinic acid was not significantly different from that after treatment with cimetidine (*Schenk J et al. Controlled trial of carbenoxolone sodium vs. cimetidine in duodenal ulcer. Scand J Gastroenterol Suppl 65:103-7, 1985*).

Experimental Double-blind Study: 31 pts. with duodenal ulcer were treated with glycyrrhetinic acid and 29 with cimetidine. Endoscopy after 6 weeks of therapy showed healing in 61% of pts. receiving glycyrrhetinic acid and 72% in those receiving cimetidine (*Cook PJ et al. Carbenoxolone (Duogastrone) and cimetidine in the treatment of duodenal ulcer—a therapeutic trial. Scand J Gastroenterol Suppl 65:93-101, 1980*).

Experimental Double-blind Study: 24 pts. with gastric ulcer and 46 pts. with duodenal ulcer received either glycyrrhetinic acid (300 m/dg for the first week, followed by 150 mg/d over the next 6 weeks. Endoscopic assessment showed a healing rate of over 70% in both gastric and duodenal ulcer, healing occurred usually between 3-5 weeks. About 36% placebo healing was observed in both types of ulcer. The preparations were well tolerated and side-effects seldom observed (*Loginov AS. The effectiveness of carbenoxolone in the treatment of gastro-duodenal ulcer patients. Scand J Gastroenterol Suppl.65:85-91, 1980*).

Experimental Double-blind Study: 54 pts. with endoscopically diagnosed benign gastric ulcer were allocated at random to treatment with either cimetidine 800 mg daily for 6 weeks or glycyrrhetinic acid 300 mg daily for one week then 150 mg daily for 5 weeks. Ulcers were reassessed by endoscopy at the end of the trial. The endoscopist was unaware of the treatment and did not take part in the clinical care of the pts.. 21 of the 27 pts. (78%) given cimetidine and 14 of the 27 (52%) given glycyrrhetinic acid had healed ulcer (*La Brooy SJ et al. Controlled comparison of cimetidine and carbenoxolone sodium in gastric ulcer. Br Med J 19;1(6174):1308-9, 1979*)

Experimental Double-blind Study: 40 pts. with an endoscopically confirmed, symptomatic duodenal ulcer were allocated at random to treatment with either glycyrrhetinic acid sodium or placebo. Endoscopic review of ulcer healing after six weeks' treatment showed that 12 pts. (60%) receiving glycyrrhetinic acid had healed ulcers, compared with 5 (25%) receiving placebo (p). Symptomatic remission occurred by the fourth week in 17 pts. (85%) receiving glycyrrhetinic acid, compared with 6 (30%) receiving placebo (p). The mean (geometric) serum glycyrrhetinic acid level in pts. with healed ulcers was 31.11 mgm/mL compared with 17.75 mgm/mL in those with unhealed ulcers (p). Side effects of glycyrrhetinic acid therapy were observed, but they did not necessitate withdrawal of the drug and were readily controlled in every instance. These results confirm the therapeutic efficacy of glycyrrhetinic acid sodium in duodenal ulcer.

In addition, a relationship between serum glycyrrhetinic acid levels and the occurrence of ulcer healing was observed (*Young GP, St John DJ, Coventry DA. Treatment of duodenal ulcer with carbenoxolone sodium: a double-masked endoscopic trial. Med J Aust 1(1):2-5, 1979*).

Experimental Double-blind Study: 20 pts. with chronic gastric ulcers and 20 pts. with superficial erosions of the stomach were given either glycyrrhetinic acid (50 mg 3 times daily) or placebo along with antacids in fixed dosage for 6 weeks. No difference was seen between glycyrrhetinic acid and placebo groups with regard to the healing rate of the ulcers of disappearance of the erosions. The subjective symptoms subsided significantly faster in the treatment groups than in the control groups. No cardiovascular side effects were evident during the treatment with glycyrrhetinic acid. One patient needed potassium supplements. Glycyrrhetinic acid had no effect on the pentagastrin-stimulated gastric acid secretion nor on the serum gastrin values (*Lehtola J, Karvonen AL, Tunturi-Hihnala H. Double-blind study of carbenoxolone in gastric ulcer and erosions. Ann Clin Res 10(1):19-23, 1978*).

Experimental Double-blind Study: 44 pts. with duodenal ulcers were given either glycyrrhetinic acid or placebo and were evaluated by endoscopy over a period of 6 weeks. The 2 groups were adequately matched with the exception that larger ulcers predominated in the glycyrrhetinic acid group. 14 of the 21 pts. in the glycyrrhetinic acid group and 7 of the 23 in the placebo group showed endoscopic evidence of complete healing (p). Side effects of glycyrrhetinic acid therapy in the form of weight gain, rise in diastolic blood pressure and hypokalaemia were observed, but no patient suffered any ill effects (*Nagy GS. Evaluation of carbenoxolone sodium in the treatment of duodenal ulcer. Gastroenterol 74(1):7-10, 1978*).

Experimental Double-blind Study: Complete ulcer healing occurred in a significantly greater number of pts. receiving glycyrrhetinic acid (200 mg/d) than placebo, the significance being greater after four and eight weeks treatment than at 12 weeks. While significant symptomatic improvement also was achieved, but only after 12 weeks on glycyrrhetinic acid, there was much closer correlation between ulcer healing and symptom relief, 69% on glycyrrhetinic acid returning to normal, compared with 22% of controls. Rise of systolic blood pressure and reduction in serum potassium levels, especially during the last four treatment weeks, were the most common side effects noted in pts. taking glycyrrhetinic acid, and 5 pts. required thiazide diuretics and potassium supplements. Higher serum glycyrrhetinic acid levels were found in pts. with healed ulcers as well as in those with more marked side-effects (*Davies WA, Reed PI. Controlled trial of Duogastrone in duodenal ulcer. Gut 18(1):78-83, 1977*).

See Also:

> **Experimental Double-blind Study:** *Hadzic N, Vrhovac B, Kallai L. Controlled double blind trial of carbenoxolone in gastric and duodenal ulcer. Int J Clin Pharmacol 10(4):309-18, 1974.*

> **Experimental Double-blind Study:** *Geismar P, Mosbech J, Myren J. A double-blind study of the effect of carbenoxolone sodium in the treatment of gastric ulcer. Scand J Gastroenterol 8(3):251-6, 1973.*

Experimental Double-blind Study: *Brown P et al. Double-blind trial of carbenoxolone sodium capsules in duodenal ulcer therapy, based on endoscopic diagnosis and follow-up. Br Med J 3(828):661-4, 1972.*

Experimental Double-blind Study: *Brown P et al. A double blind trial of carbenoxolone sodium (Duogastrone) in duodenal ulcer therapy with endoscopic diagnosis and follow up. Gut 13(4):324, 1972.*

Experimental Double-blind Study: *Cliff JM, Milton-Thompson GJ. A double-blind trial of carbenoxolone sodium capsules in the treatment of duodenal ulcer. Gut 11(2):167-70, 1970.*

- Deglycyrrhizinated Licorice (DGL):

In the treatment of peptic ulcers, DGL offers the benefits of licorice and glycyrrhetinic acid without the risk of side effects.

> *Note: In order to be effective in healing peptic ulcers, it appears that DGL must mix with saliva. DGL may promote the release of salivary compounds which stimulate the growth and regeneration of stomach and intestinal cells. DGL in capsule form has not been shown to be effective (Bardhan et al. Clinical trial of deglycyrrhizinised liquorice in gastric ulcer. Gut 19:779-82, 1978; Multicentre Trial. Treatment of duodenal ulcers with glycyrrhinizin acid-reduced liquorice. Br Med J 3(773):501-3,1973).*

The standard dosage for DGL is two to four 380 mg. chewable tablets between or 20 minutes before meals. DGL should be continued for 8 to 16 weeks, depending on the response.

> *Note: DGL tablets must be chewed before meals. Giving DGL after meals is associated with poor results (Feldman H, Gilat T. A trial of deglycyrrhizinated liquorice in the treatment of duodenal ulcer. Gut 12:499-51, 1971).*

DGL may protect the gastric mucosa by increasing mucus production.

Animal Experimental Study: Administration of DGL to rats with peptic ulcers increased the number of mucus-secreting glands and the number of mucus-secreting cells per gland *(van Marle J et al. Deglycyrrhizinised liquorice (DGL) and the renewal of rat stomach epithelium. Eur J Pharmacol 72:219-25, 1981).*

DGL improves mucosal blood flow *(Johnson B, McIssac R. Effect of some anti-ulcer agents on mucosal blood flow. Br J Pharmacol 1:308, 1981).*

Administration may promote healing.

Experimental Double-blind Study: 82 pts. with endoscopically healed gastric ulcer were treated for 2 years with either DGL (380 mg b.i.d.) or cimetidine (400 mg at bedtime). During the first year, 4/34 (12%) in the DGL gp. and 4/41 (10%) in the cimetidine gp. had an ulcer recurrence. By the second year the recurrence rate was 9/31 (29%) and 8/32 (25%), respectively. When maintenance therapy was stopped, only 2/22 DGL pts. had recurrences compared to 7/23 pts. treated with cimetidine. Therapy for pts. with dyspeptic symptoms or elderly pts. should be for life (*Morgan AG et al. Maintenance therapy: A two year comparison between Caved-S and cimetidine treatment in the prevention of symptomatic gastric ulcer. Gut 26:599-602, 1985*).

Experimental Controlled Study: 874 pts. with endoscopically confirmed chronic duodenal ulceration received either DGL, antacids, geranylferensylacetate or cimetidine. 91% of all ulcers healed within 12 wks., and there was no significant difference in healing rate in the 4 groups. However, in the DGL gp., there were fewer relapses (8.2%) compared to the anacids gp. (16.4%), the geranylferensylacetate gp. (15.5%) and the cimetidine gp. (12.9%), suggesting that it may be the superior treatment (*Kassir ZA. Endoscopic controlled trial of four drug regimens in the treatment of chronic duodenal ulceration. Ir Med J 78:153-6, 1985*).

Experimental Studies: 1.) 100 pts. received either DGL (Caved-S) 760 mg 3 times daily between meals or cimetidine 200 mg 3 times daily and 400 mg at bedtime. The percentage of ulcers healed after 6 and 12 wks. were similar in both groups. 56 pts. 2.) 56 pts. received maintenance treatment for 1 yr. with DGL (760 mg 2 times daily) or cimetidine (400 mg at bedtime). The number of recurrences were identical in each group (14%) (*Morgan AG et al. Comparison between cimetidine and Caved-S in the treatment of gastric ulceration, and subsequent maintenance therapy Gut 23:545-51, 1982*).

Experimental Study: DGL was as effective as rantidine in the treatment of gastric ulcers (*Glick L. Deglycrrhizinated liquorice in peptic ulcer. Lancet ii:817, 1982*).

Experimental Study: 40 pts. with chronic duodenal ulcers of 4-12 yrs. duration and over 6 relapses during the previous yr. received DGL. Half received 3 gm daily for 8 wks.; the other half received 4.5 gm daily for 16 weeks. All 40 displayed substantial improvement, usually within 5-7 days, and none required surgery during a 1-yr. follow-up. The higher dosage was significantly more effective (*Tewari SN, Wilson AK. Deglycyrrhizinated liquorice in duodenal ulcer. Practitioner 210:820-5, 1972*).

Experimental Double-blind Study: 33 gastric ulcer pts. received either DGL 760 mg 3 times daily or placebo. After 1 mo., there was a significantly greater reduction in ulcer size in the DGL group. Complete healing occurred in 44% of those receiving DGL, but in only 6% of controls (*Turpie AG et al. Clinical trial of deglycyrrhizinate liquorice in gastric ulcer. Gut 10:299-303, 1969*).

Experimental Double-blind Crossover Study: Ulcer pts. received DGL or placebo and were permitted to use anacids in between doses. Duodenal ulcers showed marked symptomatic improvement. In some cases, radiological healing was demonstrated, with disappearance of the ulcer crater 2-5 wks. after treatment initiation. All gastric ulcers showed extensive healing (*Tewari SN et al. Some experience with deglycyrrhizinated licorice in the treatment of gastric and duodenal ulcers with special reference to its spasmolytic effect. Gut 9:48-51, 1968*).

See Also:

Balakrishnan V et al. Deglycyrrhizinated liquorice in the treatment of chronic duodenal ulcer. J Assoc Physicians Ind 26:811-14, 1978

Administration may reduce the gastric bleeding caused by aspirin.

Experimental Study: Fecal blood loss induced by 975 mg aspirin orally 3 times a day was less when 350 mg DGL was given with each dose of aspirin (*Rees WDW et al. Effect of deglycyrrhizinated liquorice on gastric mucosal damage by aspirin. Scand J Gastroenterol 14:605-7, 1979*).

Animal Experimental Study: Gastric mucosal damage induced by giving 60 mg aspirin orally to rats was reduced by simultaneous administration of 100-500 mg DGL (*Rees WDW et al. Effect of deglycyrrhizinated liquorice on gastric mucosal damage by aspirin. Scand J Gastroenterol 14:605-7, 1979*).

Rhubarb (*Rheum* spp.):

Administration may reduce bleeding.

Experimental Double-blind Study: 3 kinds of alcohol-extracted rhubarb tablets were studied (*Rheum officinale Baill*; *Rheum palmatum L.*; *Rheum tanguticum Maxim ex Balf*). Their efficacies in regard to a gp. of 312 cases of bleeding gastric and duodenal ulcers were 90.7%, 93.7%, and 92.8%, respectively. The time taken for the stool occult blood to change from positive to negative was 57.1, 53.4, and 56 hrs., respectively ($p > 0.05$) (*Zhou H, Jiao D. [312 cases of gastric and duodenal ulcer bleeding treated with 3 kinds of alcoholic extract rhubarb tablets.] Chung Hsi I Chieh Ho Tsa Chih 10(3):150-1, 131-2, 1990*) (*in Chinese*).

See Also:

Experimental Double-blind Study: *Jiao DH. [Alcoholic extract tablet of rhubarb in treating acute upper gastrointestinal hemorrhage.] Chung Hsi I Chieh Ho Tsa Chih 8(6):344-6, 324-5, 1988 (in Chinese)*

Experimental Study: *Sun DA [Clinical evaluation of crude rhubarb powder and cimetidine in upper gastrointestinal tract bleeding.] Chung Hsi I Chieh Ho Tsa Chih 6(8):458-9, 451, 1986 (in Chinese)*

S-methylmethionine ('Vitamin U'):

Found in trace amounts in certain raw foods, particularly cabbage and other green vegetables.

Administration may be beneficial.

Animal Experimental Study: S-methylmethionine was found to protect dogs against experimental ulcers (*Szabo S, Vargha G. Unhtersuchung de Wirkungswiese des sogenannten "Vitamin U" mit histochemischen Reaktionen. Arzneimittelforsch 10:23-8, 1960*) (*in German*).

Experimental Placebo-controlled Study: Pts. were treated with conventional milk diet therapy. In addition, 26 pts. were treated with concentrated cabbage juice, while 19 controls received a facsimile which contained no cabbage juice. After 3 wks., x-rays showed healing in 24/26 (92%) of treated pts. compared to 6/19 (32%) of controls (*Cheney G. Calif Med, January, 1956*).

Experimental Study: 55 pts. with gastric, duodenal or jejunal peptic ulcers were treated with vitamin U (raw cabbage juice 1 liter daily). All but 3 were symptomatically relieved in 2-5 days, and those 3 pts. had chronic, penetrating duodenal ulcers which led to surgery for 2 of them. Healing time of the craters as judged by x-ray evidence and symptom relief averaged 11.5 days (range of 8-23 days) (*Cheney G. Vitamin U therapy of peptic ulcer. Calif Med 77(4):248-52, 1952*).

Experimental Study: 86% of 100 pts. with gastric or duodenal peptic ulcers treated with vitamin U (raw cabbage juice 1 liter daily) experienced pain relief without the continued use of drug therapy and without frequent food feedings. They also showed accelerated healing time (*Cheney G. Rapid healing of peptic ulcers in patients receiving fresh cabbage juice. Calif Med 70:10-14, 1949*).

See Also:

Tsimmerman IaS, Mikhaïlovskaia LV. [Effect of sea buckthorn oil on various pathophysiologic mechanisms and the course of peptic ulcer.] Klin Med (Mosk) 65(2):77-82, 1987 (in Russian)

Noess K. [Ulcer-fiber-cabbage and vitamin U.] Letter. Tidsskr Nor Laegeforen 106(8):693-4, 1986 (in Norwegian)

Trusov VV, Vakhrushev IaM. [Therapeutic use of vitamin U in gastroenterological practice.] Vrach Delo (10):101-4, 1978 (in Russian)

Tsimmerman IaS, Golovanova ES. [Clinical effect and an analysis of the mechanism of action of vitamin U (S-methylmethioninesulfonium chloride) in peptic ulcer of the stomach and duodenum.] Ter Arkh 48(3):29-35, 1976 (in Russian)

Cheney G. Anti-peptic ulcer dietary factor. J Am Diet Assoc 26:668-72, 1950

Gianelli VJ, Belafiore V. The fundamental importance of diet in the treatment of peptic ulcer in an Army general hospital, with special reference to vitamin U therapy. Med Clin North Am 29:706, 1945

PERIODONTAL DISEASE

See Also: INFLAMMATION

<u>Centella asiatica</u>:

Centella asiatica (Gotu kola) exerts wound healing properties (*See: 'WOUND HEALING'*) that may be useful in severe periodontal disease (*Benedicenti A, Galli D, Merlini A. [The clinical therapy of periodontal disease, the use of potassium hydroxide and the water-alcohol extract of Centella in combination with laser therapy in the treatment of severe periodontal disease]. Parodontol Stomatol 24(1):11-26, 1985*) (*in Italian*).

<u>Licorice Root</u> (*<u>Glycyrrhiza glabra</u>*):

Toothpastes containing glycyrrhizin from licorice root may be helpful in reducing gingival plaque.

Negative Experimental Double-blind Study: 40 male and female volunteers brushed their teeth twice daily with a toothpaste containing 0.25% and 0.50% glycyrrhizin, or a control toothpaste, respectively. All 3 toothpastes contained sodium lauryl sulfate as detergent. The subjects of the 3 groups were examined at days 0, 7, 14, 28, 35 and 42 for plaque, gingival and bleeding indices. None of the brushing regimens with the experimental toothpastes induced significant changes in the examined indices, that were distinct from those observed with the control toothpaste. The decrease (insignificant) in the indices of the study period from 0 to 14 days may be considered as an increased oral hygiene awareness by the subjects examined. Possible explanations for the lack of efficacy in improvement of plaque, gingival and bleeding indices may have been an insufficient glycyrrhizin concentration and/or chemical incompatibility in a toothpaste containing a mixture of an anionic detergent and an organic antibacterial surface agent (*Goultschin J et al. Effect of glycyrrhizin-containing toothpaste on dental plaque reduction and gingival health in humans. A pilot study. J Clin Periodontol 18(3):210-2, 1991*).

Experimental Study: A split-mouth technique of glycyrrhizin application was used in 21 volunteers. Subjects were instructed to discontinue all oral hygiene procedures, but no dietary modifications were imposed. After 3 days a highly significant reduction in plaque was detected in the upper central incisors on the experimental sides compared with the control sides of students' mouths. Comparing all teeth, less plaque was found on experimental sides than on control sides of the mouth. This difference demonstrated a tendency towards statistical significance. After 4 days the quantitative differences between the two halves of the mouths (less plaque on experimental sides) were greater than after 3 days. This pilot study might indicate the potential of glycyrrhizin in controlling dental plaque (*Steinberg D et al. The anticariogenic activity of glycyrrhizin: preliminary clinical trials. Isr J Dent Sci 2(3):153-7, 1989*).

Sanguinaria canadensis (bloodroot):

An alcoholic extract of *Sanguinaria* containing a mixture of benzophenanthridine alkaloids, but chiefly sanguanarine is available in commercial toothpastes and mouth rinses.

Sanguinarine demonstrates properties useful in preventing dental plaque formation.

Review Article: Sanguinarine has broad antimicrobial activity as well as antiinflammatory properties. *In vitro* studies indicate that the anti-plaque action of sanguinaria is due to its ability to inhibit bacterial adherence. The MIC of sanguinarine ranges from 1 to 32 micrograms/mL for most species of plaque bacteria. Electron microscopic studies of bacteria exposed to sanguinarine demonstrate that bacteria aggregate and become morphologically irregular *(Godowski KC. Antimicrobial action of sanguinarine. J Clin Dent 1(4):96-101, 1989).*

Topical use of the extract in toothpastes and mouth rinses may be beneficial.

Experimental Double-blind Study: This study compared the clinical efficacy of three mouthrinses containing either 0.12% chlorhexidine, phenolic compounds, or sanguinarine, which were used unsupervised, in a placebo-controlled, double-blind study of 6 months' duration in 481 adults. Compared to placebo at 6 months, the group rinsing with 0.12% chlorhexidine had significantly less gingivitis (31% reduction), gingival bleeding (39% reduction), and plaque (49% reduction) and was significantly better than any of the other treatment groups. Both the phenolic and sanguinarine groups showed moderate, yet significant, reductions in plaque compared to placebo (24% and 12% respectively) yet were significantly less effective than the 0.12% chlorhexidine rinse. However, neither the phenolic nor sanguinarine rinses were significantly different than placebo in their effects on gingivitis or gingival bleeding *(Grossman E et al. A clinical comparison of antibacterial mouthrinses: effects of chlorhexidine, phenolics, and sanguinarine on dental plaque and gingivitis. J Periodontol 60(8):435-40, 1989).*

Negative Experimental Double-blind Study: 120 adult volunteers used a dentifrice contained 750 mcg/g of sanguinaria extract or a placebo for 6 months. There were no significant differences between experimental and control groups for mean 6-month changes in plaque and gingival inflammation scores *(Mauriello SM, Bader JD. Six-month effects of a sanguinarine dentifrice on plaque and gingivitis. J Periodontol 9(4):238-43, 1988).*

Experimental Placebo-controlled Study: Volunteers who refrained from any oral hygiene used either a sanguinarine or a placebo mouth rinse. After 2 wks., although the sanguinarine rinse did not prevent gingivitis and plaque formation, its results were significantly superior to those of the placebo *(Wennstrom J, Lindhe J. Clinical effectiveness of a sanguinarine mouthrinse on plaque and gingivitis. J Dent Res 63:224, 1984).*

See Also:

Experimental Placebo-controlled Study: *Wennstrom J, Lindhe J. The effect of mouthrinses on parameters characterizing human periodontal disease. J Clin Periodontol 13:86-93, 1986*

Negative Experimental Placebo-controlled Study: *Siegrist BE et al. Efficacy of supervised rinsing with chlorhexidine digulconate in comparison to phenolic and plant alkaloid compounds. J Periodont Res 21:60-73, 1986*

- with Zinc Chloride:

Experimental Placebo-controlled Study: 60 pts. with moderate plaque and gingivitis were given toothpaste and oral rinse which randomly contained either sanguinaria extract and zinc chloride or placebo and were followed for 28 weeks. Active gp. scores were significantly lower (p<0.001) than placebo scores at each post-baseline time point for all indices, with the exception of plaque at 2 weeks. The 28-wk. active gp. scores were 21% lower than the controls for bleeding on probing. 3/30 active gp. pts. exhibited minor soft tissue irritations that resolved spontaneously without discontinuation of product use (*Harper DS et al. Clinical efficacy of a dentifrice and oral rinse containng sanguinaria extract and zinc chloride during 6 months of use. J Periodontol 61(6):352-8, 1990*).

Negative Placebo-controlled Experimental Study: 94 pts. randomly received a dentifrice with or without sanguinarine and zinc chloride while continuing their usual methods of oral hygiene. After 26 wks., there were no significant differences in plaque and gingivitis index scores between gps. (*Palcanis KG et al. Longitudinal evaluation of the effect of sanguinarine on plaque and gingivitis. Gen Dent 38(1):17-9, 1990*).

Experimental Study: 59 young adults aged 18-30 either performed supervised brushing with a sanguinaria and zinc chloride dentifrice, a sodium fluoride dentifrice, or rinsed daily with a sodium fluoride solution. After 7, 14, and 21 days both gps. using dentifrices had significantly less plaque and gingivitis than the gp. using the rinse, and there were no significant differences between the 2 gps. using either of the 2 dentifrices (*Mallatt ME et al. Clinical effect of a sanguinaria dentifrice on plaque and gingivitis in adults. J Periodontol 60(2):91-5, 1989*).

Experimental Single-blind Crossover Study: Pts. with initially plaque-free tooth surfaces received test rinses containing various doses of sanguinaria extract and zinc chloride and placebo rinses, both without oral hygiene, for 2 wks. each. Results suggest that the effects of sanguinaria rinses on developing plaque and gingivitis are influenced more by sanguinaria concentrations than the presence or absence of the zinc ion, but that the zinc ion may provide a mild enhancement of sanguinaria effectiveness (*Southard GL et al. The relationship of sanguinaria extract concentration and zinc ion to plaque and gingivitis. J Clin Periodontol 14(6):315-9, 1987*).

See Also:

> **Negative Experimental Controlled Study:** *Etemadzadeh H, Ainamo J. Lacking anti-plaque efficacy of 2 sanguinarine mouthrinses. J Clin Periodontol 14:176-80, 1987*

> **Experimental Double-blind Study:** *Klewansky P, Roth D. Sanguinaria in the control of bleeding in periodontal patients. Compend Contin Educ Dent Suppl 7:S218-20, 1986*

PERIPHERAL VASCULAR DISEASE
(including THROMBOPHLEBITIS and VARICOSE VEINS)

See Also: ATHEROSCLEROSIS
VASCULAR FRAGILITY

Bilberry (_Vaccinium myrtillus_):

Bilberry or European blueberry contains flavonoid compounds known as anthocyanosides. Bilberry anthocyanosides are potent antioxidants that improve the microcirculation and protect the vascular endothelium. Bilberry anthocyanosides exert similar effects to procyanidolic oligomers (_see below_). (_See: 'RETINOPATHY'; 'VASCULAR FRAGILITY'_)

The standard dose for Vaccinium myrtillus extract (VME) is based on its anthocyanoside content, as calculated by its anthocyanidin percentage. Most studies have used a bilberry extract standardized for an anthocyanidin content of 25% at a dosage of 160 mg to 480 mg daily.

Administration of VME may increase prostacyclin activity and promote the release of endothelium-derived relaxing factor (EDRF).

> Note: Prostacyclin prevents platelet aggregation and EDRF reduces the tension of blood vessel walls.

Ex vivo Study: Bettini V et al. _Vasodilator and inhibitory effects of Vaccinium myrtillus on the contractile responses of coronary artery segments to acetylcholine: role of the prostacyclins and of the endothelium-derived relaxing factor. Fitoter 42(1):15-28, 1991_

Animal Experimental Study: Morazzoni P, Magistretti MJ. _Effects of Vacciuium myrtillus anthocyanosides on prostacylcin-like activity in rat arterial tissue. Fitoter 42:11-4, 1986_

Administration of VME may promote improved arterial function.

Animal Experimental Study: VME improves vascular tone and blood flow in the microcirculation and ameliorates microvascular disturbances by promoting and enhancing arterioral rhythmic redistribution of microvascular blood flow and interstitial fluid formation (_Colantuoni S et al. Effects of Vaccinium myrtillus anthocyanosides on arterial vasomotion. Arzneim Forsch 41(9):905-9, 1991_).

Administration of VME may be effective in improving <u>peripheral arterial and venous insufficiency</u>.

Experimental Study: 15 pts. with polyneuritis due to peripheral vascular insufficiency were given VME (480 mg/d). Significant improvements were noted due to improved microcirculatory function as demonstrated by capillographic examinations of the ungual bed by plethysmography and thermographic techniques (*Pennarola R et al. [The therapeutic action of the anthocyanosides in microcirculatory changes due to adhesive-induced polyneuritis].* <u>Gazz Med Ital</u> *139:485-91, 1980*) (*in Italian*).

Experimental Study: 47 pts. with venous diseases were treated with VME (480 mg/d). Significant improvements (p<0.01) were found abnormal capillary permeability, edema, feelings of heaviness, paresthesia, pain, and skin dystrophy and dyschromia. Bilberry anthocyanosides improve the function of arterio-venous anastomoses by reducing capillary flow, converting richly anastomized vascular units into terminal units, and eliminating microstagnation and blood stasis as determined by foot biopsy (*Ghiringhelli C, Gregoratti F, Marastoni F. [Capillarotropic activity of anthocyanosides in high doses in phlebopathic stasis].* <u>Min Cardioangiol</u> *26:255-76, 1978*) (*in Italian*).

See Also:

> *Alcocer A, Gil Cabello C, Cervantes M. [Anthocyanosides in the symptomatic treatment of varicose veins].* <u>Prensa Med Mex</u> *37(9):390-3, 1973 (in Spanish)*

Administration of VME may be effective in preventing and treating <u>varicose veins of pregnancy</u> (*Grismond GL.[Treatment of pregnancy-induced phlebopathies.]* <u>Minerva Ginecol</u> *33:221-30, 1981*) (*in Italian*).

Bromelain:

Bromelains are sulfur-containing proteolytic enzymes or proteases obtained from the stem of the pineapple plant (*Ananas comosus*). The fibrinolytic activities of bromelain may be useful in thrombophlebitis, deep vein thrombosis, and varicose veins. (*See: '<u>INFLAMMATION</u>'*)

The standard dosage of bromelain (1,800-2,000 m.c.u.) is 125-450 mg 3 times daily on an empty stomach.

Administration may be beneficial in <u>thrombophlebitis</u>.

Review Article: Bromelain was introduced as a medicinal agent in 1957, and since that time over 400 scientific papers on its therapeutic applications have appeared in medical literature. Bromelain has been reported in these scientific studies to exert a wide variety of beneficial effects, including reducing inflammation in cases of arthritis, sports injury or trauma and prevention of swelling after trauma or surgery. Bromelain has been shown to be useful in a number of other health conditions including thrombophlebitis (*Taussig S, Batkin S. Bromelain, the enzyme complex of pineapple (Ananas comosus) and its clinical application. An update.* <u>J Ethnopharmacol</u> *22:191-203, 1988*).

Review Article: The cardiovascular applications of bromelain are presented including results from several uncontrolled trials in angina, hypertension, and thrombophlebitis. Bromelain inhibits platelet aggregation, exerts anti-anginal activity, promotes fibrinolysis, and relaxes vasoconstriction. These actions make it particularly useful in angina and thrombophlebitis (*Taussig S and Nieper H. Bromelain: Its use in prevention and treatment of cardiovascular disease present status. J Int Assoc Prev Med 6:139-51, 1979*).

Experimental Double-blind Study: For 73 pts. with acute thrombophlebitis, bromelain, as an adjunct to analgesics, was shown to reduce all the symptoms of inflammation: pain, edema, redness, tenderness, elevated skin temperature, and disability. The percentage of pts. improved, calculated as the mean percentages for each symptom, was 85.3% in the bromelain gp. and 71.1% for the placebo (*Seligman B. Oral bromelains as adjuncts in the treatment of acute thrombophlebitis. Angiology 20:22-6, 1969*).

Experimental Study: Of 11 pts. with thrombophlebitis, 8 (72%) showed good to excellent results after taking only 80 to 160 mg of enteric-coated bromelain per day (*Giacca S. [Clinical experiments with bromelain in peripheral venous diseases and chronic bronchitis]. Minerva Med 56(Suppl.98):3925-32, 1965*) (*in Italian*).

Administration may be effective for treating varicose veins.

Review Article: Individuals with varicose veins have a decreased ability to break down fibrin. Vein walls are an important source of plasminogen activator, which promotes the breakdown of fibrin. Veins that have become varicosed have decreased levels of plasminogen activator leading to the deposition of fibrin in the tissue near the varicose veins causing the surrounding skin to become hard and 'lumpy'. Decreased fibrinolytic activity increases the risk of thrombus formation, which may result in thrombophlebitis, myocardial infarction, pulmonary embolism, or stroke. Bromelain acts in a similar manner to plasminogen activator to cause fibrin breakdown (*Ako H, Cheung A, Matsura P. Isolation of a fibrinolysis enzyme activator from commercial bromelain. Arch Int Pharmacodyn 254:157-67, 1981*).

Experimental Controlled Study: In a series of 180 consecutive operations for varices, bromelain was given to alternate pts. at a dose of 40 mg 4 times daily from the first to the third postoperative day and 20 mg 4 times daily from the fourth to the seventh day, as a prophylactic treatment of hematomas. The number of hematomas and infiltrations were significantly lower in the treated group. After 2 weeks 65/90 treated pts. had no hematomas compared to only 32/90 in untreated pts. (*Durant JH, Waibel PP. [Prevention of hematoma in surgery of varices]. Praxis 61:950-1, 1972*) (*in German*).

Centella asiatica:

Most research on Centella has been performed with either the total triterpenoid fraction of *Centella asiatica* (TTFCA) or isolated triterpenoids. TTFCA has also been referred to as the 'titrated extract of *Centella asiatica*' or TECA. Both extracts are composed of a mixture of 3 triterpenes: asiatic acid (30%), madecassic acid (30%) and asiaticoside (40%). (*See:* '*WOUND HEALING*')

TTFCA appears to exert regulatory effects on the connective tissue of the vascular wall.

Experimental Study: The effects were studied of TTFCA on serum levels of the uronic acids and lysosomal enzymes involved in mucopolysaccharide metabolism (beta-glycuronidase, beta-N-acetylglucosaminidase, arylsulfatase) in pts. with varicose veins. The basal levels of uronic acids (467.7 mcg/ml) and of lysosomal enzymes (beta-glycuronidase 1.8 mM/min/l, beta-N-acetylglucosaminidase 23.1 mM/min/l, arysulfatase 0.078 mM/min/l) were elevated, indicating an increased mucopolysaccharide turnover in subjects with varicose veins. During treatment with *Centella asiatica* extract (60 mg/day for 3 mo.), these levels fell progressively. At the end of treatment the serum uronic acid (231.8 mcg/ml), beta-glycuronidase (1.2 mM/min/l), beta-N-acetyl-glucosaminidase (17.7 mM/min/l) and arysulfatase (0.042 mM/min/l) levels were highly significantly lower than the basal levels ($p<0.01$) (*Arpaia MR et al. Effects of Centella asiatica extract on mucopolysaccharide metabolism in subjects with varicose veins. Int J Clin Pharmacol Res 10(4):229-33, 1990*).

Serum levels of TTFCA are higher with chronic administration and asiaticoside is converted to asiatic acid *in vivo*. Better results are observed the longer TTFCA is used.

Experimental Crossover Study: A new HPLC assay method was used to investigate the pharmacokinetics of asiatic acid after oral administration of the TTFCA in single doses (30 or 60 mg) and after a 7-day treatment (30 or 60 mg twice daily). 12 healthy volunteers received each treatment following a randomized cross-over design with trials separated by a 3-week interval. The time of peak plasma concentration was not affected by dosage difference or by treatment scheme. Differences in peak plasma concentration and area under the concentration vs. time curve from 0 to 24 h calculated after 30 or 60 mg administration (single dose) were accounted for by the different dose regimen. However, after chronic treatment with both 30 and 60 mg, peak plasma concentrations, absorption rates, and half-life were significantly higher than those observed after the corresponding single dose administration. This phenomenon could be explained by asiaticoside being transformed into asiatic acid *in vivo* (*Grimaldi R et al. Pharmacokinetics of the total triterpenic fraction of Centella asiatica after single and multiple administrations to healthy volunteers. A new assay for asiatic acid. J Ethnopharmacol 28(2):235-41, 1990*).

Administration of TTFCA may be effective in reducing venous insufficiency.

Review Article: TTFCA is effective in venous insufficiency, reducing ankle edema, foot swelling, capillary filtration rate and by improving microcirculatory parameters. TTFCA displays a significant activity in venous hypertensive microangiopathy and its effects are dose-dependent (*Cesarone MR et al. [Activity of Centella asiatica in venous insufficiency]. Minerva Cardioangiol 40(4):137-43, 1992*) (*in Italian*).

Review Article: Centella has shown positive results in clinical trials in venous insufficiency. Centella's primary effects are to enhance the connective tissue structure of the perivascular sheath, reduce sclerosis, and improve blood flow through the affected limbs (*Kartnig T. Clinical applications of Centella asiatica (L.) Urb. Herbs Spices Med Plants 3:146-73, 1988*).

Experimental Double-blind Study: 94 pts. with venous insufficiency of the lower limbs randomly received titrated extract of *Centella asiatica* (TECA) 120 mg/d, TECA 60 mg/d or placebo. After 2 mo., a significant difference ($p<0.05$) was shown in favor of TECA for the symptoms of heaviness in the lower limbs and edema, as well as for the overall evaluation by the patient. Slightly better results were found for the higher dosage, but the difference in clinical improvement was not significant. In addition, the venous distensibility measured by a mercury strain gauge plethysmograph at 3 occlusion pressures was improved for the TECA gps. but aggravated for the placebo gp. (*Pointel JP, Boccalon H, Clarec M, et al. Titrated extract of Centella asiatica (TECA) in the treatment of venous insufficiency of the lower limbs. Angiology 38:46-50, 1987*).

Experimental Study: An extract of *Centella asiatica* was compared with that of tribenoside (ethyl-3,4,6-tri-O-benzyl-D-glucofuranoside) for the treatment of venous disease of the lower extremities. After 1 mo., both treatments caused a highly significant regression of venous insufficiency. Rheographic investigations indicated improved venous flow in 80% of pts. treated with *Centella asiatica* and in 73% of pts. treated with tribenoside. However, the extract of *Centella asiatica* was significantly more easily tolerated (*Marastoni F et al. Centella asiatica extract in venous pathology of the lower limbs and its evaluation as compared to tribenoside. Minerva Cardioangiol 30(4):201-7, 1982*) (*in Italian*).

See Also:

> *Allegra C [Comparative capillaroscopic study of certain bioflavonoids and total triterpenic fractions of Centella asiatica in venous insufficiency]. Clin Ter 110(6):555-9, 1984 (in Italian)*

> *Cospite M et al. [Study about pharmacologic and clnical activity of Centella asiatica titrated extract in the chronic venous deficiency of the lower limbs: Valuation with strain gauge plethismography]. G Ital Angiol 4(3):200-5, 1984 (in Italian)*

> *Cappelli R. [Clinical and pharmacological study on the effect of an extract of Centella asiatica in chronic venous insufficiency of lower limbs.] G Ital Angiol 3(1):44-8, 1983 (in Italian)*

> *Mariani G, Patuzzo E. [Treatment of venous insufficiency with extract of Centella asiatica]. Clin Eur (Italy) 22(1):154-8, 1983 (in Italian)*

> *Marastoni F et al. [Centella asiatica extract in venous pathology of the lower limbs and its evaluation as compared with tribenoside]. Minerva Cardioangiol 30(4):201-7, 1982 (in Italian)*

> *Allegra C. [Centella asiatica extract in venous disorders of the lower limbs. Comparative clinical and instrumental trial against a placebo]. Clin Ter 99(5):507-13, 1981 (in Italian)*

> *Bartella S et al. [Results with Centella asiatica in chronic venous insufficiency]. Gazz Med Ital 140(1):33-5, 1981 (in Italian)*

Administration of TTFCA may reduce damage to vascular endothelium in post-phebitis syndrome.

Experimental Study: A study was performed in order to assess the number of circulating endothelial cells (EC) in normal subjects and in pts. with postphlebitic syndrome (PPS), and the effect of treatment with TTFCA. Pts. with PPS showed an increased number of circulating EC in comparison to normal subjects (3.8 versus 1.5 cells per counting chamber). Treatment for three weeks with TTFCA caused a significant reduction (p<0.0001) of circulating EC (1.80 cells per counting chamber) *(Montecchio GP et al. Centella Asiatica Triterpenic Fraction (CATTF) reduces the number of circulating endothelial cells in subjects with post phlebitic syndrome. Haematologica 76(3):256-9, 1991).*

Ginkgo biloba:

The standard dose of *Ginkgo biloba* extract standardized to contain 24% ginkgoflavonglycosides is 40 mg three times daily.

Administration may protect against arterial hypoxia. *(See: 'CEREBROVASCULAR DISEASE')*

Experimental Double-blind Study: *Schaffler VK, Reeh PW. [Double-blind study of the hypoxia-protective effect of a standardized ginkgo bilobae preparation after repeated administration in healthy volunteers.] Arzneimittelforsch 35:1283-6, 1985 (in German)*

Administration may be beneficial in peripheral vascular insufficiency.

Meta-Analysis: 5 placebo-controlled clinical trials with GBE in patients with peripheral arterial disease were reviewed. In all studies treatment effect was quantified by the increase of walking distance (measured in standardized treadmill exercise test). The effect value of treatment was expressed by the standardized mean difference in walking distance increase between GBE and placebo, standardized by the standard deviation. This effect was homogeneous in all trials. The global effect size was estimated as 0.75. This means that the mean increase in walking distance achieved by GBE is 0.75 times of the standard deviation higher than that achieved by placebo *(Schneider B. [Ginkgo biloba extract in peripheral arterial diseases. Meta-analysis of controlled clinical studies]. Arzneim Forsch 42(4):428-36, 1992) (in German).*

Review Article: Because of a multitude of vascular effects, GBE may offer effective treatment for the signs, symptoms, and underlying pathophysiology of cerebral and peripheral vascular insufficiency. More than 40 and 9 double-blind studies have shown it be effective in cerebral and peripheral vascular insufficiency, respectively. GBE acts as an antioxidant, inhibits platelet aggregation and platelet activating factor, exerts vasoregulating activity, improves blood flow to ischemic areas, and enhances energy production during ischemia *(Kleijnen J, Knipschild P. Ginkgo biloba. Lancet 340:1136-9, 1992).*

Experimental Placebo-controlled Study: 37 pts. with stage 2 peripheral vascular disease randomly received GBE (Tanakan) or placebo. Scores on a visual analog scale of pain severity were significantly improved after 24 wks. only in the experimental group. Claudication distance was significantly increased by GBE, and increased only insignificantly in the control group. However, A/B ratio, Doppler ankle responses to exercise and post-exercise recovery time failed to show significant changes *(Thomson GJ et al. A clinical trial of Gingkco Biloba Extract in patients with intermittent claudication. Int Angiol 9(2):75-8, 1990).*

Experimental Double-blind Study: 64 pts. with intermittent claudication and pain at rest were given GBE (200 mg/d) or placebo for 8 days. 51% of pts. taking GBE noted a decrease of pain intensity compared to 25% in the placebo group (*Saudreau F et al. [Efficacy of Ginkgo biloba extract in the treatment of lower limb obliterative artery disease at stage III of the Fontaine classification]. J Mal Vasc 14:177-82, 1989*) (*in French*).

Experimental Double-blind Crossover Study: In an acute trial, an intravenous application of GBE (35 mg) was tested on pts. with intermittent claudication. With GBE the pts. were able to sustain exercise longer; the lactate pyruvate quotient was lower; blood viscosity was significantly reduced; and perfusion to affected limbs was greatly improved (*Rudofsky VG. [The effect of Ginkgo biloba extract in cases of arterial occlusive disease. A randomized placebo controlled double-blind cross-over study]. Fortschr Med 105:397-400, 1987*) (*in German*).

Experimental Study: 27 pts. with peripheral occlusive arterial disease received GBE 120 mg daily for 3 years. The maximum walking distance of pts. after exercise quadrupled, regardless of whether this was originally poor or relatively good. There was also a very impressive increase in ankle pressure after exercise (*Bauer U. Long-term treatment of peripheral occlusive arterial disease with Ginkgo biloba extract (GBE). A three year study. Vasa Suppl 15:26, 1986*).

Experimental Double-blind Study: 79 pts. (ave. age 61) with peripheral arterial insufficiency randomly received either GBE or placebo. After 24 wks., those receiving GBE demonstrated significantly greater pain-free and maximum walking distance, as well as improved plethysmographic and doppler measurements in the affected limb after exercise. Subsequently, 36 pts. receiving GBE continued the extract on an open trial basis for 65 weeks. Its beneficial effects were found to be stable over time and there were no significant side effects (*Bauer U. [Ginkgo biloba extract in the treatment of arteriopathy of the lower limbs. Sixty-five week study.] Presse Médicale 15(31):1546-9, 1986; Bauer U. 6-month double-blind randomized clinical trial of ginkgo biloba extract versus placebo in two parallel groups in patients suffering from peripheral arterial insufficiency. Arzneim Forsch 34:716-21, 1984*).

Experimental Double-blind Crossover Study: 26 pts. (ave. age 66) with peripheral arterial insufficiency received GBE and placebo in random order. After 6 wks. on GBE, pts. demonstrated a 75% increase in pain-free walking distance compared to when they were on placebo (*Salz H. Therap d Gegenward 119:1345, 1980*).

Experimental Double-blind Crossover Study: 40 pts. aged 41-90 with peripheral arterial insufficiency received GBE and placebo in random order. After 4 wks. on GBE, pts. demonstrated a 46% increase in pain-free walking distance compared to when they were on placebo (*Courbier R et al. Etude a double insu coissee du Tanakan dans les arteriopathies des membres inferierurs. Medit Med 126:61-4, 1977*).

See Also:

> *DeFeudis FV. Ginkgo Biloba Extract (EGb 761). Pharmacological Activities and Clinical Applications. Paris, Elsevier, 1991*

> *EW Funfgeld, Ed. Rokan (Ginkgo Biloba). Recent Results in Pharmacology and Clinic. New York, Springer-Verlag, 1988*

Hawthorn (*Crataegus* spp.):

Hawthorn extracts concentrated for procyanidins may produce similar benefit to procyanidolic oligomers (*see below*). (*See: 'ATHEROSCLEROSIS'*)

> **Experimental Study:** Injection of Crataegus extract improved blood flow and walking distance in 20 pts. with intermittent claudication (*Di Renzi L et al. [On the use of injectable crataegus extracts in therapy of disorders of peripheral arterial circulation in subjects with obliterating arteriopathy of the lower extremities]. Boll Soc Ital Cardiol (1969) 14(4):577-85, 1969*) (*in Italian*).

Horsechestnut (*Aesculus hippocastanum*):

Horsechestnut seeds have a long folk history of use in the treatment of varicose veins and hemorrhoids. The active component is escin (syn. aescin).
Escin exerts venotonic, anti-edema and anti-inflammatory properties as well as decreases capillary permeability by reducing the number and size of the small pores of the capillary walls. (*See: 'VASCULAR FRAGILITY'*)

The oral dosage is based upon escin content with 50 mg of escin three times daily.

> *Note: Although horsechestnut ingestion can produce significant toxicity, it appears to be reasonably safe for adults and the usual therapeutic dosages. Preparations should be kept out of the reach of children, however.*

Horsechestnut or escin preparations may be effective in <u>venous insufficiency</u>, both when taken internally and when applied topically.

> **Review Article:** Horsechestnut extracts standardized to contain 50 mg of aescin per dose exert tonic effects on the veins, and decrease venous and capillary permeability. The mechanism of action is not fully understood, although there is recent evidence suggesting that they may attenuate lysosomal proteoglycan destructing enzymes, which show increase activity in pts. with chronic venous insufficiency. In several double-blind randomized cross-over studies, subjective complaints were diminished and objective paramaters improved. Horsechestnut extracts are well tolerated (*Hitzenberger G. [The therapeutic effectiveness of chestnut extract]. Wien Med Wochenschr 139(17):385-9, 1989*) (*in German*).

> **Experimental Double-blind Study:** Horse chestnut has an inhibitory effect on edema formation via a decrease in transcapillary filtration and thus improves edema-related symptoms in venous diseases of the legs. 22 pts. with proven chronic venous insufficiency determined by measuring the capillary filtration coefficient and the intravascular volume of the lower leg by venous-occlusion plethysmograph were given a horse chestnut seed extract (600 mg providing 50 mg aescin) or a placebo. Three hours after administration, the capillary filtration coefficient had decreased by 22% in the treated gp., whereas in the placebo gp. the coefficient actually rose. The difference in the effect of horse chestnut extract and placebo was statistically significant ($p=0.006$) (*Bisler H et al. [Effects of horse-chestnut seed extract on transcapillary filtration in chronic venous insufficiency]. Dtsch Med Wochenschr 111(35):1321-9, 1986*) (*in German*).

See Also:

> **Experimental Study:** *Pedrini L, Cifiello BI. [Modification of venous function after pharmacologic treatment. Plethysmographic study.] Clin Ter 106(4):271-7, 1983 (in Italian)*

The efficacy of escin in the treatment of varicose veins and capillary fragility may be due to its ability to prevent destruction of glycosaminoglycans by enzymes.

> **Experimental Double-blind Study:** The serum activity of 3 lysosomal glycosaminoglycan hydrolases were studied in 18 healthy subjects and 15 pts. with varicose veins. In pts. with varicose veins elevated levels of b-glucuronidase (+70%), beta-N-acetylglucosaminidase (+63.5%), and arylsulphatase (+121.7%) were found. In the 15 pts. with varicosities, after 12 days of treatment with horsechestnut extract 300 mg (containing 50 mg escin) 3 times daily, the enzymes were significantly reduced by 29.1%, 25.7%, and 28.7%, respectively, compared to placebo *(Kreysel HW, Nissen HP, Enghoffer E. A possible role of lysosomal enzymes in the pathogenesis of varicosis and the reduction in their serum activity by venostasin. VASA 12:377-82, 1983).*

Escin appears to exert a tonic effect on human saphenous vein.

> **In vitro Experimental Study:** Histologically normal segments of human saphenous veins were stimulated with escin. Stimulation always induced an increase in venous tone which was constant for a given dose and stable for some time. The increase was maintained for as long as one hour after removal of the substance from the bath *(Annoni F et al. Venotonic activity of escin on the human saphenous vein. Arzneim Forsch 29:672-5, 1975).*

Procyanidolic oligomers:

Procyanidolic oligomers (PCOs), also known as leukocyanidins or pycnogenols) are complexes of flavonoids (polyphenols). Most commercial preparations use PCOs extracted from grape seed skin (*Vitis vinifera*), although PCOs can also be extracted from the bark of Landes' pine, the bracts of the lime tree, and the leaves of the hazel-nut tree. (*See: 'VASCULAR FRAGILITY'*)

The standard therapeutic dosage of PCOs is 150 to 300 mg per day.

PCOs stabilize collagen and ground substance, including collagen structures that support blood vessels.

> **Review Article:** PCOs increase intracellular vitamin C levels, decrease capillary permeability and fragility, scavenge oxidants and free radicals, and possess a unique ability to bind to collagen structures directly as well as inhibit destruction of collagen. Collagen, the most abundant protein of the body, is responsible for maintaining the integrity of "ground substance" as well as the integrity of tendons, ligaments, and cartilage. Collagen also is the support structure of the dermis and blood vessels. Leukocyanidins and other flavonoids are remarkable in their effect in supporting collagen structures and preventing collagen destruction. They affect collagen metabolism in several ways. They have the unique ability to crosslink collagen fibers, resulting in reinforcement of the natural crosslinking of collagen that forms the so-called collagen matrix of

connective tissue (ground substance, cartilage, tendon, etc.). They prevent free radical damage with their potent antioxidant and free radical scavenging action. They inhibit enzymatic cleavage of collagen by enzymes secreted by white blood cells during inflammation, and microbes during infection. They prevent the release and synthesis of compounds that promote inflammation, such as histamine, serine proteases, prostaglandins, and leukotrienes. These effects on collagen are put to good use in the treatment of capillary fragility, easy bruising, and varicose veins (*Masquelier J. [Procyanidolic oligomers (leucocyanidins)]. Parfums Cosmet Arom 95:89-97, 1990*) (*In French*).

Animal Experimental Study: PCOs bound to insoluble elastin markedly affect its rate of degradation by elastases. Insoluble elastin pretreated with PCOs was resistant to the hydrolysis induced by both porcine pancreatic and human leukocyte elastases. The quantitative adsorption of pancreatic elastase was similar on either untreated or PCO-treated elastin suggesting that the binding of this compound to elastin increases the non-productive catalytic sites of elastase molecules. PCOs bind to skin elastic fibres when injected intradermally into young rabbits. As a result, these elastic fibres were found more resistant to the hydrolytic action of porcine pancreatic elastase when injected to the same site emphasizing their potential effect preventing elastin degradation by elastases as occurred in inflammatory processes (*Tixier JM et al. Evidence by in vivo and in vitro studies that binding of pycnogenols to elastin affects its rate of degradation by elastases. Biochem Pharmacol 33(24):3933-9, 1984*).

Animal Experimental Study: PCOs of grape seed skin (*Vitis vinifera*) were found to have an affinity for the collagen structures that support arteries, capillaries, and veins (*Harmand MF, Blanquet P. The fate of total flavonolic oligomers (OGFT) extracted from "Vitis vinefera L." in the rat. Eur J Drug Metab Pharmacokin 1:15-30, 1978*).

See Also:

> *Masquelier J et al. [Stabilization of collagen with procyanidolic oligomers]. Acta Therapeutica 7:101-5, 1981 (In French)*

> *Masquelier J. Pycnogenols: Recent advances in the therapeutic activity of procyanidins, in Natural Products as Medicinal Agents, vol. 1. Stuttgart, Hippokrates Verlag, 1981:243-56*

> *Masquelier J et al. Flavonoids and pycnogenols. Int J Vit Nutr Res 49:307-11, 1979*

Administration may reduce veno-lymphatic insufficiency (*Henriet JP. [Veno-lymphatic insufficiency. 4,729 pts. undergoing hormonal and procyanidol oligomer therapy]. Phlebologie (1993 Apr-Jun) 46(2):313-25, 1993*) (in French).

Administration may reduce the symptoms of varicose veins (*Gomez Trillo JT. [Varicose veins of the lower extremities. Symptomatic treatment with a new vasculotrophic agent]. Prensa Med Mex 38(7):293-6, 1973 (In Spanish)*

Ruscus aculeatus:

Ruscus aculeatus (Butcher's broom) is a sub-shrub of the lily family that grows in the Mediterranean region. The rhizome from butcher's broom has a long history of use in treating venous disorders such as hemorrhoids and varicose veins.

The active ingredients in butcher's broom are known as ruscogenins. These compounds have demonstrated a wide range of pharmacological actions, including anti-inflammatory and vasoconstrictor effects.

The standard dosage of Ruscus is based on the ruscogenin content. For best results the dosage of any Ruscus preparation should supply 16.5 to 33 mg of ruscogenins 3 times daily.

Most clinical research has employed a Ruscus extract standardized for ruscogenin in combination with trimethyl hesperidine chalcone and ascorbic acid.

Administration may be effective for venous insufficiency.

- with Hesperidine methylchalcone:

Experimental Double-blind Study: In 20 healthy volunteers, the efficacy of the combination of Ruscus extract and hesperidine methylchalcone (HMC) was determined by comparing the effectiveness of the individual substances, the combination and a placebo on the venous hemodynamics and the volume of the foot. Ruscus extract augmented the tonicity of the venous wall. This is expressed by a decrease in venous capacity, a reduction in the blood pool in the lower leg under orthostatic conditions, and a decrease in tissue volume of the foot and ankle. HMC lowered the capillary filtration rate but augmented the blood pool. The increase in blood volume can be explained by dehydration of the tissue of the lower leg lowering the pressure of tissue on the venous system and increasing the blood pool in the limb. After administration of the combination, the blood volume was between the Ruscus and HMC volumes, while the effects on filtration rate, venous capacity and tissue volume corresponded to the changes seen after administration of HMC and Ruscus extract alone (*Rudofsky G. [Improving venous tone and capillary sealing. Effect of a combination of Ruscus extract and hesperidine methyl chalcone in healthy probands in heat stress].* Fortschr Med *107(19):52, 55-8, 1989*) (*in German*).

- with Hesperidin and Vitamin C:

Experimental Double-blind Crossover Study: The effectiveness and tolerability of a venotropic drug (RAES) composed of an extract of *Ruscus aculeatus* (16.5 mg), hesperidin (75 mg) and ascorbic acid (50 mg) were evaluated in 40 pts. (30 female, 10 male) aged between 28 and 74 years, suffering from chronic venous insufficiency of the lower limbs. Symptoms of edema, itching, paraesthesia, leg heaviness, and cramps decreased significantly more with treatment. Phlethysmography results also demonstrated significant improvement with RAES compared to placebo. No side effects were reported (*Cappelli R, Nicora M, Di Perri T. Use of extract of Ruscus aculeatus in venous disease in the lower limbs.* Drugs Exp Clin Res *14(4):277-83, 1988*).

- with <u>Trimethylhesperidine chalcone</u> and <u>Vitamin C</u>:

> **Experimental Double-blind Study:** 50 pts. suffering from trunk or branch varicosis were orally treated with either a commercial preparation of Ruscus extract, trimethyl hesperidine chalcone and ascorbic acid (Phlebodril), or a placebo over 2 weeks. Changes of the venous tonus were measured by means of venous occlusion plethysmography in rest position (venous capacity, venous distensibility) as well as during (active) exercise (expelled blood volume). All parameters showed a tendency towards improvement in the treated gp. However, the course of the study suggests that the period of treatment was too short to obtain the full pharmacologic effect (*Weindorf N, Schultz-Ehrenburg U. [Controlled study of increasing venous tone in primary varicose veins by oral administration of Ruscus aculeatus and trimethylhespiridinchalcone].* <u>Z Hautkr</u> *62(1):28-38, 1987*) (*in German*).

See Also:

> *Elbaz C, Nebot F, Reinharez D. [Venous insufficiency of the lower limbs. Controlled study of the action of Cyclo 3].* <u>Phlebologie</u> *29(1):77-84, 1976 (in French)*

Topical application may be effective for <u>venous insufficiency</u>.

> **Experimental Double-blind Study:** The venoconstrictive action of the topical application of Ruscus extract was evaluated using duplex B-scan ultrasonography. Within 2 1/2 hours of the application of 4 to 6 g of a cream containing 64 to 96 mg Ruscus extract, the diameter of the femoral vein decreased by an average (median) of 1.25 mm, while placebo (base of the cream) was associated with a diameter increase of 0.5 mm (means) ($p=0.014$). The decrease in venous diameter reflects good percutaneous absorption of the active substance (*Berg D. [Venous constriction by local administration of ruscus extract].* <u>Fortschr Med</u> *108(24):473-6, 1990*) (*in German*).

See Also:

> *Marcelon G et al. Effect of Ruscus aaculeatus on isolated cutaneous veins.* <u>Gen Pharmacol</u> *14:103, 1983*

- -

COMBINATION TREATMENT

<u>Padma 28</u>:

Padma 28 is a commercial product based on an ancient Tibetan (lamaistic) formula. It contains a mixture of 28 different herbs.

Administration may reduce <u>intermittent claudication</u>.

> **Experimental Double-blind Study:** 36 pts. (median age 67 yrs.) with intermittent claudication for a median duration of 5 yrs. randomly received either Padma 28 (two 380 mg tablets twice daily) or placebo. After 4 months, the pts. receiving Padma 28 attained a significant increase in pain-free walking distance from 52 m to 86 m and a significant increase in maximal walking distance from 115 m to 227 m. No significant

changes were noted in the placebo gp.   (*Drabaek H, Mehlsen J, Himmelstrup H, Winther K. A botanical compound, Padma 28, increases walking distance in stable intermittent claudication. Angiology 44(11):863-7, 1993*).

Experimental Double-blind Study: 43 pts. with intermittent claudication were given either Padma 28 or placebo. The pts. had a disease history of at least 8 months, a steady state for symptoms (maximum walking distance below 250 m), and were distributed randomly in the two gps. After 16 weeks the pts. treated with Padma 28 exhibited on standardized ergometry an increase of nearly 100% in the maximum as well as painfree walking distance. The control pts. showed increases of 21% in maximum and 46% in painfree walking distance. Padma 28 was well tolerated and no side effects were reported (*Schrader R, Nachbur B, Mahler F. [Effects of the Tibetan herbal preparation Padma 28 in intermittent claudication]. Med Wochenschr 115(22):752-6, 1985*) (*in German*).

PREGNANCY-RELATED ILLNESS

See Also: **DIABETES MELLITUS**
HYPERTENSION
NAUSEA AND VOMITING

Bilberry (*Vaccinium myrtillus*):

Bilberry or European blueberry contains flavonoid compounds known as anthocyanosides. Bilberry anthocyanosides are potent antioxidants that improve the microcirculation and protect the vascular endothelium. Bilberry anthocyanosides exert similar effects to procyanidolic oligomers (*see below*). (*See: 'RETINOPATHY'; 'VASCULAR FRAGILITY'*)

The standard dose for Vaccinium myrtillus extract (VME) is based on its anthocyanoside content, as calculated by its anthocyanidin percentage. Most studies have used a bilberry extract standardized for an anthocyanidin content of 25% at a dosage of 160 mg to 480 mg daily.

Administration of VME may be effective in preventing and treating varicose veins of pregnancy (*Grismond GL. [Treatment of pregnancy-induced phlebopathies.] Minerva Ginecol 33:221-30, 1981*) (*in Italian*).

Ginger (*Zingiber officinale*):

Administration may treat hyperemesis gravidarum (severe nausea & vomiting).

Experimental Double-blind Crossover Study: 27 women with hyperemesis gravidarum requiring hospitalization received powdered ginger root 250 mg 4 times daily and a lactose placebo, each for 4 days, with a 2-day washout period. Significantly greater symptom relief occurred after ginger compared to placebo. 70.4% of the women felt better taking ginger than taking placebo (p=0.003). Specifically, ginger appeared to reduce the degree of nausea and the number of attacks of vomiting. There were no side effects (*Fischer-Rasmussen W et al. Ginger treatment of hyperemesis gravidarum. Eur J Obstet Gynaecol Reprod Biol 38:19-24, 1990*).

Clinical Observations: Ginger root capsules were effective in reducing or eliminating pregnancy nausea in >75% of cases. The most successful pts. took 3-8 caps before arising, and then 3-5 more at the first hint of nausea. There was no evidence of side effects (*Mowrey DB. The Scientific Validation of Herbal Medicine. Cormorant Books, 1986, p. 199*).

Case Report: A woman experienced severe hyperemesis gravidarum through the full term of her first pregnancy, most of which she spent in the hospital. Six yrs. later, halfway through her second, equally devastating pregnancy, she began to ingest ginger in 500 mg capsules (up to 20/d to "keep ahead of that queasy feeling"). Treatment was strikingly effective and her symptoms remained under control throughout her pregnancy. Since then she has completed 2 more successful pregnancies while consuming ginger without experiencing significant hyperemesis gravidarum (*Roach B. Townsend Letter for Doctors July, 1983, September, 1984 & June, 1986*).

Jasmine Flowers:

Fresh jasmine flowers stringed into cotton thread are used by Indian women for hair adornment. Applying fresh jasmine flowers to the breast is also an old folk remedy for suppression of breast milk.

Experimental Study: 60 women requiring suppression of lactation because of stillbirth or neonatal death were divided into 2 gps. Gp. I was given bromocriptine, gp. II were treated with jasmine flowers. Each breast had 50 cm. of stringed flowers applied to it. The flowers were held in place by adhesive tape. Clinical assessment (breast engorgement, mild production, and analgesic intake) demonstrated both treatments are equally effective. Both treatments lowered serum prolactin levels, bromocriptine more than jasmine flowers (*Shrivastav P et al. Suppression of puerperal lactation using jasmine flowers (Jasminum sambac). Aust NZ J Obstet Gynaecol 28:68-71, 1988*).

PROSTATITIS

Pygeum africanum:

A tropical African evergreen tree.

Administration of extracts of the bark (standardized to contain 14% beta-sitosterol and 0.5% n-docosanol) may be beneficial at a dosage of 50-100 mg twice daily. (*See: 'BENIGN PROSTATIC HYPERPLASIA'*)

Experimental Study: 18 pts. with benign prostatic hypertrophy or chronic prostatitis and, simultaneously, sexual disturbances, received an extract of *Pygeum africanum* (Tadenan®, Roussel-Pharma) 200 mg daily. After 60 days, the extract had improved all the urinary parameters that were investigated. Also, sexual behavior was reported to be improved despite a lack of change in the levels of sex hormones or in nocturnal penile tumescence and rigidity. No side effects were observed (*Carani C, Salvioli V, Scuteri A, et al. [Urological and sexual evaluation of treatment of benign prostatic disease using Pygeum africanum at high doses.] Arch Ital Urol Nefrol Androl 63(3):341-5, 1991*) (*in Italian*).

- -

COMBINATION TREATMENT

Flower Pollen:

Administration of a standardized extract of flower pollen (Cernilton®, Cernitin SA, Lugano, Switzerland) may be beneficial.

Note: In vitro studies suggest that Cernilton® is a potent cyclo-oxygenase and lipoxgenase inhibitor and a smooth muscle relaxant (Buck AC, Rees RW, Ebeling L. Treatment of chronic prostatitis and prostatodynia with pollen extract. Br J Urol 64(5):496-9, 1989).

Experimental Study: 90 pts. with chronic prostatitis received Cernilton N one tablet 3 times daily. After 6 mo., in the 72 pts. without complicating factors (urethral strictures, prostatic calculi or bladder neck sclerosis), 56 (78%) had a favorable response; 26 (36%) were cured of their signs and symptoms and 30 (42%) improved significantly with an increase in flow rate, a reduction in leukocyturia in the post-prostate massage urine and a decrease in complement C3/ceruloplasmin in the ejaculate. In the 18 pts. with complicating factors, however, only 1 pt. showed a response; thus complicating factors should be considered in pts. who fail to respond to treatment within 3 months. The extract was well tolerated by 97% of pts. (*Rugendorff EW, Weidner W, Ebeling L, Buck AC. Results of treatment with pollen extract (Cernilton N) in chronic prostatitis and prostatodynia. Br J Urol 71(4):433-8, 1993*).

Experimental Study: 25 pts. with chronic prostatitis received Cernilton tablets. Improvement of subjective symptoms and objective findings was noted in 96% and 76%, respectively. Sonographic finding showed 33-100% improvement in 4 objective parameters. No side effects were observed (*Suzuki T, Kurokawa K, Mashimo T, et al. [Clinical effect of Cernilton in chronic prostatitis.] Hinyokika Kiyo 38(4):489-94, 1992*) (*in Japanese*).

Experimental Study: 13/15 pts. with chronic prostatitis and prostodynia with a mean duration of 3.3 yrs. were treated with Cernilton, 2 tabs twice daily. 7 had complete and lasting symptom relief, while 6 had marked improvement. Most pts. who responded (11/13) did not start to show improvement until 3 mo. after starting treatment, and symptoms recurred in 2 pts. who stopped treatment. No adverse reactions were seen (*Buck AC, Rees RW, Ebeling L. Treatment of chronic prostatitis and prostatodynia with pollen extract. Br J Urol 64(5):496-9, 1989*).

Experimental Study: 32 pts. with chronic prostatitis received Cernilton 6 tabs daily. After an average of 6 wks., improvement of subjective symptoms and objective findings was noted in 74.2% and 65.6%, respectively. The effective rate was 75%. No subjective side effects or abnormal changes in laboratory data were observed (*Jodai A, Maruta N, Shimomae E, et al. [A long-term therapeutic experience with Cernilton in chronic prostatitis.] Hinyokika Kiyo 34(3):561-8, 1988*) (*in Japanese*).

Experimental Double-blind Study: Based on a grading system using both objective and subjective measures, of 14 pts. with non-gonorrheal prostatitis and urethritis given Cernilton 4 tabs daily, it was 'effective' in 10 (71%), and 'slightly effective' in 3 (21%). Of 16 pts. given placebo, it was 'effective' in 7 (44%) and 'slightly effective' in none. Subjective symptoms disappeared in 10 pts. (71%) and diminished in 4 (29%) while the rest had some degree of improvement in the Cernilton group. In the placebo gp., subjective symptoms disappeared in 5 pts. (31%), diminished in 2 (13%), and worsened in 2 (13%). In the Cernilton gp., there was normalization of the urinary sediment in 5 pts. (36%), improvement in 1 (7%), persistence of the abnormal state in 2 (14%), exacerbation in 1 (7%), and continuation of the normal state in 4 (29%) (the result in 1 pt. is unknown). In the placebo gp., there was normalization in 3 pts. (19%), improvement in 2 (13%), persistence of the abnormal state in 3 (13%) and persistence of the normal state in 8 (50%). For the Cernilton gp., urinary bacteria following prostatic massage disappeared in 3 pts. (21%), failed to change in 2 (14%), and remained normal in 9 (64%). For the placebo gp., bacteria disappeared in 1 pt. (6%), failed to change in 2 (13%), reappeared in 1 (6%) and remained normal in 12 (75%). There were no notable subjective or objective side effects (*Ohkoski M, Kawamura N, Nagakubo I. [Clinical evaluation of Cernilton in chronic prostatitis.] Rev Med Suiza 2(16):436-9, 1970*) (*in Spanish*).

See Also:

Kato T, Watanabe H, Takahashi H, et al. [Clinical experience on treatment of chronic prostatitis with Cernilton tablet.] Hinyokika Kiyo 16(4):192-5, 1970

Ask-Upmark E. Prostatitis and its treatment. Acta Med Scand 181(3):355-7, 1967

Diamant B. [Pollen?] Lakartidningen 64(11):1100-2, 1967 (in Swedish)

Andersson A, Linden W van der. [The treatment of chronic prostatitis with pollen.]
Z Urol Nephrol 59(6):437-40, 1966 (in German)

PSORIASIS

Capsaicin:

Capsaicin is the active component of cayenne pepper (*Capsicum frutescens*). When topically applied, capsaicin is known to stimulate and then block small-diameter pain fibers by depleting them of the neurotransmitter substance P. Substance P is thought to be the principal chemomediator of pain impulses from the periphery. In addition, substance P has been shown to activate inflammatory mediators in psoriasis.

Commercial ointments containing 0.025% or 0.075% capsaicin are available over-the-counter.

Topical application may be beneficial.

> **Experimental Double-blind Study:** Pts. applied capsaicin 0.025% cream (n=98) or vehicle (n=99) 4 times a day for 6 weeks. Efficacy was based on a physician's global evaluation and a combined psoriasis severity score including scaling, thickness, erythema, and pruritus. Capsaicin-treated pts. demonstrated significantly greater improvement in global evaluation (p=0.024 after 4 weeks and p=0.030 after 6 weeks) and in pruritus relief (p=0.002 and p=0.060, respectively), as well as a significantly greater reduction in combined psoriasis severity scores (p=0.030 and p=0.036, respectively). The most frequently reported side effect in both treatment gps. was a transient burning sensation at application sites (*Ellis CN et al. A double-blind evaluation of topical capsaicin in pruritic psoriasis. J Am Acad Dermatol 29(3):438-42, 1993*).

> **Experimental Double-blind Study:** 44 pts. with symmetrically distributed lesions applied topical capsaicin to one side of their body and a placebo to the other side. After 3-6 wks., significantly greater reductions in scaling and erythema accompanied capsaicin application. Burning, stinging, itching, and skin redness were noted by nearly half of the pts. initially but diminished or vanished upon continued application (*Bernstein JE et al. Effects of topically applied capsaicin on moderate and severe psoriasis vulgaris J Am Acad Dermatol 15(3):504-7, 1986*).

Oleum Horwathiensis:

Oleum Horwathiensis (Prosicur®) is a commercial product in Hungary that contains yarrow, garlic, calendula, dandelion, nettles, and veronica.

Topical application may be beneficial.

> **Experimental Double-blind Study:** The efficacy and tolerability of topically applied oleum horwathiensis were evaluated in a study of 42 pts. with chronic stable psoriasis. Both gps. of pts., 19 receiving oleum horwathiensis treatment and 23 receiving placebo treatment for 12 weeks, showed clinically relevant effects of treatment. Oleum hor-

wathiensis was more effective than placebo throughout the treatment period but the difference was not statistically significant at any time. No changes in laboratory values attributable to treatment were recorded. The symptoms of the oleum horwathiensis-treated gp. continued to be less severe than those of the placebo-treated gp. throughout the 12 weeks of follow- up. The follow-up period, however, occurred partly during the summer and since the clinical status of the pts. may have been affected by climate the difference between the treatment gps. was not analysed statistically. The tolerability and cosmetic acceptance of oleum horwathiensis were remarkably good, and good clinical efficacy in scalp lesions—which was not the subject of this study—was sponta-neously reported by several pts. (*Lassus A, Forsstrom S. A double-blind study compar-ing oleum horwathiensis with placebo in the treatment of psoriasis. J Int Med Res 19(2):137-46, 1991*).

Psoralea coryliforia:

For over 3000 years, the furocoumarin group of compounds (psoralens) combined with natu-ral sunlight have been used to treat skin disease (*McEnvoy MT, Stern RS. Rsoralens and related compounds in the treatment of psoriasis. Pharmac Ther 34:75-97, 1987*).

> *Note: Although psoralens (furocoumarins) occur naturally in Psoralea corylifolia and in certain other plants, the drugs available for therapeutic use in PUVA therapy (psoralen + ultraviolet light A) and other photochemotherapy are synthetic compounds (methoxsalen and trioxsalen).*

Sarsaparilla:

Sarsaparilla (*Smilax sarsaparilla*) contains saponins or steroid-like molecules which may bind to gut endotoxins and improve psoriasis.

Individuals with psoriasis have been shown to have high levels of circulating endotoxins (lipopolysaccharide components of the cell walls of gram negative bacteria). Binding of endotoxin in the gut is associated with clinical improvement in these individuals (*Juhlin L, Vahlquist C. The influence of treatment and fibrin microclot generation in psoriasis. Br J Dermatol 108:33-7, 1983*).

> **Experimental Controlled Study:** In a controlled study of 92 patients, an endotoxin-binding saponin (sarsaponin) from sarsaparilla greatly improved the psoriasis in 62% of the patients and resulted in complete clearance in 18%. Sarsaponin was more effective in the chronic, large plaque forming variety of psoriasis (*Thurman FM. The treatment of psoriasis with sarsaparilla compound. N Engl J Med 227:128-33, 1942*).

Silymarin:

Silymarin, the flavonolignan complex of milk thistle (*Silybum marianum*), has been reported to be of value in the treatment of psoriasis (*Weber G, Galle K. [The liver, a therapeutic target in dermatoses]. Med Welt 34:108-11, 1983*) (*in German*).

Its efficacy is likely to be due to its ability to improve liver function, inhibit inflammation, and reduce excessive cellular proliferation. (*See: 'HEPATITIS'*)

RETINOPATHY
Including MACULAR DEGENERATION and RETINITIS PIGMENTOSA

See Also: DIABETES MELLITUS

<u>Bilberry:</u>

Bilberry or European blueberry (*Vaccinium myrtillus*) contains flavonoid compounds known as anthocyanosides, potent antioxidants that improve the microcirculation and promote the formation of visual purple. (*See: 'PERIPHERAL VASCULAR DISEASE'*)

The standard dose for *Vaccinium myrtillus* extract (VME) is based on its anthocyanoside content, as calculated by its anthocyanidin percentage. Most studies have used a bilberry extract standardized for an anthocyanidin content of 25% at a dosage of 160 mg to 480 mg daily.

Administration of VME may be beneficial.

Experimental Study: 31 pts. with various types of retinopathy (20 with <u>diabetic retinopathy</u>; 5 with <u>retinitis pigmentosa</u>; 4 with <u>macular degeneration</u>; 2 with <u>hemorrhagic retinopathy</u> due to anti-coagulant therapy) were treated with VME. A tendency towards reduced permeability and tendency to hemorrhage was observed in all pts., expecially those with diabetic retinopathy (*Scharrer A, Ober M. [Anthocyanosides in the treatment of retinopathies]. <u>Klin Monatsbl Augenheilkd</u> 178:386-9, 1981*) (*in German*).

See Also:

> Bonanni R, Molinelli G. *[Clinical study of the action of myrtillin alone or associated with beta-carotene on normal subjects and on patients with degenerative changes of the fundus oculi.] <u>Atti Accad Fisiocrit Siena [Med Fis]</u> 17(2):1470-88, 1968 (in Italian)*

Administration of VME may improve visual function in <u>retinitis pigmentosa</u>. (*See: 'VISUAL DYSFUNCTION'*)

Negative Experimental Study: 6 pts. with retinitis pigmentosa were given a single oral dose of 200 mg of *Vaccinium myrtillus* anthocyanosides. Based on electro-retinography, the results were inconclusive (*Caselli L. Clinical and electroretinographic study on activity of anthocyanosides. <u>Arch Med Int</u> 37:29-35, 1985*).

- with <u>Beta-carotene</u>:

Experimental Study: 33 pts. (11 emmetropic, 11 ametropic, 11 with retinitis pigmentosa) administered 400 mg/day of *Vaccinium myrtillus* anthocyanosides and

20 mg/day of beta-carotene demonstrated improved adaptation to light and night vision, and enlargement of the visual field (*Fiorni G, Biancacci A, Graziano FM. [Perimetric and adaptometric modifications of anthocyanosides and beta-carotene.] Ann Ottal Clin Ocul 91:371-86, 1965*) (*in Italian*).

Ginkgo biloba:

The usual dose of *Ginkgo biloba* extract (GBE) standardized to contain 24% ginkgoflavonglycosides is 40 mg three times daily.

Administration of extracts of *Ginkgo biloba* leaves may be beneficial.   (*See: 'CEREBROVASCULAR DISEASE' ; 'PERIPHERAL VASCULAR DISEASE'*)

Experimental Double-blind Study: The chronic cerebral retinal insufficiency syndrome in elderly patients is an organ specific expression of a generalized vascular cerebral deficiency. In this study, retinal blood flow measurements were made on 24 pts. (4 men and 20 women with an age of 74.9 +/- 6.9 years). The effect of *Ginkgo biloba* extract (GBE) on the reversibility of visual field disturbances was tested using a randomized and double blind study-design in two phases and with two dose levels. The main parameter investigated in this study was the change in the luminous density difference threshold after therapy with GBE. In group B (GBE dose 160 mg/day) a significant increase in retinal sensitivity was seen within 4 weeks (p less than 0.05). In the lower dose (80 mg GBE/day) group (A), this change in retinal sensitivity was first seen after increasing the dose to 160 mg/day (p<0.01). The relative sensitivity of damaged retinal areas was more strongly influenced than 'healthy' areas. The assessment by both doctors and patients of the general condition of the patients showed a significant improvement after the course of therapy (*Raabe A, Raabe M, Ihm P. [Therapeutic follow-up using automatic perimetry in chronic cerebroretinal ischemia in elderly patients. Prospective double-blind study with graduated dose ginkgo biloba treatment (EGB 761)]. Klin Monatsbl Augenheilkd 199(6):432-8, 1991*) (*in German*).

Experimental Double-blind Study: 10 pts. with macular degeneration received either *Ginkgo biloba* extract 80 mg twice daily or placebo. Drug efficacy was assessed by fundoscopy and by measurements of visual acuity and visual field. After 6 mo., a statistically significant improvement in long-distance visual acuity was observed (*Lebuisson DA et al. [Treatment of senile macular degeneration with Ginkgo biloba extract. A preliminary double-blind drug vs. placebo study.] Presse Med 15(31):1556-8, 1986*) (*in French*).

Experimental Study: 46 pts. with, in most cases, severe vascular degenerative retinochoroidal circulatory disturbances or with glaucomatous visual field defects were treated with *Ginkgo biloba* extract 160 mg/day for 4 weeks, then 120 mg/day. Treatment success was assessed monthly by measuring visual acuity, visual field, funduscopy, pulse rate and blood pressure, sometimes including intraocular pressure, fluorescence angiography and ODG. Mild improvements were noted, but were deemed relevant due to the largely bad prognosis of these serious disorders (*Merte HJ, Merkle W. [Long-term treatment with Ginkgo biloba extract of circulatory disturbances of the retina and optic nerve.] Klin Monatsbl Augenheilkd 177(5):577-83, 1980*) (*in German*).

Procyanidolic Oligomers:

Procyanidolic oligomers (PCOs), also known as leukocyanidins or pycnogenols) are complexes of flavonoids (polyphenols). Most commercial preparations use PCOs extracted from grape seed skin (*Vitis vinifera*), although PCOs can also be extracted from the bark of Landes' pine, the bracts of the lime tree, and the leaves of the hazel-nut tree. (*See: 'PERIPHERAL VASCULAR DISEASE'*)

The standard therapeutic dosage of PCOs is 150 to 300 mg per day.

PCOs are potent antioxidants.

In vitro Study: PCOs from *Vitis vinifera* were found to be the most active of flavonoids tested for protection against superoxide and lipid peroxidation (*Meunier MT, Duroux E, Bastide E. [Free radical scavenger activity of procyanidolic oligomers and anthocyanosides with respect to superoxide anion and lipid peroxidation]. Plant Med Phytother 23(4):267-74, 1989) (in French)*.

Administration may be effective in diabetic retinopathy.

Experimental Study: *Soyeux A et al. [Endotelon. Diabetic retinopathy and hemorheology (preliminary study)]. Bull Soc Ophtalmol Fr 87(12):1441-4, 1987) (in French)*

RHEUMATOID ARTHRITIS

<u>Bromelain:</u>

Bromelain is a mixture of sulfur containing proteolytic enzymes or proteases obtained from the stem of the pineapple plant (*Ananas comosus*). (*See: 'INFLAMMATION'*).

The standard dosage of bromelain (1,800-2,000 m.c.u.) is 125-450 mg 3 times daily on an empty stomach.

Administration may be effective in reducing inflammation and the amount of corticosteroids needed.

Experimental Study: 25 pts. with stages II or III RA, along with 1 pt. with both RA and osteoarthritis, 2 pts. with OA alone and 1 pt. with gout had residual joint swelling and impairment in mobility following long-term corticosteroid therapy. Their doses were tapered to small maintenance doses and they received enteric-coated bromelain 20-40 mg 3-4 times daily with each mg equal to 2500 Rorer units of activity. In most pts. residual joint swelling was significantly reduced (p<0.01) and joint mobility was increased soon after supplementation was started. After 3 wks.- 13 mo. of observation, 8/29 (28%) had excellent results, 13/29 (45%) good results, 4/29 (14%) fair results and 4/29 (14%) poor results. The pt. with gout had poor results. One of the OA pts. had good results; the other fair results. It seemed that smaller amts. of steroids were needed when bromelain was given concurrently. There were no side effects (*Cohen A, Goldman J. Bromelains therapy in rheumatoid arthritis. <u>Pennsyl Med J</u> 67:27-30, June 1964*).

<u>Capsaicin:</u>

Capsaicin is the active component of cayenne pepper (*Capsicum frutescens*). When topically applied, capsaicin is known to stimulate and then block small-diameter pain fibers by depleting them of the neurotransmitter substance P. Substance P is thought to be the principal chemomediator of pain impulses from the periphery. In addition, substance P has been shown to activate inflammatory mediators into joint tissues in osteoarthritis and rheumatoid arthritis.

Commercial ointments containing 0.025% or 0.075% capsaicin are available over-the-counter.

Administration may be effective in relieving pain.

Experimental Double-blind Study: 70 pts. with osteoarthritis (OA) and 31 with rheumatoid arthritis (RA) received capsaicin or placebo for four weeks. The pts. were instructed to apply 0.025% capsaicin cream or its vehicle (placebo) to painful knees four times daily. Pain relief was assessed using visual analog scales for pain and relief, a categorical pain scale, and physicians' global evaluations. Most of the pts. continued to receive concomitant arthritis medications. Significantly more relief of pain was reported by the capsaicin-treated pts. than the placebo pts. throughout the study; after four weeks of capsaicin treatment, RA and OA pts. demonstrated mean reductions in pain of 57% and 33%, respectively. These reductions in pain were statistically significant compared with those reported with placebo (p=0.003 and p=0.033, respectively). According to the global evaluations, 80% of the capsaicin-treated pts. experienced a reduction in pain after two weeks of treatment. Transient burning was felt at the sites of application by 23 of the 52 capsaicin-treated pts.; two pts. withdrew from treatment because of this side effect *(Deal CL et al. Treatment of arthritis with topical capsaicin: a double-blind trial. Clin Ther 13(3):383-95, 1991).*

Topically-applied capsaicin may be more effective in osteoarthritis than rheumatoid arthritis.

Experimental Double-blind Study: 21 pts. with either RA (n=7) or OA (n=14) with painful involvement of the hands received applied either capsaicin 0.075% or vehicle-only cream to the hands 4 times daily. Assessments of pain (visual analog scale), functional capacity, morning stiffness, grip strength, joint swelling and tenderness (dolorimeter) were performed before randomization. Treatment was applied to each painful hand joint 4 times daily with reassessment at 1, 2 and 4 weeks after entry. Capsaicin reduced tenderness (p) and pain (p) associated with OA, but not RA as compared with placebo. A local burning sensation was the only adverse effect noted *(McCarthy GM, McCarty DJ. Effect of topical capsaicin in the therapy of painful osteoarthritis of the hands. J Rheumatol 19(4):604-7, 1992).*

Curcumin:

Curcumin is the yellow pigment and active component of turmeric *(Curcuma longa)*. *Curcuma longa* has been used in Ayurvedic medicine, the indigenous systems of medicine of India, both locally and internally, in the treatment of sprains and inflammation. *(See: 'INFLAMMATION')*

The recommended dosage for curcumin as an anti-inflammatory agent is 400 to 600 mg three times a day. To achieve a similar amount of curcumin using turmeric would require a dosage of 8,000 to 60,000 mg.

Experimental Double-Blind Study: Pts. received either curcumin (1,200 mg per day) or phenylbutazone (300 mg per day). The improvements in the duration of morning stiffness, walking time, and joint swelling were comparable in both groups. However, while phenylbutazone is associated with significant adverse effects, curcumin has not been shown to produce any side effects at the recommended dosage level *(Deodhar SD et al. Preliminary studies on antirheumatic activity of curcumin (diferuloyl methane). Ind J Med Res 71:632-4, 1980).*

Devil's Claw *(Harpagophytum procumbens)*:

Devil's claw is an herb native to Africa that has a long history of use in the treatment of arthritis.

May exhibit anti-inflammatory activity comparable to phenylbutazone *(Kampf R. Schweizerische Apotheker-Zeitung 114:337-42, 1976).*

Eicosanoid metabolism may not be involved in its mechanism of action.

> **Experimental Study:** Healthy volunteers took 4 capsules of 500 mg *H. procumbens* daily for 21 days. No biochemical effects on arachidonic acid or eicosanoid metabolism were noted (*Moussard C et al. A drug used in traditional medicine, Harpagophytum procumbens: No evidence for NSAID-like effect on whole blood eicosanoid production in human. Prostaglan Leukotri Essent Fatty Acids 46:283-6, 1992*).

Administration may be beneficial.

> **Experimental Study:** 43 pts. with various types of arthritis received Harpagophytum capsules (Arkopharma) 1.5 g daily for 60 days. 89% noted decreased pain intensity; 84% noted increased range of motion, and 86% noted decreased time for morning stiffness to wear off. Improvement was noted by the 8th day of treatment and gradually increased. Side effects were limited to slight digestive discomfort in 2 pts. (*Pinget M, Lecomte A. [The effects of Harpagophytum captules (Arkocaps) in degenerative rheumatology.] Médecine Actuelle 12(4):65-67, 1985*).

> **Experimental Study:** 72% of 84 pts. who received Harpagophytum reported good to very good results (*Dahout C. J Pharm Belg 35(2):143-49, 1980*).

The equivocal research results of Devil's claw in experimental models may reflect: a mechanism of action that is inconsistent with current anti-inflammatory drugs; a lack of quality control (standardization) of the Devil's claw preparations used; or inactivation of inflammatory principles during the process of digestion.

> **Animal Experimental Study:** An aqueous extract of *Harpagophytum procumbens* exhibited significant and dose dependent anti-inflammatory effects. The main iridoid glycoside, harpagoside, exerted no anti-inflammatory effect. Also, the anti-inflammatory effect of *H. procumbens* could be eliminated after an acid treatment similar to the physio-chemical conditions found in the stomach (*Lanhers MC et al. Anti-inflammatory and analgesic effects of an aqueous extract of Harpagophytum procumbens. Planta Med 58:117-23, 1992*)

> **Negative Animal Experimental Study:** At doses 100 times or greater than the recommended daily dose for humans, *H. procumbens* was completely ineffective in reducing rat hind foot edema. *H. procumbems* was also ineffective in inhibiting prostaglandin synthesis *in vitro* (*Whitehouse LW, Znamirowski M, Paul CJ. Devil's claw (Harpagophytum procumbens): no evidence for anti-inflammatory activity in the treatment of arthritic disease. Can Med Assoc J 129:249-51, 1983*).

> **Negative Animal Experimental Study:** No anti-inflammatory effect was noted for *H. procumbens* (*McLeod DW, Revell P, Robinson BV. Investigations of Harpagophytum procumbens (Devil's claw) in the treatment of experimental inflammation and arthritis in the rat. Br J Pharmacol 66:140P-141P, 1979*).

Feverfew (*Tanacetum parthenium*):

Feverfew has a long history of folk use in rheumatoid arthritis. It has been shown to inhibit the release of blood vessel dilating substances from platelets (serotonin and histamine) and inhibit the production of inflammatory substances (leukotrienes, serine proteases, etc.).

Commercial sources providing assurance of botanical identity and minimum required level of parthenolides are needed (*Awang DVC. Feverfew. Can Pharm J 122:266-70, 1989*).

The dosages of feverfew used in migraine studies (*See: 'HEADACHE'*) *were 25 mg of the freeze-dried pulverized leaves twice daily or 82 mg of dried powdered leaves once daily. While these low dosages may be effective in preventing a migraine attack, a higher dose (1 to 2 grams) appears to be necessary to reduce inflammation in rheumatoid arthritis.*

> *Note: The efficacy of feverfew is dependent upon adequate levels of parthenolide, the active ingredient. (The preparations used in successful clinical trials have a parthenolide content of 0.4-0.66%.)*

> > **Animal Ex vivo Study:** Extracts of fresh feverfew caused a dose- and time-dependent, irreversible inhibition of the contractile response of rabbit aortic rings to all receptor-acting agonists tested. The presence of potentially SH reacting parthenolide and other sesquiterpene alpha-methylenebutyrolactones in these extracts, and the close parellelism of pure parthenolide, suggest that the inhibitory effects are due to these compounds. Extracts of the dry leaves were not inhibitory and actually caused potent and sustained contractions of aortic smooth muscle; these extracts were found to be devoid or parthenolide or butyrolactones (*Barsby RWJ, Salan U, Knight BW, Hoult JRS. Feverfew and vascular smooth muscle: Extracts from fresh and dried plants show opposing pharmacological profiles, dependent upon sesquiterpene lactone content. Planta Medica 59:20-5, 1993*).

> > **Chemical Analysis:** The parthenolide content of over 35 different commercial preparations of feverfew was determined by bioassay, 2 HPLC methods, and NMR. The results indicate a wide variation in the amts. of parthenolide in commercial preparations. The majority of products contained no parthenolide or only traces (*Heptinstall S et al. Parthenolide content and bioactivity of feverfew (Tanacetum parthenium (L.) Schultz-Bip.). Estimation of commercial and authenticated feverfew products. J Pharm Pharmacol 44:391-5, 1992*).

> WARNING: No long-term toxicity studies have been conducted. While feverfew is extremely well-tolerated and no serious side effects have ever been reported, chewing the leaves can result in small ulcerations in the mouth and swelling of the lips and tongue in about 10% of users (*Awang DVC. Feverfew. Can Pharm J 122:266-70, 1989*).

This lack of parthenolide may explain the poor results in the following clinical study:

> **Negative Experimental Double-blind Study:** 41 female pts. randomly received either dried, chopped feverfew 70-86 mg or placebo capsules daily. After 6 wks., no important differences between clinical or laboratory variables between the 2 gps. were found (*Pattrick M et al. Feverfew in rheumatoid arthritis: a double blind, placebo controlled study. Ann Rheum Dis 48(7):547-9, 1989*).

Ginger (*Zingiber officinale*):

Administration may be beneficial.

> **Experimental Study:** 28 pts. with rheumatoid arthritis who had been taking powdered ginger for periods ranging from 3 months to 2.5 years were evaluated. Based on clinical observations, 75% of pts. experienced relief in pain or swelling. The recommended dosage was 500 to 1,000 mg per day, but many pts. took 3 to 4 times this amount. Pts. taking the higher dosages reported quicker and better relief. None reported side effects (*Srivastava KC, Mustafa T. Ginger (Zingiber officinale) in rheumatism and musculoskeletal disorders. Med Hypothesis 39:342-8, 1992*).

> **Experimental Study:** 7 pts. in whom conventional treatment had provided only temporary or partial relief with treated with ginger. One took 50 g/d of lightly cooked fresh ginger, while the other 6 took either 5 g fresh or 0.1-1 g of powdered ginger daily. All reported substantial improvement, including pain relief, better joint movement, and a decrease in swelling and morning stiffness. Two pts. also reported improvement in muscle stiffness (*Srivastava KC, Mustafa T. Ginger (Zingiber officinale) and rheumatic disorders. Med Hypotheses 29:25-8, 1989*).

Tripterygium wilfordi:

The root of *Tripterygium wilfordi* may be helpful, but should be used with great caution in children and either men or women of reproductive years as it may lead to amenorrhea or impaired spermatogenesis, respectively. Both of these side effects eventually disappear with discontinued use.

Several components exert anti-inflammatory action, but immunomodulation is thought to be the major mechanism of action. In the case of rheumatoid arthritis, ankylosing spondylitis, and other autoimmune disorders, *Tripterygium wilfordi* appears to act as an immunosuppressor, although its benefits occur faster than other disease modifying or immunosuppressive drugs. (*See: 'LUPUS'*)

The glycoside extract of the decorticated root is regarded as being better tolerated and less harmful to reproductive function than crude *Tripterygium wilfordi* preparations.

Administration may be effective in both rheumatoid arthritis and ankylosing spondylitis.

> **Experimental Double-blind, Crossover Study:** A glycoside extract of *Tripterygium wilfodii* hook F (TWH) with a code name of T2 was used in a double-blind, controlled, cross-over study on the treatment of 70 patients. T2 (60 mg daily) exhibited an overall effectiveness rate of 90% in Gp. A and 80% in Gp. B after 12 weeks of treatment. Side effects were common. Skin rash and cheilosis occurred in 55.5% of pts. in Gp. A and 28% in Gp. B. Amenorrhea occurred in 31% of women of child-bearing age in Gp. A and 5.5% in Gp. B. Postmenopausal vaginal bleeding occurred in 1 patient. Other side effects were GI discomfort, nausea, and mild abdominal pain. These side effects occurred early and disappeared spontaneously after a few days (*Tao XL et al. A prospective, controlled, double-blind, cross-over study of tripterygium wilfodii hook F in treatment of rheumatoid arthritis. Chin Med J 102(5):327-32, 1989*).

Experimental Study: In 144 pts. treated with the glycoside extract of *Tripterygium wilfordi*, the overall effective rate was 93.3% with 17.6% having total clinical remission, 37.5% effective treatment, and 37.5% noting improvement. The criteria of effectiveness were: 'clinical remission' if symptoms disappeared, articular function was recovered, and laboratory findings were normal; 'effective' treatment if joint pain was alleviated and there was a complete recovery of function, ESR became normal, and RF became negative; 'improvement' if joint pain was alleviated with increased mobility, and ESR decreased but not to normal; and 'no improvement' if symptoms, signs, and laboratory findings remained unchanged. Of 132 pts. with severe joint pain before therapy, 124 said the pain was reduced or gone. Most pts. noted benefit within the first 2 weeks of therapy. Side effects were common. Poor appetite was reported in 20%, dry mouth 18.7%, skin rash 15.9%, hyperpigmentation 13.2%, and nausea 6.9%. Gynecomastia occurred in 2 males and 23% of the women experienced amenorrhea or other menstrual disturbance (*Deyong Y. Clinical observation of 144 cases of rheumatoid arthritis treated with glycoside of radix Tripterygium wilfordii. J Trad Chin Med 3(2):125-9, 1983*).

Experimental Study: 95 pts. with rheumatoid arthritis and 38 pts. with ankylosing spondylitis were treated with a tincture of *Tripterygium wilfordi* root at a dose of 15-30 ml (equivalent to 1.8-3.6 g of crude root) daily in divided doses from 2 months to 2 years. Relief of joint pain to various degrees was accomplished in 98%. Some reduction of joint swelling and improved joint function was noted in 87%. Most pts. noted benefit within the first 2 weeks of therapy. Side effects were common, but were not serious. In menstruating women, 47% experienced amenorrhea or other menstrual disturbance (*Deyong Y. Clinical observation of 144 cases of rheumatoid arthritis treated with glycoside of radix Tripterygium wilfordii. J Trad Chin Med 3(2):125-9, 1983*).

Yucca Saponin Extract:

Administration may be beneficial.

Experimental Double-blind Study: 149 arthritis pts., 41.1% with a positive RA fixation test, were randomly given either yucca saponin extract ('Desert Pride Herbal Food Tablets') 4 daily (range of 2 - 8) or placebo in periods ranging from 1 wk. to 15 mo. before re-evaluation. 61% noted less swelling, pain and stiffness versus 22% on placebo. Some improved in days, some in wks., and some in 3 mo. or longer (*Bingham R et al. Yucca plant saponin in the management of arthritis. J Appl Nutr 27:45-50, 1975*).

- -

COMBINATION TREATMENT

Phytodolor N:

Phytodolor N is a commercial product available in Germany that contains hydroalcoholic extracts of European aspen or poplar (*Populus tremula*), goldenrod (*Solidago virgaurea*) and European ash (*Fraxinus excelsior*).

Animal Experimental Study: Aqueous/alcoholic extracts of *Populus tremula, Solidago virgaurea* and *Fraxinus excelsior* (components of Phytodolor N) were tested individually and in 3 different combinations for anti-inflammatory activity using carrageenan-induced edema and/or adjuvant-induced arthritis of the rat paw. The tested combinations as well as the individual extracts significantly reduced the paw edema to varying degrees and also dose-dependently inhibited the arthritic paw volume. The anti-inflammatory activity of the combinations was respectively comparable to the tested doses of diclofenac (*el-Ghazaly M et al. Study of the anti-inflammatory activity of Populus tremula, Solidago virgaurea and Fraxinus excelsior. Arzneim Forsch 42(3):333-6, 1992*).

Experimental Double-blind Study: In 40 pts. hospitalized with painful degenerative diseases, the additional requirement for nonsteroidal anti-inflammatory drugs (NAIDs) to obtain results identical with a given daily dose of either 3 x 30 drops of Phytodolor N or placebo administered over 3 weeks was investigated. Under Phytodolor N, a total of 100 mg of diclofenac and 1 tablet (500 mg) of paracetamol were additionally administered in 18 pts.; under placebo, 2,400 mg of diclofenac and 3 tablets of paracetamol. Additional medication was required on 3 days in the Phytodolor gp., and on 47 days in the placebo group. Under Phytodolor N, the improvements obtained were identical to those in the gp. receiving considerably higher doses of NSAIDs and placebo. Clinical improvements were marked and major improvements (p) occurred after only 1 week, with improvement being progressive. No side effects were observed (*Huber B. [Therapy of degenerative rheumatic diseases. Need for additional analgesic medication with Phytodolor N]. Fortschr Med 109(11):248-50, 1991*) (*in German*).

SCLERODERMA

Bromelain:

Bromelain is a mixture of proteolytic enzymes or proteases obtained from the stem of the pineapple plant (*Ananas comosus*). (*See: 'INFLAMMATION'*)

The standard dosage of bromelain (1,800-2,000 m.c.u.) is 125-450 mg 3 times daily on an empty stomach.

Administration may be beneficial.

> **Case Report:** A 32 year-old woman demonstrated clinical improvement with bromelain therapy. After 3 months she was once again able to clench her fist, eat normal portions of food, and sleep in reclining position (*Pierce HE. Pineapple proteases in the treatment of scleroderma - A case report. J Natl Med Assoc 56(3):272-3, 1964*).

Centella asiatica:

Centella asiatica (Gotu kola) has a long history of use in Chinese and Ayurvedic medicine. The primary active constituents of *Centella asiatica* are known to be triterpenoid acids.

Most research on Centella has been performed with either the total triterpenoid fraction of *Centella asiatica* (TTFCA) or isolated triterpenoids. TTFCA has also been referred to as the 'titrated extract of *Centella asiatica*' or TECA. Both extracts are composed of a mixture of 3 triterpenes: asiatic acid (30%), madecassic acid (30%) and asiaticoside (40%).

Administration of TTFCA may be beneficial.

> **Experimental Study:** 13 female pts. were treated with TTFCA (Madecassol®) 2 times weekly with 20 mg doses intramuscularly or 3 times weekly with 20 mg doses orally. Treatment was very successful in 3/13, successful in 8/13 and unsuccessful in 2/13. Improvement consisted of decreased skin induration, lessened arthralgia and improved finger mobility (*Sasaki S et al. Studies on the mechanism of action of asiaticoside (Madecassol) on experimental granulation tissue and cultured fibroblasts and its clinical application in systemic fibroblasts and its clinical application in systemic scleroderma. Acta Diabetol Lat 52:141-50, 1972; Sasaki S et al. Experimental and clinical effects of asiaticoside (Madecassol) on fibroblasts, granulomas, and scleroderma. Jap J Clin Dermatol 25:585-93, 1971*).

See Also:

> **Experimental Study:** *Szczepanski A, Dabrowska H, Blaszczyk M. [Madecassol in the treatment of scleroderma (preliminary study).] Przegl Dermatol 61(5):701-3, 1974 (in Polish)*

- -

COMBINATION TREATMENT

Piasclédine:

The total unsaponifiable extract from avocado and soy bean oils in an alcohol solution.

Administration may be beneficial.

> **Animal Experimental Study:** As piasclédine (Pharmascience, France) is said to be beneficial in scleroderma, the skin of rats fed on the extract was examined. Analysis showed the very probable presence of phystosterols and richer proportion of cholesterol precursors, particularly methostenol, compared to controls (*Chevallier F, Lutton C, Sulpice JC, D'Hollander F. [Influence of the daily ingestion of a total unsaponifiable extract from avocado and soy bean oils on cholesterol metabolism in the rat. Pathol Biol (Paris) 23(3):225-30, 1975) (in French).*

> **Experimental Study:** 50 pts. (17 males; 33 females), 12 of whom with scleroderma of infancy, were treated. Dermatological manifestations were predominant except for 6 pts. who had associated esophageal symptoms and 1 pt. who had pulmonary sclerosis with repeated episodes of pneumothorax. Following at least 1 year's treatment with piasclédine (Pharmascience, Paris) 300 mg daily, 50% showed favorable clinical or biological changes. All of the 14 pts. with Raynaud's syndrome responded; they had better finger movement and better cold adaptation during the winter as well as a reduction in the frequency and severity of necrotic ulcers. 5 had 'good results' and 9 had 'partial success'. 4/6 pts. with esophageal reflux were 'quite improved' in regard to the amt. of reflux and the level of pain with the passage of food. Pts. have been followed for up to 7 yrs. and no toxicity has been found (*Lamberton JN. [Antisclerotic therapy of scleroderma: insaponifiable oils of avocado and soya. 50 clinical applications of H. Thiers treatment.] Presse Med 78(27):1235-6, 1970) (in French).*

See Also:

> *Petrova IL, Shakhnes IE. [Treatment of scleroderma with piasclédine]. Vestn Dermatol Venerol (10):46-8, 1979 (in Russian)*

> *Szczepanski A, Dabrowska H, Moskalewska K. [Effect of piasclédine treatment of scleroderma.] Przegl Dermatol 62(4):555-8, 1975 (in Polish)*

> *Szczepanski A, Dabrowska H, Moskalewska K. [Piasclédine in the treatment of scleroderma.] Przegl Dermatol 61(4):525-7, 1974 (in Polish)*

> *Chaze J. [Treatment of hypodermatitis of the leg with unsaponifiable extracts of avocado and soya.] Phlebologie 25(3):315-18, 1972 (in French)*

> *Coget J-M, Mosca P, Merlen J-F. [Treatment of sclerodermic states by an unsaponifiable extract of avocado and soybean.] Gaz méd Fr No. 20, May 21, 1971 (in French)*

Lamberton JN. [An "anti-sclerotic" therapy of scleroderma: an unsaponifiable extract of avocado and soy oils.] Gaz méd Fr No. 24, September 25, 1970 (in French)

Lattes GA. [Clinical study of the action of an unsaponifiable extract of soybean and avocado in stomatology.] Rev Stomatol (Paris) 71:577-80, 1970 (in French)

Thiers H et al. [A group of new therapeutic agents: the unsaponifiable extract of vegetable oils, their carotenoids, their phytosterols and their indeterminates administered in an alcoholic solution.] Thérapie 16:235-51, 1961 (in French)

SPORTS INJURIES

See Also: WOUND HEALING

Bromelain:

Bromelain is a mixture of sulfur containing proteolytic enzymes or proteases obtained from the stem of the pineapple plant (*Ananas comosus*). (*See: 'INFLAMMATION'*).

The standard dosage of bromelain (1,800-2,000 m.c.u.) is 125-450 mg 3 times daily on an empty stomach.

Administration may speed healing of contusions, sprains, ecchymoses, hematomas and other soft tissue injuries.

Review Article: Bromelain was introduced as a medicinal agent in 1957, and since that time over 400 scientific papers on its therapeutic applications have appeared in medical literature. Bromelain has been reported in these scientific studies to exert a wide variety of beneficial effects, including reducing inflammation in cases of arthritis, sports injury or trauma and preventing swelling after trauma or surgery (*Taussig S, Batkin S. Bromelain, the enzyme complex of pineapple (Ananas comosus) and its clinical application. An update. J Ethnopharmacol 22:191-203, 1988*).

Animal Experimental Study: Traumatic edema was induced in the hindlegs of rats. While the parenteral administration of bromelain had only a minimal effect, enteral administration produced a significant reduction in edema, supporting the observation that enzymes can be absorbed by the gut without losing their biological properties (*Uhlig G, Seifert J. [The effect of proteolytic enzymes (Traumanase) on posttraumatic edema.] Fortschr Med 99(15):554-6, 1981) (in German*).

Clinical Observations: 1.) 219 pts. with inflammation and edema associated with traumatic injuries, postoperative tissue reactions, cellulitis, and certain types of ulceration were given bromelain in the form of enteric-coated tablets (40 mg 4 times daily) in addition to standard treatment. 75% of the pts. were rated as showing excellent or good responses (substantially better than expected based on previous experience with similar cases). There were no undersirable effects. 2.) The median time from admission to discharge for 150 pts. treated with bromelains was 8 days compared to 100 pts. with similar diagnoses not given bromelains whose median time was 16 days (*Cirelli MG. Five years of clinical experience with bromelains in therapy of edema and inflammation in postoperative tissue reaction, skin infections and trauma. Clin Med 74(6):55-9, 1967*).

Clinical Observation: 90% of 71 pts. with contusions, sprains, post-operative swellings and hematomas had 'favorable results' from the administration of bromelain

(Weisskirchen H, el-Salamouny AR. [Treatment of post-traumatic and postoperative swellings with proteolytic enzymes.] Med Welt 52:3211-12, 1967) (in German).

Experimental Double-blind Study: 90% of 42 pts. with surgical and non-surgical trauma who received bromelain had good responses, while 10% had fair responses. Among placebo-treated controls, 10% had good responses, 20% fair responses and 70% poor responses. In most instances, resolution of edema and ecchymoses required a third to a half as many days for treated pts. compared to controls *(Seltzer AP. EENT 43:54, 1964).*

Experimental Placebo-controlled Study: 74 boxers with numerous bruises received bromelain, while 72 controls received placebo. For 58/74 (78%) of the treated boxers, all signs of bruising cleared within 4 days; clearance for the remaining subjects took 8-10 days. Among controls, only 10/72 (14%) had healing within 4 days, and the remainder took 7-14 days to heal *(Blonstein J. Control of swelling in boxing injuries. Practitioner 203-6, 1960).*

VASCULAR FRAGILITY

See Also: PERIPHERAL VASCULAR DISEASE

Bilberry (*Vaccinium myrtillus*):

Bilberry or European blueberry contains flavonoid compounds known as anthocyanosides. Bilberry anthocyanosides are potent antioxidants that improve the microcirculation and protect the vascular endothelium.

The standard dose for *Vaccinium myrtillus* extract (VME) is based on its anthocyanoside content, as calculated by its anthocyanidin percentage. Most studies have used a bilberry extract standardized for an anthocyanidin content of 25% at a dosage of 160 mg to 480 mg daily.

Administration of VME may reduce capillary permeability.

Experimental Study: Following oral administration of anthocyanosides, pts. with varicose veins and ulcerative dermatitis had a substantial drop in capillary leakage. Anthocyanosides were found to protect altered capillary walls by increasing the endothelium barrier-effect through stabilization of membrane phospholipids, and by increasing the biosynthetic processes of the acid mucopolysaccharides of the connective ground substance through restoration of the altered mucopolysaccharidic pericapillary sheath (*Mian E, Curri SB, Lietti A, Bombardelli E. [Anthocyanosides and the walls of microvessels: further aspects of the mechanism of action of their protective effect in syndromes due to abnormal capillary fragility.] Minerva Med 68(52):3565-81, 1977*).

Animal Experimental Study: VME demonstrated significant vasoprotective and antiedema properties in rabbits and cats. Their activity in reducing capillary permeability was more lasting than that of rutin (*Lietti A, Cristoni A, Picci M. Studies on Vaccinium myrtillus anthocyanosides. I. Vasoprotective and antiinflammatory activity. Arzneim Forsch 26(5):829-32, 1976*).

Ginkgo biloba:

Extracts of *Ginkgo biloba* leaves standardized to contain 24% ginkgoflavonglycosides may be effective.

The standard dose of *Ginkgo biloba* extract (GBE) is 40 mg 3 times daily.

Administration may be beneficial in idiopathic cyclic edema.

Experimental Study: Idiopathic cyclic edema is characterized by water and sodium retention with secondary hyperaldosteronism. The syndrome is due to capillary hyperpermeability which can be measured by Landis' labelled albumin test. In all 10 pts.

given *Ginkgo biloba* extract orally, and in all 5 pts. given IV *Ginkgo biloba* extract, the biological anomaly was fully corrected by administration of the extract *(Lagrue G et al. Idiopathic cyclic edema. The role of capillary hyperpermeability and its correction by Ginkgo biloba extract. Presse Med 15 (31):1550-3, 1986).*

Horsechestnut (*Aesculus hippocastanum*):

Horsechestnut seeds have a long folk history of use in the treatment of varicose veins and hemorrhoids. The active component is escin (syn. aescin).

Escin exerts venotonic, anti-edema and anti-inflammatory properties as well as decreases capillary permeability by reducing the number and size of the small pores of the capillary walls.

> *Note: Although horsechestnut ingestion can produce significant toxicity, the usual therapeutic doses appear to be reasonably safe for adults. Preparations should be kept out of the reach of children, however.*

Review Article: Horsechestnut extracts standardized to contain 50 mg of aescin per dose exert tonic effects on the veins, and decreased venous and capillary permeability. The mechanism of action is not fully understood, although there is recent evidence suggesting they may attenuate lysosomal proteoglycan destructing enzymes, which show increased activity in pts. with chronic venous insufficiency. In several double-blind randomized cross-over studies, subjective complaints were effectively diminished and objective paramaters improved. Horsechestnut extracts are well tolerated *(Hitzenberger G. [The therapeutic effectiveness of chestnut extract]. Wien Med Wochenschr 139(17):385-9, 1989) (in German).*

The efficacy of escin in the treatment of capillary fragility may be due to its ability to prevent destruction of glycosaminoglycans by enzymes.

> **Experimental Double-blind Study:** The serum activity of 3 lysosomal glycosaminoglycan hydrolases were studied in 18 healthy subjects and 15 pts. with varicose veins. In pts. with varicose veins elevated levels of b-glucuronidase (+70%), beta-N-acetylglucosaminidase (+63.5%), and arylsulphatase (+121.7%) were found. In the 15 pts. with varicosities, after 12 days of treatment with horsechestnut extract (300 mg containing 50 mg escin 3 times daily), the enzymes were significantly reduced by 29.1%, 25.7%, and 28.7%, respectively, compared to placebo *(Kreysel HW, Nissen HP, Enghoffer E. A possible role of lysosomal enzymes in the pathogenesis of varicosis and the reduction in their serum activity by venostasin. VASA 12:377-82, 1983).*

Procyanidolic Oligomers:

Procyanidolic oligomers (PCOs), also known as leukocyanidins or pycnogenols, are complexes of flavonoids (polyphenols). Most commercial preparations use PCOs extracted from grape seed skin (*Vitis vinifera*), although PCOs can also be extracted from the bark of Landes' pine, the bracts of the lime tree, and the leaves of the hazel-nut tree.

The standard therapeutic dosage of PCOs is 150 to 300 mg per day.

Review Article: PCOs increase intracellular vitamin C levels, decrease capillary permeability and fragility, scavenge oxidants and free radicals, and posess a unique ability to bind to collagen structures directly as well as inhibit destruction of collagen. Collagen, the most abundant protein of the body, is responsible for maintaining the integrity of "ground substance" as well as the integrity of tendons, ligaments, and cartilage. Collagen also is the support structure of the dermis and blood vessels. Leukocyanidins and other flavonoids are remarkable in their effect in supporting collagen structures and preventing collagen destruction. They affect collagen metabolism in several ways. They have the unique ability to crosslink collagen fibers, resulting in reinforcement of the natural crosslinking of collagen that forms the so-called collagen matrix of connective tissue (ground substance, cartilage, tendon, etc.). They prevent free radical damage with their potent antioxidant and free radical scavenging action. They inhibit enzymatic cleavage of collagen by enzymes secreted by white blood cells during inflammation, and microbes during infection. They prevent the release and synthesis of compounds that promote inflammation, such as histamine, serine proteases, prostaglandins, and leukotrienes. These effects on collagen are put to good use in the treatment of capillary fragility, easy bruising, and varicose veins (*Masquelier J. [Procyanidolic oligomers (leucocyanidins)]. Parfums Cosmet Arom 95:89-97, 1990) (in French)*.

See Also:

> **Review Article:** *Masquelier J. Pycnogenols: Recent advances in the therapeutic activity of procyanidins, in Natural Products as Medicinal Agents, vol. 1. Stuttgart, Hippokrates Verlag, 1981:243-56.*

> **Review Article:** *Masquelier J et al. Flavonoids and pycnogenols. Int J Vit Nutr Res 49:307-11, 1979.*

Administration may reduce capillary fragility in diabetics and hypertensives.

Experimental Double-blind Study: The effects of 150 mg/d of procyanidol oligomers on capillary resistance disorders in hypertensive and diabetic pts. were studied in a double-blind trial versus placebo in 25 patients. Capillary resistance rose from 14.6 cm Hg to 18 cm Hg in the treated gp., while no significant variation was observed in the placebo gp. (*Lagrue G, Olivier-Martin F, Grillot A. [A study of the effects of procyanidol oligomers on capillary resistance in hypertension and in certain nephropathies.] Sem Hop Paris 57(33-6):1399-401, 1981) (in French)*.

Experimental Study: The effects of 150 mg/d of procyanidol oligomers on capillary resistance disorders in hypertensive and diabetic pts. were studied in 28 pts. in an open trial. Capillary resistance rose from 15.4 cm Hg to 18.1 cm Hg. (*Lagrue G, Olivier-Martin F, Grillot A. [A study of the effects of procyanidol oligomers on capillary resistance in hypertension and in certain nephropathies.] Sem Hop Paris 57(33-6):1399-401, 1981) (in French)*.

VISUAL DYSFUNCTION
Including MYOPIA AND NIGHT BLINDNESS

Bilberry:

Bilberry or European blueberry (*Vaccinium myrtillus*) contains flavonoid compounds known as anthocyanosides, potent antioxidants that improve the microcirculation and promote the formation of visual purple.

The standard dose for *Vaccinium myrtillus* extract (VME) is based on its anthocyanoside content, as calculated by its anthocyanidin percentage. Most studies have used a bilberry extract standardized for an anthocyanidin content of 25% at a dosage of 160 mg to 480 mg daily.

Administration of VME may improve visual function.

Experimental Study: 22 pts. suffering from myopia (n=8), glaucoma (n=8), or retinitis pigmentosa (n=6) were given a single oral dose of 200 mg of *Vaccinium myrtillus* anthocyanosides. Improvement was noted based on electro-retinography in pts. with glaucoma and myopia, but results in retinitis pigmentosa were inconclusive (*Caselli L. Clinical and electroretinographic study on activity of anthocyanosides. Arch Med Int 37:29-35, 1985*).

Experimental Study: VME administration improved the absolute visual threshold by 2 log. units in 80% of treated pts. (*Gloria E, Perla A. Activity of anthocyanosides on absolute visual threshold. Ann Ottalm Clin Ocul 92:595-605, 1966*).

Experimental Study: 33 pts. (11 emmetropic, 11 ametropic, 11 with retinitis pigmentosa) administered 400 mg/day of *Vaccinium myrtillus* anthocyanosides and 20 mg/day of beta-carotene demonstrated improved adaptation to light and night vision, and enlargement of the visual field (*Fiorni G, Biancacci A, Graziano FM. [Perimetric and adaptometric modifications of anthocyanosides and beta-carotene.] Ann Ottal Clin Ocul 91:371-86, 1965*) (*in Italian*).

See also:

Experimental Study: *Sala D, Rolando M, Rossi PL, Pissarello L. Effect of anthocyanosides on visual performances at low illumination. Minerva Oftalmol 21:283-5, 1979 (in Italian)*

Experimental Study: *Wegmann R, Maeda K, Tronche P, Bastide P. Effects of anthocyanosides on photoreceptors. Cytoenzymatic aspects. Ann Histochim 14:237-56, 1969*

Experimental Study: *Urso G. [Effect of Vaccinium myrtillus anthocyanosides associated with betacarotenes on light sensitivity.] Ann Ottalmol Clin Ocul 3(9):930-8, 1967 (in Italian)*

Administration of VME may improve myopia.

- with <u>Vitamin E</u>:

Experimental Study: 8 myopic pts. were given a single oral dose of 200 mg of *Vaccinium myrtillus* anthocyanosides. Improvement was noted as based on electro-retinography (*Caselli L. Clinical and electroretinographic study on activity of anthocyanosides. Arch Med Int 37:29-35, 1985*).

Experimental Study: 36 pts. with progressive myopia were treated with a Difrarel, a product containing anthocyanosides and vitamin E. After an observation period of 14.5 months an ave. increase of myopia by 0.53 dpt per eye was demonstrated. The final examination of 29 pts. showed a stabilization of the fundus-alterations, as well as a stable, or an improved visual acuity respectively. In 7 pts. a moderate deterioration of the partial or overall medical findings occured (*Politzer M. [Experiences in the medical treatment of progressive myopia.] Klin Monatsbl Augenheilkd 171(4):616-9, 1977*) (*in German*).

See Also:

Korzekwa A, Szymankiewiczowa S. [Treatment of progressive myopia in children by saddamine and calcium iontophoresis and difrarel.] Klin Oczna 87(8):322-3, 1985 (in Polish)

Barradah MA, Shoukry I, Hegazy M. Difrarel 100 in the treatment of retinal vascular disorders and high myopia. Bull Ophthalmol Soc Egypt 60(64):251-2, 1967

<u>Procyanidolic Oligomers</u>:

Procyanidolic oligomers (PCOs), also known as leukocyanidins or pycnogenols) are complexes of flavonoids (polyphenols). Most commercial preparations use PCOs extracted from grape seed skin (*Vitis vinifera*), although PCOs can also be extracted from the bark of Landes' pine, the bracts of the lime tree, and the leaves of the hazel-nut tree.

The standard therapeutic dosage of PCOs is 150 to 300 mg per day.

Administration may improve visual function.

Experimental Double-blind Study: 100 normal volunteers with no retinal disorder received 200 mg/d PCOs or placebo for five weeks and a control group received no treatment. The group receiving PCOs demonstrated significant improvement in visual performance in the dark and after glare compared to the placebo group (*Corbe C, Boissin JP, Siou A. [Light vision and chorioretinal circulation. Study of the effect of procyanidolic oligomers (Endotelon)]. J Fr Ophtalmol 11(5):453-60, 1988*).

Experimental Double-blind Study: 100 pts. received either PCOs (Endotelon[®]) 200 mg/d or a placebo for 6 weeks. Using a Comberg's nictometer and Ergovision, a statistically significant (p>0.0001) improvement in recovery from dazzling was noted in the PCOs gp. *(Boissin JP, Corbe C, Siou A. [Chorioretinal circulation and dazzling: use of procyanidol oligomers (Endotelon)]. Bull Soc Ophtalmol Fr 88(2):173-4, 177-9, 1988).*

Experimental Study: 40 myopic pts. received either PCOs (150 mg/d) or placebo for 30 days. In 14 pts. in the PCOs gp. with low LED VEP's, 12 (85.7%) demonstrated significant improvement compared to 0/17 in the placebo gp. (p<0.0001). Significant electroretinographic improvements were noted in 8 pts. (40%) in the PCOs gp. and 0 pts. in the placebo gp. (p<0.0001) *(Proto F et al. Electrophysical study of Vitis vinifera procyanoside oligomers effects on retinal function in myopic subjects. Ann Ott Clin Ocul 114:85-93, 1988).*

VITILIGO

Khella (*Ammi visnaga*):

Khella is an ancient medicinal plant native to the Mediterranean region which contains khellin. Khellin is structurally similar to psoralen, a plant extract which can be isolated from the roots of *Psoralea Drupacae Bge U* (*Kartashkina IN, Shamsutdinov RI, Shakirov TT. [A method of isolation of psoralen from roots of Psoralea Drugacae Bge U.] Med Prom SSSR 29(5):38-40, 1966*).

Note: Oral or topical use of psoralen compounds, with subsequent exposure to UVA radiation, stimulates melanin synthesis and repigmentation in about one-third of patients (Drug Evaluations Subscription. Chicago, American Medical Association, Summer, 1993). "The major advantage of khellin is that it does not lead to phototoxic skin erythema and thus can be considered safe for home treatment. Because of its photochemisty it may be considered less hazardous than psoralens regarding mutagenicity and carcinogenicity" (Ortel B, Tanew A, Honigsmann H. Treatment of vitiligo with khellin and ultaviolet A. J Am Acad Dermatol 18(4 Pt 1):693-701, 1988).

Administration may be beneficial.

WARNINGS: At higher doses (120-160 mg per day) khellin preparations are associated with mild side effects such as insomnia, anorexia, nausea, and dizziness. Khellin may also markedly increase liver transaminases (*Duschet P, Schwarz T, Pusch M, Gschnait F. Marked increase of liver transanimases after khellin and UVA therapy. Letter. J Am Acad Dermatol 21(3 Pt 1):592-4, 1989*) and can produce a pseudoallergic reaction (*Jung EG, Fingerhut W. Pseudoallergic reaction from Khellin in photochemotherapy of vitiligo: a case report. Photodermatol 5(5):235-6, 1988*).

Note: Khella extracts standardized for khellin content (typically 12%) are available.

Experimental Study: 25 pts. received khellin orally and 3 with treated topically. Treatment were given 3 times weekly. While khellin induced repigmentation similar to psoralens, it did not induce the skin ptototoxicity with UVA associated with psoralens. More than 70% repigmentation was achieved in 41% of pts. who received 1-200 treatments, a success rate comparable to that obtained with psoralens. 7 pts. had a mild elevation of liver transaminases early in treatment and their treatments were discontinued. No long-term organ or skin toxicity was observed (*Ortel B, Tanew A, Honigsmann H. Treatment of vitiligo with khellin and ultaviolet A. J Am Acad Dermatol 18(4 Pt 1):693-701, 1988*).

Experimental Double-blind Study: Khellin (100 mg/d) was orally administered to 30 vitiligo pts. for 4 months with subsequent exposure to natural sunlight. At the end of the trial period, 5 pts. out of 30 (16.6%) repigmented 90-100%; 7 cases (23.3%) repigmented 50-60% of the vitiliginous areas treated; 11 (36.6%) repigmented 25% or less, and 7 subjects (23.3%) showed negative response. 30 control subjects failed to repigment at all. The achieved repigmentation was stable after drug cessation for a period of 1 year. No side effects were reported (*Abdel-Fattah A et al. An approach to the treatment of vitiligo by khellin. Dermatologica 165(2):136-40, 1982*).

See Also:

> *Morliere P, Honigsmann H, Averbeck D, et al. Phototherapeutic, photobiologic, and photosensitizing properties of khellin. J Invest Dermatol 90(5):720-4, 1988*

Topical administration appears to be ineffective.

> **Negative Experimental Controlled Study:** 41 pts. had macules on one side painted with a 2% solution of khellin in acetone and propylene glycol (90 and 10%, respectively) and exposed to sunlight for a period of 4 months with 3 weekly applications and with exposure times up to 90 min. The macules of the other side were treated in 36 of the 41 pts. with acetone and propylene glycol only and sun-exposed with the same schedule, while in the remaining 5 pts. they were neither treated with khellin or placebo nor sun-exposed. No significant difference was evidenced between the khellin and placebo-treated sides: no excellent result (repigmentation more than 75% of the affected area) was found, and good results (repigmentation more than 50%) were found in 24.9% of khellin- plus sunlight-treated macules and in 22.3% of placebo-plus sunlight-treated macules (*Orecchia G, Perfetti L. Photochemotherapy with topical khellin and sunlight in vitiligo. Dermatology 184(2):120-3, 1992*).

Psoralea coryliforia:

For over 3000 years, the furocoumarin group of compounds combined with natural sunlight have been used to treat skin disease. In ancient India, physicians and herbalists used naturally occurring plant furrocoumarins by having patients either ingest or apply an extract of *Psoralen corylifolia* before exposing them to natural sunlight to treat vitiligo (*McEnvoy MT, Stern RS. Rsoralens and related compounds in the treatment of psoriasis. Pharmac Ther 34:75-97, 1987*).

> *Note: Although psoralens (furocoumarins) occur naturally in Psoralea corylifolia and in certain other plants, the drugs available for therapeutic use in PUVA therapy (psoralen + ultraviolet light A) and other photochemotherapy are synthetic compounds (methoxsalen and trioxsalen).*

WOUND HEALING

Aloe vera:

The topical effects of _Aloe vera_ appear to be due to a combination of enhancement of wound healing along with anti-inflammatory, moisturizing, emollient, and antimicrobial actions.

Aloe vera gel has been shown to stimulate fibroblast and connective tissue formation as well as stimulate the epidermal growth and repair process, presumably due to its polysaccharides.

> WARNING: _Aloe vera_ gel has been shown to delay wound healing in cases of surgical wounds such as those produced during laparotomy or cesarean delivery. _Aloe vera_ should not be used in treating deep vertical wounds (_Schmidt JM, Greenspoon JS. Aloe vera dermal wound gel is associated with a delay in wound healing. Obstet Gynecol 78:115-7, 1991_).

Experimental Study: The wound healing effects of _Aloe vera_ were demonstrated in preventing progressive dermal ischemia caused by burns, frostbite, electrical injury, and intra-arterial drug abuse. _In vivo_ analysis of these injuries showed that the primary mediator of progressive tissue damage was thromboxane A2 (TX2). Aloe was subsequently shown to inhibit the formation of TX2. Burn pts. treated with Aloe healed without tissue loss as did those with frostbite (p=0.001). In intra-arterial drug abuse pts., Aloe reversed tissue necrosis (_Heggers JP, Pelley RP, Robson MC. Beneficial effects of Aloe in wound healing. Phytother Res 7:S48-52, 1993_).

Review Article: _Aloe vera_ is known to contain several pharmacologically active ingredients, including a carboxypeptidase which inactivates bradykinin, salicylates, and a thromboxane inhibitor. Scientific studies also exist that support an antibacterial and antifungal effect for substances in Aloe. Studies and case reports provide support for the use of Aloe in the treatment of radiation ulcers and statis ulcers while animal studies indicate that Aloe may be useful in burns and frostbite (_Klein AD, Penneys NS. Aloe vera. J Amer Acad Dermatol 18:714-9, 1988_).

Experimental Study: _Aloe vera_ gel was used quite successfully in three patients with chronic leg ulcers of 5, 7, and 15 years duration. The gel was applied to the ulcers on gauze bandages. A rapid reduction in ulcer size was noted in all 3 subjects and complete resolution occurred in 2 (_el Zawahry M, Hegazy MR, Helal M. Use of aloe in treating leg ulcers and dermatoses. Int J Dermatol 12:68-73, 1973_).

See Also:

> **Review Article:** _Shelton RW. Aloe vera, its chemical and therapeutic properties. Int J Dermatol 30:679-83, 1991_

Review Article: *Grindlay D, Reynolds T. The aloe vera leaf phenomena: A review of the properties and modern use of the leaf parenchyma gel. J Ethnopharm 16:117-51, 1986*

Bromelain:

Bromelain is a mixture of proteolytic enzymes or proteases obtained from the stem of the pineapple plant (*Ananas comosus*). (*See: 'INFLAMMATION'*)

The standard dosage of bromelain (1,800-2,000 m.c.u.) is 125-450 mg 3 times daily on an empty stomach.

Administration may be beneficial.

Review Article: Bromelain was introduced as a medicinal agent in 1957, and since that time over 400 scientific papers on its therapeutic applications have appeared in medical literature. Bromelain has been reported in these scientific studies to exert a wide variety of beneficial effects, including reducing inflammation in cases of arthritis, sports injury or trauma and prevention of swelling after trauma or surgery (*Taussig S, Batkin S. Bromelain, the enzyme complex of pineapple (Ananas comosus) and its clinical application. An update. J Ethnopharmacol 22:191-203, 1988*).

Experimental Double-blind Study: 158 primigravidae with mediolateral episiotomies randomly received either enteric coated bromelain tablets (Ananase®, Rorer) 40 mg 4 times daily or placebo. No significant differences could be found between groups, although the rate of reduction of edema and bruising was more rapid in pts. on bromelain, especially when edema and bruising were severe (*Howat RCL, Lewis GD. The effect of bromelain therapy on episotomy wounds - A double blind controlled clinical trial. J Obstet Gynaecol Br Commonw 79:951-3, 1972*).

Experimental Single-blind Study: 74 boxers with bruises of the face and hematomas of the orbits, lips, ears, chest and arms received bromelains (Ananase®, Rorer) 40 mg 4 times daily for 4 days or until all signs of bruising had disappeared, while 72 boxers received placebo. All signs of bruising cleared completely in 4 days in 58/74 treated boxers; the remainder completely cleared in 8-10 days. This compared to clearing in 4 days in only 10/72 controls and 7-14 days for the remainder to completely clear (*Blonstein JL. Control of swelling in boxing injuries. Practitioner 203:206, 1969*).

Clinical Observations: 1.) 219 pts. with inflammation and edema associated with traumatic injuries, postoperative tissue reactions, cellulitis, and certain types of ulceration were given bromelain in the form of enteric-coated tablets (Ananase®, Rorer) 40 mg 4 times daily in addition to standard treatment. 75% of the pts. were rated as showing excellent or good responses (substantially better than expected based on previous experience with similar cases). There were no undersirable effects.   2.) The median time from admission to discharge for 150 pts. treated with bromelain was 8 days compared to 100 pts. with similar diagnoses not given bromelain whose median time was 16 days. 3.) 62.5% of 339 adult pts. for whom bromelain was added due to poor responses to conventional treatments were judged to have made accelerated recoveries (*Cirelli MG. Five years of clinical experience with bromelains in therapy of edema and inflammation in postoperative tissue reaction, skin infections and trauma. Clin Med 74(6):55-9, 1967*).

Clinical Observations: 90% of 71 pts. with contusions, sprains, post-operative swellings and hematomas had 'favorable results' from administration of bromelain (*Weisskirchen H, Elsalmouny AR. Med Welt 52:3211, 1967*).

Experimental Double-blind Crossover Study: 16 pts. with multiple tooth impactions were randomly provided with either bromelain (Ananase®, Rorer) 40 mg 4 times daily or placebo starting 72 hrs. prior to the first surgical procedure. Following recovery, they were crossed over for their second surgical procedure. 24 hrs. after surgery, 12/16 (75%) of pts. on bromelain had mild or no inflammation compared to 3/16 (19%) of pts. on placebo. 72 hrs. after surgery, 14/16 (85%) of pts. on bromelain compared to 7/16 (44%) were considered to have mild or no swelling. Treated pts. had post-surgical pain for 5.1 days compared to 8.1 days for pts. on placebo, and swelling disappeared in 3.8 days for bromelain pts. vs. 7 days for placebo cases (*Tassman G et al. A double-blind crossover study of a plant proteolytic enzyme in oral surgery. J Dent Med 20:51-4, 1965*).

Experimental Double-blind Study: 90% of 42 pts. with surgical and non-surgical trauma who received bromelain had good responses, while 10% had fair responses. Among placebo-treated controls, 10% had good responses, 20% fair responses and 70% poor responses. In most instances, resolution of edema and ecchymoses required a third to a half as many days for treated pts. compared to controls (*Seltzer AP. EENT 43:54, 1964*).

See Also:

> **Experimental Double-blind Study:** *Cowie DH et al. A double-blind trial of bromelains as an adjunct to vaginal plastic repair operations. J Obstet Gynaecol Br Commonw 77(4):365-68, 1970*

Centella asiatica (Gotu kola):

Centella asiatica has a long history of use in Chinese and Ayurvedic medicine. The whole plant is used medicinally.

The primary active constituents of *Centella asiatica* are known to be triterpenoid acids. The concentration of triterpenes in Centella can vary between 1.1 and 8 percent, with most samples yielding a concentration between 2.2 and 3.4 percent.

Most research on Centella has been performed with either the total triterpenoid fraction of *Centella asiatica* (TTFCA) or isolated triterpenoids. TTFCA has also been referred to as the titrated extract of *Centella asiatica* or TECA. Both extracts are composed of a mixture of 3 triterpenes: asiatic acid (30%), madecassic acid (30%) and asiaticoside (40%).

The standard dosage for TTFCA is 60 to 120 mg/d. Using TTFCA or extracts standardized for triterpenoid acids may produce more reliable results compared to crude preparations. The concentration of triterpenoids in Centella can vary between 1.1% and 8%, with most samples yielding a concentration between 2.2-3.4% percent. To achieve a similar dosage of triterpenoids compared to TTFCA with the crude plant would require 2 to 4 grams per day, although it is not known if this would still correlate with the clinical efficacy noted for TTFCA.

Note: Do not confuse gotu kola with cola nut. Gotu kola is not related to the cola nut (Cola nitida or C. acuminata), nor does it contain any caffeine.

Administration of TTFCA may promote wound healing.

In vitro Study: TTFCA increased the collagen synthesis in a dose-dependent fashion whereas a simultaneous decrease in the specific activity of neosynthesized collagen was observed. Asiatic acid was found to be the only component responsible for collagen synthesis stimulation. TTFCA and all three terpenes increased the intracellular free proline pool. This effect was independent of the stimulation of collagen synthesis (*Maquart FX et al. Stimulation of collagen synthesis in fibroblast cultures by a triterpene extracted from Centella asiatica. Connect Tissue Res 24(2):107-20, 1990*).

Review Article: Centella has shown positive results in clinical trials. The types of wounds healed include surgical wounds such as episiotomies and ENT surgeries, skin ulcers due to arterial or venous insufficiency, traumatic injuries to the skin, gangrene, skin grafts, schistosomiasis lesions, and perineal lesions produced during childbirth. The outcome of Centella's complex actions is a balanced multiphasic effect on cells and tissues participating in the process of healing, particularly connective tissues. Enhanced development of normal connective tissue matrix is perhaps the prime mechanism of action (*Kartnig T. Clinical applications of Centella asiatica (L.) Urb. Herbs Spices Med Plants 3:146-73, 1988*).

In vitro Study: The mechanism of action of the total triterpenoid fraction extracted from *Centella asiatica* (TTFCA) was evaluated using human skin fibroblasts cultures as the experimental system. In particular its influence on the biosynthesis of collagen, fibronectin and proteoglycans was considered. The presence of TTFCA (25 mug/ml) does not seem to affect cell proliferation, total protein synthesis or the biosynthesis of proteoglycans in a significant way. A statistically important increase was observed in the percentage of collagen and, as revealed by immunofluorescence measurements, in cell layer fibronectin. This effect on collagen and fibronectin may help to explain the action of TTFCA in promoting wound healing, and suggests an interesting working hypothesis for its action on basal endothelia (*Tenni et al. Effect of the triterpenoid fraction of Centella asiatica on macromolecules of the connective matrix in human skin fibroblast cultures. Ital J Biochem 37(2):69-77, 1988*).

Experimental Study: Asiaticoside (Madecassol) 25 mg IM accelerated wound healing. The invasion of capillary branches favored the formation of granulation tissue (*Kiesswetter H. Erfahrungsbericht über behandlung von wunden mit asiaticosids (Madecassol). Wien Med Wschr 114:124-6, 1964*).

See Also:

Collonna d'Istria J. Research on healing action of Madecassol in cervical and laryngeal surgery after ionizing radiations. J Fr Otorhinolaryngol 19:507-10, 1970

Castellani C et al. Asiaticoside and cicatrization of episiotomies. Bull Fed Soc Gynecol Obstet 18:184-6, 1966

Sevin P. Some observations on the use of asiaticoside (Madecassol) in general surgery. Progr Med (France) 90:23-4, 1962

Boiteau P, Ratsimamanga AR. Asiaticoside extracted from Centella asiatica, its therapeutic uses in the healing of experimental or refractory wounds, leprosy, skin tuberculosis, and lupus. Therapie 11:125-49, 1956

Administration of TTFCA may prevent keloid formation.

Experimental Double-blind Study: Administration of *Centella asiatica* (Madecassol) both orally and topically was found to be of clinical value in stopping the inflammatory phase of hypertrophic scars and keloids. Its effect on other forms of connective tissue abnormalities was similar, gradually bringing scars to the maturation phase. It also had a preventive effect on burn and postoperative hypertrophic scars, and compares favorably with compression bandaging, and gave more lasting results than intralesional cortisone or radiation therapy. Its placebo effect of 29% was well within acceptable limits. Side effects appeared to be limited to occasional mild gastric intolerance and allergic reactions (*Bossë JP et al. Clinical study of a new antikeloid agent. Ann Plast Surg 3(1):13-21, 1979*).

Administration of TTFCA intramuscularly may promote the healing of second- and third-degree burns (*Boiteau P, Ratsimamanga AR. Important cicatrizants of vegetable origin and the biostimulins of Filatov. Bull Soc Sci Bretagne 34:307-15, 1959; Gravel JA. Oxygen dressings and asiaticoside in the treatment of burns. Laval Med 36(5):413-15, 1965*).

Administration of TTFCA may assist the healing of skin ulcers.

Negative Experimental Double-blind Study: No difference could be detected in the healing success, clinical appearance or histological findings of 13 pts. with ulcus cruris treated orally with asiaticoside or placebo (*Mayall RC et al. U'lceras tróficas - Arbo cicatricial do extrato titulado da Centella asiatica. Rev Bras Med 32:26-9, 1975*).

Experimental Study: Pts. with ulcus cruris of different causes had extraordinary healing when treated with 20 mg asiaticoside intramuscularly (*Mayall RC. Oasiaticoside comom cicaytrizante de ulceraçoes. Hospital (Rio) 64:1065-74, 1963*).

See Also:

Vittori F. [The treatment of ulcus cruris.] J Med Lyon 63(1372):429-32, 1982

Delaunay MM. [Management of perforating ulcer of the sole of the foot.] Bordeaux Med 10(21):1453-4, 1977

Huriez CL. [Action of the titrated extract of Centella asiatica upon cicatrization of leg ulcers (10 mg tablets). Apropos of 50 cases.] Lille Med 17(suppl 3):574-9, 1972

Hadida E et al. [Association of Medecassol (asiaticoside), neomycin and hydrocortisone in the treatment of leg ulcers.] Bull Soc Fr Dermatol Syph 77(4):522-5, 1970

Hanna LK et al. Trophic ulcers and their treatment with Madecassol Afr Med 8(69):315-18, 1969

Chamomile (*Matricaria chamomilla*):

Topical chamomile preparations may accelerate the healing of scrapes and dermabrasion.

Experimental Double-blind Study: A topical chamomile preparation was shown to decrease the length of the healing and drying process after dermabrasion of tattoos (*Glowania HJ, Raulin C, Swoboda M. [Effect of chamomile on wound healing—a clinical double-blind study]. Z Hautkr 62(17):1262, 1267-71, 1987*) (*in German*).

Echinacea spp:

Echinacea may inhibit hyaluronidase activity and activate fibroblasts to produce hyaluronic acid (*Busing KH. [Inhibition of hyaluronidase by Echinacin.] Arzneimittelforsch 2:467-72, 1952* (*in German*).

> *Note: Hyaluronic acid helps to bind cells together.*

Administration may promote wound healing.

Animal Experimental Study: Echinacin B, a polysaccharide in Echinacea, was shown to promote wound healing in experimental animals by forming a complex with hyaluronic acid that is resistant to attack by hyaluronidase (*Bonadeo I et al. [Echinacin B: Active polysaccharide from Echinacea.] Riv Ital Essenze Profumi Piante 53:281-95, 1971*) (*in Italian*).

Human and Animal Experimental Studies: After the placement of hetero- and homogeneous fibrin grafts, the grafts were transformed under the influence of leukocytic enzymes into components of connective tissue substance. Echinacea appeared to have a protective action towards the mesenchymal glycosaminoglycans produced by fibrocytes, as larger quantities of glycosaminoglycans were found in echinacin-fibrin grafts causing accelerated wound healing (*Tunnerhoff FK, Schwabe HK. [Studies in human beings and animals on the influence of Echinacea extracts on the formation of connective tissue following the implantation of fibrin.] Arzneimittelforsch 6:330-4, 1956*) (*in German*).

Topical application may promote wound healing.

Animal Experimental Study: The rate of healing of wounds of the skin in guinea pigs treated with Echinacin® ointment was increased. On the 6th and 9th days, wounds treated with Echinacin® ointment were significantly smaller than those of controls (*Kinkel HJ, Plate M, Tullner U. [Effect of Echinacin ointment in healing of wound]. Med Klin 79(21):580-3, 1984*) (*in German*).

Papain:

A proteolytic enzyme from collected from the unripe green papaya (*Carica papaya*). May possess properties similar to those of bromelain.

Administration may be beneficial.

Experimental Double-blind Study: 69 obstetrical pts. requiring episiotomies received either a highly purified and standardized extract of proteolytic enzymes from *Carica papaya* (Papase® tablets, Warner-Chilcott) 1 tab every 2 waking hrs. for 48 hrs., then 1 tab every 3-4 hrs. until discharge, or placebo. By the fourth postpartum day, edema was either absent or nearly absent in a much higher percentage of enzyme-treated pts. than in placebo-treated pts. (79% vs. 32%). Improvement at the time of discharge was either marked or moderate about twice as often in pts. who received the enzymes than in those who received placebo, and their results were superior (p>0.001). 59% vs. 21% of pts. were asymptomatic at the time of discharge. There were no side effects *(Pollack PJ. Oral administration of enzymes from Carica papaya: Report of a double-blind clinical study. Curr Ther Res 4(5):229-37, 1962).*

Procyanidolic Oligomers:

Procyanidolic oligomers (PCOs), also known as leukocyanidins or pycnogenols) are complexes of flavonoids (polyphenols). Most commercial preparations use PCOs extracted from grape seed skin (*Vitis vinifera*), although PCOs can also be extracted from the bark of Landes' pine, the bracts of the lime tree, and the leaves of the hazel-nut tree. *(See: 'PERIPHERAL VASCULAR DISEASE'; 'VASCULAR FRAGILITY')*

The standard therapeutic dosage of PCOs is 150 to 300 mg per day.

Review Article: PCOs increase intracellular vitamin C levels, decrease capillary permeability and fragility, scavenge oxidants and free radicals, and possess a unique ability to bind to collagen structures directly as well as inhibit destruction of collagen. Collagen, the most abundant protein of the body, is responsible for maintaining the integrity of 'ground substance' as well as the integrity of tendons, ligaments, and cartilage. Collagen also is the support structure of the dermis and blood vessels. Leukocyanidins and other flavonoids are remarkable in their effect in supporting collagen structures and preventing collagen destruction. They affect collagen metabolism in several ways. They have the unique ability to crosslink collagen fibers, resulting in reinforcement of the natural crosslinking of collagen that forms the so-called collagen matrix of connective tissue (ground substance, cartilage, tendon, etc.). They prevent free radical damage with their potent antioxidant and free radical scavenging action. They inhibit enzymatic cleavage of collagen by enzymes secreted by white blood cells during inflammation, and microbes during infection. They prevent the release and synthesis of compounds that promote inflammation, such as histamine, serine proteases, prostaglandins, and leukotrienes. These effects on collagen are put to good use in the treatment of capillary fragility, easy bruising, and varicose veins *(Masquelier J. [Procyanidolic oligomers (leucocyanidins)]. Parfums Cosmet Arom 95:89-97, 1990) (In French).*

PCOs may reduce postoperative edema *(Baruch J. [Effect of Endotelon in postoperative edema. Results of a double-blind study versus placebo in 32 female patients]. Ann Chir Plast Esthet 29(4):393-5, 1984) (in French).*

Tea Tree oil (*Melaleuca alternifolia*):

Tea tree is a small tree native to only one area of the world - the northeast coastal region of New South Wales, Australia. Its leaves are the source of tea tree oil.

The medical world's first mention of tea tree appeared in the Medical Journal of Australia in 1930 when a surgeon in Sydney reported impressive results from a solution of tea tree oil for cleaning surgical wounds (*Humphery E. A new Australian germicide. Med J Australia 1:417-8, 1930*).

Tea tree oil possesses significant antiseptic properties and is regarded by many as the ideal skin disinfectant. It is active against a wide range of organisms, possesses good penetration, and is non-irritating to the skin.

Review Article: Topical application of tree oil has been used in the following conditions: acne, apthous stomatitis (canker sores), athlete's foot, boils, burns, carbuncles, corns, empyema, gingivitis, herpes, impetigo, infections of the nail bed, insect bites, lice, mouth ulcers, psoriasis, root canal treatment, ringworm, sinus infections, sore throat, skin and vaginal infections, tinea, thrush, and tonsilitis (*Altman PM. Australian tea tree oil. Australian J Pharmacy 69:276-8, 1988*).

GLOSSARY

Abortifacient - A substance which induces abortion.

Acrid - A pungent biting taste which causes irritation.

Acute - Having a rapid onset, severe symptoms, and a short course; not chronic.

Adaptogen - A substance which is safe, increases resistance to stress, and has a balancing effect on body functions.

Adjuvant - A substance which enhances the effect of the medicinal agent or increases the antigenicity of a cancer cell.

Alkaloids - Naturally occurring amines (nitrogen containing compounds), arising from heterocyclic and often complex structures, that display pharmacological activity. Their trivial names usually end in -ine. They are usually classified according to the chemical structure of their main nucleus: phenylalkylamines (ephedrine), pyridine (nicotine), tropine (atropine, cocaine), quinoline (quinine), isoquinolone (papaverine), phenanthrene (morphine), purine (caffeine), imidazole (pilocarpine), and indole (physostigmine, yohimbine).

Allopathy - A term that describes the conventional method of medicine which combats disease by using substances and techniques specifically against the disease.

Alterative - A substance which produces a balancing effect on a particular body function.

Analgesic - A substance which reduces the sensation of pain.

Androgen - Hormones which stimulate male charateristics.

Anthelminthic - A substance which causes the elimination of intestinal worms.

Anthocyanidin - A particular class of flavonoids which gives plants, fruits, and flowers colors ranging from red to blue.

Antibody - Proteins manufactured by the body which bind to antigens to neutralize, inhibit, or destroy it.

Antidote - A substance which neutralizes or counteracts the effects of a poison.

Antigen - Any substance that when introduced into the body causes the formation of antibodies against it.

Antihypertensive - Blood pressure lowering effect.

322

Antioxidant - A compound which prevents free radical or oxidative damage.

Aphrodisiac - A substance which increases sexual desire.

Astringent - An agent which causes the contraction of tissue.

Balm - A soothing or healing medicine applied to the skin.

Benign - A mild disorder that is usually not fatal.

Carminative - A substance which promotes the elimination of intestinal gas.

Cathartic - A substance which stimulates the movement of the bowels, more powerful than a laxative.

Cholagogue - A compound which stimulates the contraction of the gallbladder.

Choleretic - A compound which promotes the flow of bile.

Cholestasis - The stagnation of bile within the liver.

Cholelithiasis - Gallstones.

Chronic - Long-term or frequently recurring.

Cirrhosis - A severe disease of the liver characterized by the replacement of liver cells with scar tissue.

Colic - Severe, spasmodic pain that occurs in waves of increasing intensity, reaches a peak, then abates for a short time before returning.

Compress - A pad of linen applied under pressure to an area of skin and held in place.

Decoctions - Teas prepared by boiling the botanical with water for a specified period of time, followed by straining or filtering.

Demulcent - A substance soothing to irritated mucous membranes.

Douche - Introduction of water and/or a cleansing agent into the vagina with the aid of a bag with a tubing and nozzle attached.

Emulsify - The dispersement of large fat globules into smaller uniformly distributed particles.

Enteric-coated - A special way of coating a tablet or capsule to ensure that it does not dissolve in the stomach so it can reach the intestinal tract.

Essential oils - Also known as volatile oils, ethereal oils or essences. They are usually complex mixtures of a wide variety of organic compounds (e.g., alcohols, ketones, phenols, acids, ethers, esters, aldehydes, oxides, etc.) that evaporate when exposed to air. They generally represent the odoriferous principles of plants.

Extracts - Concentrated forms of natural products obtained by treating crude materials containing these substances with a solvent and then removing the solvent completely or partially from the preparation. The most commonly used extracts are fluid extracts, solid extracts, powdered extracts, tinctures and native extracts.

Flavonoid - A generic term for a group of flavone-containing compounds that are found widely in nature. They include many of the compounds that account for plant pigments (anthocyanins, anthoxanthins, apigenins, flavones, flavonols, bioflavonols, etc.). These plant pigments exert a wide variety of physiological effects in the human body.

Fluid Extracts - These extracts are typically hydro-alcoholic solutions with a strength of 1 part solvent to 1 part herb. The alcohol content varies with each product. They are in essence concentrated tinctures.

Free radicals - Highly reactive molecules, characterized by an unpaired electron, that can bind to and destroy cellular compounds.

Glycosides - Sugar containing compounds composed of a glycone (sugar component) and an aglycone (nonsugar containing component) that can be cleaved on hydrolysis. The glycone portion may be glucose, rhamnose, xylose, fructose, arabinose or any other sugar. The aglycone portion can be any kind of compound, e.g., sterols, triterpenes, anthraquinones, hydroquinones, tannins, carotenoids and anthocyanidins.

Hepatic - Pertaining to the liver

Hormone - A secretion of an endocrine gland that controls and regulates body functions.

Iatrogenic - Meaning literally "physician produced," the term can be applied to any medical condition, disease, or other adverse occurrence that results from medical treatment.

Idiopathic - Of unknown cause.

Infusions - Teas produced by steeping the botanical in hot water.

In vitro - Outside a living body and in an artificial environment.

In vivo - In a living body of an animal or plant

Laxative - A substance which promotes the evacuation of the bowels.

Lesion - Any localized, abnormal change in tissue formation.

Lipotropic - Promoting the flow of lipids to and from the liver.

Malignant - A term used to describe a condition that tends to worsen and eventually causes death.

Menstrums - Solvents used for extraction, e.g. water, alcohol, acetone, etc.

Mucous membrane - The soft, pink, tissue which lines most of the bodies cavities and tubes in the body, including the respiratory tract, gastrointestinal tract, genitourinary tract, and eyelids. The mucous membranes secrete mucus.

Mucus - The slick, slimy fluid secreted by the mucous membranes which acts as a lubicant and mechanical protector of the mucous membranes.

Neoplasia - A medical term for a tumor formation, characterized by a progressive, abnormal replication of cells.

Oleoresins - Primarily mixtures of resins and volatile oils. They either occur naturally or are made by extracting the oily and resinous materials from botanicals with organic solvents (e.g., hexane, acetone, ether, alcohol). The solvent is then removed under vacuum, leaving behind a viscous, semisolid extract which is the oleoresin. Examples of prepared oleoresins are paprika, ginger, and capsicum.

Pathogen - Any agent, particularly a microorganism, that causes disease.

Pathogenesis - The process by which a disease originates and develops, particularly the cellular and physiologic processes.

Peristalsis - Successive muscular contractions of the intestines which move food through the intestinal tract.

Phytoestrogen - Plant compounds which exert estrogen effects.

Placebo - An inert or inactive substance used to test the efficacy of another substance.

Polysaccharide - A molecule composed of many sugar molecules linked together.

Powdered extract - A solid extract which has been dried as a powder.

Prostaglandin - Hormone-like compounds manufactured from essential fatty acids.

Putrefaction - The process of breaking down protein compounds by rotting.

Resins - Complex oxidative products of terpenes that occur naturally as plant exudates, or are prepared by alcohol extraction of botanicals that contain resinous principles.

Saponins - Non-nitrogenous glycosides, typically with sterol or triterpenes as the aglycone, that possess the common property of foaming, or making suds, when strongly agitated in aqueous solution.

Satiety - A feeling of fullness or gratification.

Solid Extracts - Extracts which have had all of the residual solvent or liquid removed.

Submucosa - The tissue just below the mucous membrane.

Syndrome - A group of signs and symptoms that occur together in a pattern characteristic of a particular disease or abnormal condition.

Tincture - Alcoholic or hydro-alcoholic solutions usually containing the active principles of botanicals in low concentrations. They are usually prepared by maceration, percolation or by dilution of their corresponding fluid or native extracts. The strengths of tinctures are typically 1:10 or 1:5. Alcohol content will vary.

Tonic - A substance which exerts a gentle strengthening effect on the body.

Vasoconstriction - The constriction of blood vessels.

Vasodilation - The dilation of blood vessels.

RESOURCES

Books

Felter HW, Lloyd JU. **King's American Dispensatory.** Eclectic Medical Publications, 11231 Market St., Portland, OR 97216, USA, 1983

> A reprint of a classic. First publishced in 1898. Important component in any herbal practitioner's library. (*Eclectic has reprinted several other classics.*)

Griggs B. **Green Pharmacy.** Jill Norman & Hobhouse, Ltd., London, UK, 1981

> An excellent book on the history of herbal medicine. Essential reading.

Leung AY. **Encyclopedia of Common Natural Ingredients Used in Food, Drugs and Cosmetics.** John Wiley & Sons, New York, NY, USA, 1980

> Perhaps the best reference book/dictionary. Extremely useful for researchers.

Oliver-Bever B. **Medicinal Plants in Tropical West Africa.** Cambridge University Press, Cambridge, UK, 1986

> Excellent book for the practitioner as well as the researcher.

Tyler VE, Brady LR, Robbers JE. **Pharmacognosy.** Lea & Febitger, Philadelphia, PA, USA, 1988

> The standard pharmacognosy text in the United States.

Reference Publications. **Medicinal Plants of the World.** Reference Publications, Algonac, MI, USA.

> Excellent series of books providing comprehensive reviews of the medicinal plants of particular regions. A must for the serious researcher.

Weiss RF. **Herbal Medicine.** AB Arcanum, Gothenburg, Sweden, 1985

> An indispensable modern text in botanical medicine. Plant drugs are arranged by clinical diagnoses relating to particular systems.

Williard T. **The Wild Rose Scientific Herbal.** Wild Rose College of Natural Healing, Calgary, Canada, 1992.

> Excellent book with detailed information on plant identification, constituents, mechanisms of action, historical use, dosage, and toxicity. Well referenced.

Willard T. **Textbook of Advanced Herbology.** Wild Rose College of Natural Healing, Calgary, Canada, 1992

An exellent book on pharmacognosy and clinical applications. Well referenced.

Journals and Periodicals

American Herb Association Quarterly
(*See* American Herb Association)

Australian Journal of Medical Herbalism
(*See* National Herbalists Association of Australia)

Economic and Medicinal Plant Research
Academic Press
24/28 Oval Road
London NW1, UK

HerbalGram
(*See* American Botanical Council or Herb Research Foundation)

Herbs, Spices, and Medicinal Plants: Recent Advances in Botany, Horticulture, and Pharmacology
Oryx Press
2214 North Central at Encanto
Phoenix, AZ 85004-1483, USA

Journal of Ethnopharmacology
Elsevier Scientific Publishers
Bay 15 Shannon Industrial Estate
County Clare, Ireland

Journal of Herbs, Spices, and Medicinal Plants
Haworth Press
10 Alice Street
Binghamton, NY 13904-1580, USA

Journal of Natural Products
(*See* American Society of Pharmacognosy)

Journal of Naturopathic Medicine
Journal Management Group, Inc.
10 Morgan Avenue
Norwalk, CT 06851, USA

Medical Herbalism
Paul Bergner
P.O. Box 33080
Portland, OR 97233, USA

Phytotherapy Research
>Heyden & Son, Limited
>Spectrum House
>Hillview Gardens
>London NW4 2JQ, UK

Planta Medica: The Journal of Medicinal Plant Research
>Thieme Medical Publishers, Inc.
>381 Park Avenue South
>New York, NY 10016, USA

Vis Medicatrix Naturae
>(*See* General Council and Register of Consultant Herbalists)

Organizations

Australia

National Herbalists Association of Australia
>Raymond Khoury, Secretary
>P.O. Box 65
>Kingsgrove, NSW
>02-502-2938
>02-554-3459 (fax)

>Publishes the *Australian Journal of Medical Herbalism.*

New Zealand

Herb Federation of New Zealand
>P.O. Box 33007
>Christchurch

>Sponsors a biennial conference and a quarterly publication.

United Kingdom

British Herbal Medicine Association
>P.O. Box 304
>Bournemouth
>Dorset BH7 6JZ
>0202-433691

Genral Council and Register of Consultant Herbalists
>18 Sussex Square
>Brighton, East Sussex BN2 5AA

>Publishes *Vis medicatrix Naturae*, a quarterly journal.

National Institute of Medical Herbalists
41 Hatherley Road
Winchester
Hants SO22 6RR
0962-68766

The Herb Society
The Secretary
P.O. Box 599
London SW11 4RW
Fax: 0296-625126

A registered education charity that encourages interest in and knowledge of all aspects of herbs including herbal medicine. Publications include a magazine and a newsletter.

USA

American Botanical Council
P.O. Box 201660
Austin, TX 78720
(512) 331-8868
Fax: (512) 331-1924

A non-profit organization dedicated to education. Co-publishes the *HerbalGram* with the Herb Research Foundation. Provides excellent reference materials including a series of *Classic Botanical Reprints*.

American Herb Association
P.O. Box 1673
Nevada City, CA 95959
Fax: (916) 265-9552

Membership includes a subscription to the *AHA Quarterly* which is devoted to providing information on medicinal herbs.

American Herbalist Guild
P.O. Box 1683
Soquel, CA 95073

A non-profit membership organization. Members receive a quarterly journal and discounts to seminars and workshops.

American Society of Pharmacognosy
Chicago School of Pharmacy
555 31st St.
Downers Grove, IL 60515

A non-profit membership organization. Members receive the *Journal of Natural Products*.

The Herb Research Foundation
        1007 Pearl St. #200
        Boulder, CO 80302
        (303) 449-2265
        Fax: (303) 443-0949

The foundation provides accurate and reliable information on botanicals. Co-publisher of the *HerbalGram*. Offers research and educational services.

INDEX

ORDERING INFORMATION

The following books by Melvyn R. Werbach, M.D. are available by mail:

SOURCEBOOKS OF CLINICAL RESEARCH SERIES

1. **Botanical Influences on Illness.** *(Michael T. Murray, N.D., co-author)*
   344 pages   7" x 10"   1994   **Price: $39.95**   [hard cover]

   The newest addition to the internationally acclaimed series.

2. **Nutritional Influences on Illness,** *Second* **Edition**
   700 pages   8 1/2" x 11"   1993   **Price: $64.95** [hard cover]

   Summarizes and abstracts the research in nutritional medicine for almost 100 illnesses.

   > *"An encyclopedic reference work of exceptional value and precision suitable for physicians and laypeople alike."*   East West magazine

3. **Nutritional Influences on Mental Illness**
   360 pages   7" x 10"   1991   **Price: $39.95** [hard cover]

   A unique, award-winning volume covering 16 mental disorders.

RELATED BOOKS OF INTEREST

Healing Through Nutrition   *Published by Harper/Collins (US)*
443 pages   6 1/2" x 9 1/2"   1993   **Price: $25.00** [hard cover]

> *"In this informative volume, Dr. Werbach, widely regarded as the expert on the subject of nutritional influences on illness . . . , shows how nutrition can be both the cause and the cure for our most common illnesses."*   Let's Live magazine

Third Line Medicine: Modern Treatment for Persistent Symptoms
215 pages   5" x 7 1/2"   1986   **Price: $10.95** [soft cover]

An answer for patients who fail to benefit from mainstream treatments.

> *"For this clear exposition of what has happened and where we are going, all doctors . . . ought to be grateful."*   Abram Hoffer, M.D., Ph.D., Editor-in-Chief
Journal of Orthomolecular Medicine

(over)

THIRD LINE PRESS
4751 Viviana Drive, Suite 102
Tarzana, California 91356
USA

Phone: (800) 916-0076
In CA: (818) 996-0076
FAX: (818) 774-1575

Please send:

____ copies of **Botanical Influences on Illness** @ $39.95. $_____

____ copies of **Nutritional Influences on Illness, 2nd Ed.** @ $64.95. $_____

____ copies of **Nutritional Influences on Mental Illness** @ $39.95. $_____

____ copies of **Healing Through Nutrition** @ $25.00. $_____

____ copies of **Third Line Medicine** @ $10.95. $_____

SHIPPING CHARGES
(add $3.00 for orders from outside of the US)
1 book $6.00
2 books: $7.00
3 books: $8.50
4-6 books: $10.00

Subtotal $_____

8.25% tax (CA residents) $_____

Shipping $_____

QUANTITY PRICES ON REQUEST   **TOTAL ENCLOSED** $_____

Outside of the United States:

- Beyond North America, shipping charges are for surface shipping (up to 3 months). *(airmail rates on request)*
- Payment may be made by Visa or MasterCard *(fill in the information below)*; otherwise payment must be in US dollars by a check drawn on a US bank.

Please charge my: Visa ____   MasterCard ____

Card #: _____ - _____ - _____ - _____   Expiring : _____

Signature:_____

NAME:_____

ADDRESS:_____

_____

_____

PHONE: _____   **FAX:** _____

[ ] **Please add my name to your mailing list to let me know of your latest books.**

344